Student Mastery Manual for

Clinical Procedures for Medical Assistants

Outcome-Based Education

5th Edition

Kathy Bonewit-West, B.S., M.Ed., C.M.A.

Coordinator and Instructor
Medical Assistant Technology
Hocking Technical College
Nelsonville, Ohio

Former Member, Curriculum Review Board
of the American Association
of Medical Assistants

W.B. Saunders Company
An Imprint of Elsevier Science
Philadelphia   London   New York   St. Louis   Sydney   Toronto

W.B. Saunders Company
An Imprint of Elsevier Science

The Curtis Center
Independence Square West
Philadelphia, Pennsylvania 19106-3399

Student Mastery Manual to Accompany   ISBN 0-7216-894
CLINICAL PROCEDURES FOR MEDICAL ASSISTANTS
Fifth Edition

Printed in the United States of America.

Last digit is the print number: 9 8 7 6 5 4

Preface

Outcome-based education is education directed toward preparing individuals to perform the pre-specified tasks of an occupation under "real world" conditions at a level of accuracy and speed required of the entry-level practitioner of that profession. Outcome-based education plays an important role in medical assisting programs to assist in preparing qualified individuals for careers in medical offices, clinics, and related health care facilities. *The Student Mastery Manual for Clinical Procedures for Medical Assistant* has been developed using a complete and thorough outcome-based approach. It meets the criteria stipulated by the *AAMA/CAAHEP Standards and Guidelines for an Accredited Educational Program for the Medical Assistant*. Instructors should find this workbook a valuable teaching aid for preparing well-trained students who are able to think critically and to perform competently in the clinical setting.

Each workbook chapter is organized into six sections. The Key Terminology Assessment section provides the student with an assessment of his or her knowledge of the medical terms relating to each chapter. The Self-Evaluation Questions help the student evaluate his or her progress through each chapter. Once the student has completed these questions and checked them for accuracy, they will serve as an ongoing review of the cognitive knowledge presented in the textbook. Individuals preparing for the certification examination by the American Association of Medical Assistants will find the completed Self-Evaluation sections a useful study aid for the clinical aspect of the examination.

In the Critical Thinking Skills section, the student gains experience in handling real-life situations, which enhances his or her ability to think critically. Some situations require that the student become involved in a role-playing situation; others require that the student utilize independent study in order to answer questions posed by a patient. Independent study helps the student become familiar with resources available to acquire additional knowledge and skills outside the classroom. By learning techniques of self-development, the medical assisting student may become aware of the necessity for continuing education after graduation and entrance into the medical assisting profession.

The Practice for Competency section consists of worksheets that provide the student with classroom laboratory practice in each clinical skill presented in the textbook. The instructor must designate the number of times that the student is required to practice each procedure.

The Evaluation of Competency section is divided into two parts. The first part is the Performance Objective. Its purpose is to provide an exact description of what the learner must be able to demonstrate to attain competency. A performance objective consists of the following three components: (1) the outcome, (2) conditions, (3) standards. Each Performance Objective in this workbook has been developed to correspond with the procedures presented in the textbook. The second part of the Evaluation of Competency section is the Performance

Evaluation Checklist. The Performance Evaluation Checklist provides quality control by comparing the student's performance against an established set of performance standards.

Due to the nature of the material, several medical assisting content areas are more difficult than others for the student to comprehend and perform. In particular, students have difficulty in taking patient symptoms and in calculating drug dosage. Because of this, two supplemental education sections have been incorporated into this manual. The section *Taking Patient Symptoms* provides supplemental education for Chapter 2 (The Medical Record) in the textbook; the section *Drug Dosage Calculation* provides supplemental education for Chapter 7 (Administration of Medication). In these two sections, a step-by-step, self-directed approach has been used, beginning with basic concepts and advancing to more difficult ones. The student should find that this type of approach facilitates the process of becoming proficient in these areas.

I would like to thank the staff at W.B. Saunders for their assistance and support in preparing this review manual. I would also like to express my appreciation to the following individuals who provided encouragement and friendship throughout this endeavor: Marlene Donovan, Deborah Murray, Tanya Howe, Katie West, Kim Bonewit, Rob Bonewit, Hollie Bonewit, and Hugh Bloemer.

KATHY BONEWIT-WEST, B.S., M.Ed., CMA

Message to the Student

This student manual has been designed to facilitate the attainment of competency in the clinical theory and procedures in your textbook. Each chapter of the manual has been organized into the six sections listed below. To obtain maximum benefit form this workbook, learning activities are outlined under each section along with the resource to use to accomplish each one. By completing the activities below, it is hoped that your ability to assimilate the theory and perform the clinical skills will be greatly enhanced.

1. KEY TERMINOLOGY ASSESSMENT

    A. *Textbook:* Review the Key Terminology section of your textbook.
    B. *Workbook:* Match the medical terms with the definitions.
    C. *Textbook and Workbook:* Check your work for accuracy, using your textbook.
    D. *Workbook:* Correct any errors.

2. SELF-EVALUATION QUESTIONS

    A. *Textbook*: Read the textbook chapter.
    B. *Workbook:* Complete the Self-Evaluation questions.
    C. *Textbook and Workbook:* Check your work for accuracy, using the textbook.
    D. *Workbook:* Correct any errors.

3. CRITICAL THINKING SKILLS

    A. *Workbook:* Review the Critical Thinking Skills questions.
    B. *Reference Materials:* Obtain any additional materials or resources required.
    C. *Workbook:* Complete the Critical Thinking Skills questions.

4. PRACTICE FOR COMPETENCY

    A. *Textbook:* Review the procedure in your textbook for performing the clinical skill.
    B. *Textbook and Workbook:* Practice the clinical skill and record results. Your instructor will designate the number of times that you should practice the procedure.

5. EVALUATION OF COMPETENCY: PERFORMANCE OBJECTIVE

    A. *Workbook:* Review the requirements stated in the Performance Objective.
    B. *Workbook:* Make sure that you are able to perform the skills according to the criteria stipulated under conditions and standards.
    C. *Workbook:* If directed by the instruction, obtain a peer evaluation using the performance Evaluation Checklist.

6. EVALUATION OF COMPETENCY: PERFORMANCE CHECKLIST

A. *Workbook:* Write your name and date in the space indicated on the Performance Evaluation Checklist and give it to your instructor.

B. *Workbook:* Demonstrate the proper procedure for performing the clinical skill for your instructor.

C. *Workbook:* Record results (if required) in the chart provided below the checklist.

D. *Workbook:* Obtain instructor's initials on your Outcome Assessment Record.

MESSAGE TO THE STUDENT

Once you have completed each chapter in this manual, it is suggested that you place the perforated tear–out sheet into a 3–ring notebook. This will provide you with an ongoing record of your academic progress. In addition, the notebook will be useful both as a classroom reference and as a certification examination review resource.

The author hopes that this student manual will assist your attainment of competency in clinical medical assisting procedures, and in turn, facilitate your transition from the classroom to the work place.

KATHY BONEWIT WEST, B.S., M.Ed., CMA

Outcome Assessment Record

Guidelines: This list of outcomes is used to maintain an ongoing record of classroom and externship outcome assessment. Your instructor should initial each outcome when you have performed it with competency in the classroom. When you have performed the outcome with competency at your externship facility, it should be initialed by your internship supervisor. (Note: Space is provided for three externship experiences in the event that you extern at more than one externship site.)

Name _____	Classroom Performance	Externship	Externship	Externship
MEDICAL ASEPSIS				
Wash hands.				
Adhere to the OSHA Standard.				
THE MEDICAL RECORD				
Complete a consent to treatment form.				
Assist a patient in the completion of a consent to release medical information form.				
Prepare a medical record for a new patient.				
Obtain and record patient symptoms.				
VITAL SIGNS				
Measure oral body temperature.				
Measure aural body temperature.				
Measure axillary body temperature.				
Measure radial pulse.				
Measure apical pulse.				
Measure respiration.				
Measure blood pressure.				
THE PHYSICAL EXAMINATION				
Prepare the examining room.				
Prepare the patient for a physical examination.				
Measure weight.				
Measure height.				
Position and drape an individual.				
Assist the physician with a physical examination.				

Name _____	Classroom Performance	Externship	Externship	Externship
STERILIZATION AND DISINFECTION				
Sanitize instruments.				
Wrap and label an article for autoclaving.				
Sterilize articles in the autoclave.				
Chemically disinfect contaminated articles.				
MINOR OFFICE SURGERY				
Apply and remove sterile gloves.				
Open a sterile package.				
Add a sterile article to a sterile field using a peel-apart package.				
Pour a sterile solution into a container on a sterile field.				
Change a sterile dressing.				
Remove sutures.				
Remove staples.				
Apply and remove adhesive skin closures.				
Set up a surgical tray for minor office surgery.				
Assist the physician with minor surgery.				
Apply the following bandage turns: circular, spiral, spiral-reverse, figure-eight, and recurrent.				
Apply a tubular gauze bandage.				
ADMINISTRATION OF MEDICATION				
Administer oral solid medication.				
Administer oral liquid medication.				
Reconstitute a powdered drug.				
Prepare an injection from a vial.				
Prepare an injection from an ampule.				
Administer an intradermal injection.				
Administer a subcutaneous injection.				
Locate the following intramuscular injection sites: dorsogluteal, deltoid, vastus lateralis, vertrogluteal.				
Administer an intramuscular injection.				
Administer an injection using the Z-tack method.				

Name _____	Classroom Performance	Externship	Externship	Externship
Administer a Mantoux test.				
Read and interpret Mantoux test results.				
Administer a tine test.				
Read and interpret tine test results.				
EYE AND EAR PROCEDURES				
Assess distance visual acuity.				
Assess color vision.				
Perform an eye irrigation.				
Perform an eye instillation.				
Perform an ear irrigation.				
Perform an ear instillation.				
PHYSICAL THERAPY				
Apply a hot water bag.				
Apply a heating pad.				
Apply a hot soak.				
Apply a hot compress.				
Apply an ice bag.				
Apply a cold compress.				
Apply a chemical cold pack.				
Administer an ultrasound treatment.				
Measure an individual for axillary crutches.				
Instruct an individual in mastering crutch gaits.				
Instruct an individual in the use of a cane.				
Instruct an individual in the use of a walker.				
GYNECOLOGICAL/PRENATAL CARE				
Provide instructions for a breast self-examination.				
Prepare the patient for a gynecologic examination.				
Assist with a gynecologic examination.				
Prepare the patient for a prenatal examination.				
Assist the physician with a prenatal examination.				

Name _____	Classroom Performance	Externship	Externship	Externship
PEDIATRICS				
Carry an infant in the following positions: cradle and upright.				
Measure the weight of an infant.				
Measure the length of an infant.				
Measure the head circumference of an infant.				
Measure the chest circumference of an infant.				
Plot pediatric measurements on a growth chart.				
Apply a pediatric urine collector.				
Collect a specimen for a PKU screening test.				
CARDIOPULMONARY PROCEDURES				
Record a 12-lead ECG.				
Instruct a patient in the guidelines for wearing a Holter monitor.				
Apply a Holter monitor.				
Assist with pulmonary function testing.				
COLON PROCEDURES				
Provide instructions for a fecal occult blood test.				
Develop a fecal occult blood test.				
Prepare the patient for a sigmoidoscopy.				
Assist the physician with a sigmoidoscopy.				
RADIOLOGY AND DIAGNOSTIC IMAGING				
Instruct a patient in the proper preparation required for each of the following x-ray examinations: mammogram, upper GI, lower GI, cholecystogram, and intravenous pyelogram.				
Instruct a patient in the proper preparation required for each of the following: ultrasonography, computed tomography, magnetic resonance imaging.				

Name _____	Classroom Performance	Externship	Externship	Externship
INTRODUCTION TO THE CLINICAL LABORATORY				
Use a laboratory directory.				
Complete a laboratory request form.				
Instruct the patient in advance preparation requirements for a specimen collection.				
Collect a biologic specimen.				
Properly handle and store a biologic specimen.				
Review a laboratory report.				
URINALYSIS				
Instruct a patient in clean-catch midstream urine specimen collection.				
Instruct a patient in 24-hour urine specimen collection.				
Assess the color and appearance of a urine specimen.				
Measure the specific gravity of a urine specimen.				
Perform a chemical assessment of a urine specimen.				
Prepare a urine specimen for microscopic analysis.				
Identify urine sediment structures.				
Perform a rapid urine culture test.				
Perform a urine pregnancy test.				
PHLEBOTOMY				
Perform a venipuncture using the vacuum tube method.				
Perform a venipuncture using the butterfly method.				
Perform a venipuncture using the syringe method.				
Separate serum from whole blood.				
Obtain a capillary blood specimen.				
HEMATOLOGY				
Perform a hemoglobin determination.				
Perform a hematocrit determination.				
Prepare a blood smear.				

Name _____	Classroom Performance	Externship	Externship	Externship
BLOOD CHEMISTRY AND SEROLOGY				
Perform blood chemistry testing.				
Perform a fasting blood sugar using a glucose meter.				
Perform a rapid mononucleosis test.				
MICROBIOLOGY				
Use a microscope.				
Obtain a specimen for a throat culture.				
Obtain a specimen using a collection and transport system.				
Perform a rapid strep test.				
Prepare a wet mount slide.				
Prepare a hanging drop slide.				
Prepare a microbiologic smear.				
ADDITIONAL OUTCOMES (List)				

Contents

Table of Contents

## CHAPTER 1

Medical Asepsis and Infection Control

NAME _____

Key Terminology Assessment

Directions: Match each medical term with its definition.

_____ 1. aerobe
_____ 2. anaerobe
_____ 3. asepsis
_____ 4. bloodborne pathogens
_____ 5. cilia
_____ 6. contaminate
_____ 7. exposure incident
_____ 8. infection
_____ 9. microorganism
_____10. nonintact skin
_____11. nonpathogen
_____12. occupational exposure
_____13. opportunistic infection
_____14. optimum growth temperature
_____15. pathogen
_____16. pH
_____17. regulated waste
_____18. reservoir host
_____19. susceptible
_____20. transient flora

A. A disease-producing microorganism.
B. Microorganisms that reside in the superficial skin layers and are picked up in the course of daily activities.
C. A microorganism that needs oxygen in order to live and grow.
D. Reasonably anticipated skin, eye, mucous membrane, or parenteral contact with bloodborne pathogens or other potentially infectious materials that may result from the performance of an employee's duties.
E. Free from infection or pathogens.
F. Easily affected; lacking resistance.
G. Skin that has a break in the surface.
H. The temperature at which an organism grows best.
I. The degree to which a solution is acidic or basic.
J. A specific eye, mouth, other mucous membrane, nonintact skin, or parenteral contact with blood or other potentially infectious materials that results from an employee's duties.

K. Pathogenic microorganisms capable of causing disease that are present in human blood.
L. The condition in which the body, or part of it, is invaded by a pathogen.
M. Any waste containing infectious material that would pose a substantial threat to health and safety if the public were exposed to it.
N. Slender hairlike processes.
O. A microorganism that does not normally produce disease.
P. A microscopic plant or animal.
Q. A microorganism that grows best in the absence of oxygen.
R. To soil or to make impure.
S. The organism that becomes infected by a pathogen and also serves as a source of transfer of the pathogens to others.
T. An infection resulting from a defective immune system that cannot defend the body from pathogens normally found in the environment.

Self Evaluation

Directions: Fill in each blank with the correct answer.

1. What is a microorganism?

   _____

2. List two examples of types of microorganisms.

   _____

3. What is the name given to the organism that uses organic or living substances for food?

   _____

4. Why do most microorganisms prefer a neutral pH?

   _____

   _____

5. List three examples of how microorganisms can enter the body.

   _____

   _____

6. List three examples of how a microorganism can be transmitted from one person to another.

_____

_____

_____

7. List two examples of factors that would make a host more susceptible to the entrance of a pathogen.

_____

_____

8. List five protective devices of the body that prevent the entrance of miccroorganisms.

_____

_____

_____

9. Define medical asepsis.

_____

_____

10. Explain the difference in techniques for removing resident flora and transient flora from the skin.

_____

_____

_____

11. How do each of the following handwashing agents function in cleansing the skin?
    a. soaps _____
    b. detergents _____
    c. antimicrobial agents _____

12. List six medical aseptic practices the medical assistant should follow in the medical office.

_____

_____

_____

_____

_____

_____

13. What does OSHA stand for and what is its purpose?

_____

_____

14. Define an engineering control and list three examples of engineering controls.

_____

_____

_____

15. List six guidelines that must be followed when using personal protective equipment.

_____

_____

_____

_____

_____

_____

16. What is the most likely means of contracting hepatitis B in the healthcare setting?

_____

_____

17. Why is chronic viral hepatitis considered such a serious condition?

_____

_____

_____

18. What are the symptoms of acute HIV infection?

_____

_____

19. Explain what occurs during the symptomatic period of the AIDS virus infection cycle.

_____

_____

20. What are the symptoms of AIDS?

_____

_____

21. How is HIV transmitted?

_____

_____

_____

22. List five AIDS-defining conditions.

_____

_____

_____

Critical Thinking Skills

1. Carefully review the Infection Process Cycle and the requirements for growth needed by microorganisms. Create an environment in a medical office that would work to interrupt the Infection Process Cycle and discourage the growth of pathogens.

_____

_____

_____

_____

_____

2. Using the principles outlined in the handwashing procedure, tell what might happen under the following circumstances:

   a. The medical assistant's uniform touches the sink during the handwashing procedure.

   _____

   b. The hands are not held lower than the elbows during the handwashing procedure.

   _____

   _____

   _____

   c. Friction is not used to wash the hands.

   _____

   _____

   _____

d. Water is splashed on the medical assistant's uniform during the handwashing procedure.

_____

_____

e. The medical assistant continually uses water that is too cold to wash hands.

_____

_____

_____

f. The medical assistant turns off the running water with her bare hands.

_____

_____

_____

g. The medical assistant does not clean her fingernails daily.

_____

_____

_____

h. The medical assistant's skin becomes chapped.

_____

_____

3. Which of the following situations requires the use of personal protective equipment?

_____ a. Giving an injection to an infant.

_____ b. Sanitizing operating scissors for sterilization.

_____ c. Performing a finger puncture.

_____ d. Performing a vision screening test on a school-aged child.

_____ e. Cleaning up a blood spill on a laboratory work table.

_____ f. Drawing blood from an elderly patient.

_____ g. Measuring the weight of a college student.

_____ h. Testing a blood specimen for glucose.

4. Which of the following situations violates the OSHA Standard?

    _____ a. Recapping a contaminated needle with two hands.

    _____ b. Refusing to get the hepatitis B vaccination.

    _____ c. Picking up a broken test tube with gloved hands.

    _____ d. Recapping a needle after withdrawing medication from a vial.

    _____ e. Washing your uniform, which has been splashed with blood, at home.

    _____ f. Throwing a tube of blood into the regular trash.

    _____ g. Drinking coffee in the medical office laboratory.

    _____ h. Placing a contaminated lancet in a leak-proof biohazard bag.

Practice for Competency

Assignment

A. Perform the handwashing procedure five times. List five medically aseptic steps that must be followed during this procedure.

Medically Aseptic Steps to Follow During Handwashing

1._____

_____

2._____

_____

3._____

_____

4._____

_____

5._____

_____

B. Apply and remove clean disposable gloves five times.

Evaluation of Competency

PROCEDURE 1-1: HANDWASHING

Name _____ Date _____

Evaluated By _____ Score_____

Performance Objective

Outcome: Wash hands.
Conditions: Using a sink.
      Given liquid soap or bar soap and paper towels.
Standards: Time: 5 minutes.
      Accuracy: Satisfactory score on the Performance Evaluation
      Checklist.

Performance Evaluation Checklist

Trial 1	Trial 2	Point Value	Performance Standards
		●	Removed watch or pushed it up on the forearm.
		●	Removed rings.
		▷	Is able to state the reason for removing rings.
		●	Stood at sink with clothing away from edge of sink.
		●	Turned on faucets with paper towel.
		▷	Is able to state the principle for turning on faucets with paper towel.
		●	Adjusted temperature of water.
		●	Discarded towel into trash can.
		●	Wet hands and forearms with water.
		●	Held hands lower than elbows at all times.
		▷	Is able to state the principle for holding hands lower than elbows.
		●	Did not touch the inside of sink with hands.
		●	Applied soap to hands.
		●	Washed palms and backs of hands with 10 circular motions and friction.
		▷	Is able to state why circular motions and friction are needed to wash hands.
		●	Washed fingers while interlaced, with 10 circular motions and friction.

Trial 1	Trial 2	Point Value	Performance Standards
		●	Rinsed well (keeping hands lower than elbows).
		●	Washed wrists and forearms using friction and circular motion.
		▷	Is able to state why hands are washed before wrists and forearms.
		●	Rinsed arms and hands.
		●	Cleaned fingernails using manicure stick.
		●	Repeated handwashing procedure (if necessary).
		●	Dried hands gently and thoroughly.
		▷	Is able to state the principle for drying hands gently and completely.
		●	Turned off faucets using paper towel.
		●	Did not touch sink area with bare hands.
		▷	Is able to state the principle for not touching sink area with bare hands.
		★	Completed the procedure within 5 minutes.

Evaluation of Student Performance

EVALUATION CRITERIA			COMMENTS
Symbol	Category	Point Value	
★	Critical Step	16 points	
●	Essential Step	6 points	
▷	Theory Question	2 points	

Score calculation: 100 points
−_____ points missed
_____ Score
Satisfactory score: 85 or above

AAMA/CAAHEP Competency Achieved:
☐ Perform handwashing.

Evaluation of Competency

PROCEDURE 1-2: APPLICATION AND REMOVAL OF CLEAN DISPOSABLE GLOVES

Name _____ Date _____

Evaluated By _____ Score_____

Performance Objective

Outcome:	Apply and remove clean disposable gloves.
Conditions:	Given the appropriate sized clean disposable gloves.
Standards:	Time: 5 minutes
	Accuracy: Satisfactory score on the Performance Evaluation Checklist.

Performance Evaluation Checklist

Trial 1	Trial 2	Point Value	Performance Standards
			APPLICATION OF CLEAN GLOVES
		●	Removed all rings.
		▷	Is able to state why rings should be removed.
		●	Washed the hands.
		●	Chose the appropriate sized gloves.
		●	Applied the gloves.
		●	Adjusted the gloves so that they fit comfortably.
		●	Inspected the gloves for tears.
		▷	Is able to state what to do if a glove is torn.
			REMOVAL OF CLEAN GLOVES
		●	Grasped the outside of the left glove 1 to 2 inches from the top with the gloved right hand.
		●	Slowly pulled left glove off the hand.
		●	Pulled the left glove free and scrunched it into a ball with the gloved right hand.
		●	Placed the index and middle fingers of the left hand on the inside of the right glove.
		●	Did not allow the clean hand to touch outside of the glove.

Trial 1	Trial 2	Point Value	Performance Standards
		●	Pulled the glove off the right hand enclosing the balled up left glove.
		●	Discarded both gloves in an appropriate waste container.
		●	Washed hands thoroughly.
		★	Completed the procedure in 5 minutes.

Evaluation of Student Performance

EVALUATION CRITERIA			COMMENTS
Symbol	Category	Point Value	
★	Critical Step	16 points	
●	Essential Step	6 points	
▷	Theory Question	2 points	
Score calculation: 100 points			
− _____ points missed			
_____ Score			
Satisfactory score: 85 or above			

AAMA/CAAHEP Competency Achieved:
☐ Practice Standard Precautions.

The Medical Record

## CHAPTER 2

NAME _____

Key Terminology Assessment

Directions: Match each medical term with its definition.

_____ 1. charting
_____ 2. computer-based patient record
_____ 3. consultation report
_____ 4. diagnosis
_____ 5. discharge summary report
_____ 6. familial
_____ 7. health history report
_____ 8. informed consent
_____ 9. medical impressions
_____ 10. medical record
_____ 11. objective symptom
_____ 12. physical examination report
_____ 13. problem
_____ 14. prognosis
_____ 15. objective symptom
_____ 16. symptom

A. A collection of subjective data about a patient.
B. A narrative report of an opinion about a patient's condition by a practitioner other than the attending physician.
C. Any patient condition that requires further observation, diagnosis, management, or patient education.
D. A symptom that is felt by the patient but is not observable by an examiner.
E. The process of making written entries about a patient in the medical record.
F. Consent given by a patient for a medical procedure after being informed of the procedure.
G. Any change in the body or its functioning that indicates that a disease is present.

Continued on next page

H. Conclusions drawn by the physician from an interpretation of data.

I. A medical record that is stored on a computer.

J. A brief summary of the significant events of a patient's hospitalization.

K. A written record of the important information regarding a patient.

L. A symptom that can be observed by an examiner.

M. The probable course and outcome of a disease and the prospects of patient recovery.

N. The scientific method of determining and identifying a disease.

O. A report of the objective findings from the physician's assessment of each body system.

P. Occurring or affecting members of a family more frequently than would be expected by chance.

Self-Evaluation

1. List three functions of the medical record.

   _____

   _____

   _____

2. What two general categories of information are included in a patient registration record?

   _____

3. List three uses of the health history.

   _____

   _____

   _____

4. What is the purpose of the physical examination?

   _____

   _____

5. What is the purpose of progress notes?

_____

_____

6. List three categories of medication that may be included in a medication report.

_____

_____

7. What is the purpose of home health care?

_____

_____

8. What is the purpose of a laboratory report?

_____

_____

9. What is a diagnostic procedure?

_____

_____

10. What is the purpose of a therapeutic service report?

_____

_____

11. What is physical therapy?

_____

_____

_____

12. What is the purpose of hospital documents?

_____

_____

13. What is included in a pathology report?

_____

_____

14. Why is a copy of an emergency room report sent to the patient's physician?

_____

_____

15. When is a consent to treatment form required?

_____

_____

16. What information must the patient be informed of before signing a consent to treatment form?

_____

_____

17. What does "witnessing a signature" mean? What does it not mean?

_____

_____

_____

18. What must be completed before information from a patient's medical record can be released?

_____

_____

19. How are documents organized in a source-oriented medical record?

_____

_____

20. How are documents organized in a problem-oriented medical record?

_____

_____

21. List and describe the four parts of a POR.

_____

_____

_____

_____

22. What is the purpose of a file folder?

_____

_____

23. What are the seven parts of the health history?

_____

_____

_____

_____

24. What is a chief complaint?

_____

25. What guidelines should be followed in recording the chief complaint?

_____
_____
_____
_____

26. List five examples of information included in the past history.

_____
_____
_____
_____

27. List three examples of familial diseases.

_____
_____

28. Explain the importance of the social/occupational history.

_____
_____

29. What is the purpose of the review of systems (ROS)?

_____
_____

30. List the guidelines that should be followed to ensure accurate and concise charting.

_____
_____
_____
_____
_____
_____
_____

31. List three examples of subjective symptoms.

_____
_____

32. List three examples of objective symptoms.

_____

_____

33. What is the medical term for excessive perspiration?

_____

34. What is edema?

_____

35. What is the medical term for the loss of appetite?

_____

36. What is used as a guide to determine if a patient is constipated?

_____

_____

37. What is the difference between nausea and vomiting?

_____

_____

38. What is the medical term for dizziness?

_____

39. What is the difference between a productive and nonproductive cough?

_____

_____

40. Why should the following be charted in the patient's medical record?
    a. Procedures performed on the patient.

    _____

    _____

    b. Specimens collected from the patient.

    _____

    _____

    c. Laboratory tests ordered on the patient.

    _____

    _____

    d. Instructions given to the patient regarding medical care.

_____

_____

Critical Thinking Skills

1. Refer to the Consultation Report (Figure 2-3) in your textbook and identify the following information using the corresponding letter (A, B, C, or D).

    A. Documentation that the consultant reviewed the patient's health history.

    B. Documentation that the consultant examined the patient.

    C. A report of the consultant's impressions.

    D. A report of the consultant's recommendations.

2. Refer to the radiology Report (Figure 2-5) in your textbook and answer the following questions.

    a. What type of radiologic examination was performed on Elaine Silverman?

_____

    b. Were the lungs clear?

_____

    c. Were any masses noted in the abdomen?

_____

3. Refer to the Diagnostic Imaging Report (Fig 2-6) in your textbook and answer the following questions.

    a. What type of diagnostic imaging procedure was performed on Vera Ruth?

_____

    b. What vertebrae of the spine were scanned?

_____

    c. What problem may be present with L4-5?

_____

    d. What additional tests might be scheduled for Vera Ruth?

_____

_____

4. Refer to the Discharge Summary Report (Fig 2-10) in your textbook and answer the following questions.

    a. How long was Elaine Silverman hospitalized?

    _____

    b. What was her hemoglobin level at admission?

    _____

    c. What was the admitting diagnosis?

    _____

    _____

    d. Was Elaine pregnant?

    _____

    e. What was her discharge diagnosis?

    _____

5. Refer to the Consent to Release Medical Information form (Fig 2-14) in your textbook and identify the following information using the corresponding letter (A, B, C, or D).

    A. Name of the medical practice releasing the information.

    B. Name of the facility to receive the information.

    C. Specific information to be released.

    D. Purpose of the information.

6. Create an atmosphere in a medical office that would not be conducive to taking a meaningful health history. Next create an atmosphere that would encourage communication.

    _____

    _____

    _____

    _____

    _____

    _____

    _____

7. Indicate whether each of the following statements is an incorrect (I) or correct (C) example of recording a chief complaint. If the example is incorrect, explain which recording guideline is not being followed.

    _____ a. Low back pain _____

    _____

_____ b. Sore throat and fever for the past 2 days _____

_____

_____ c. Dyspnea, paleness, and fatigue similar to that associated with anemia, which has lasted for 2 weeks _____

_____

_____ d. Poor health for the past several months _____

_____

_____ e. Weakness and fatigue related to poor eating habits and lack of exercise _____

_____

_____ f. Heart palpitations occurring after drinking coffee in the morning before work _____

_____

8. Refer to the Abbreviation Boxes on pages 67 and 68 of your textbook. Write a "make-believe" story about a patient with an illness using as many of these abbreviations as possible.

Practice for Competency

Assignment

1. Complete the health history form (pages 23 to 26) using yourself as the patient.

2. Complete the consent to treatment form (page 27) using yourself as the patient.

3. Complete the release of medical information form (page 28) using yourself as the patient.

4. Prepare a medical record.

5. Practice obtaining patient symptoms, by completing Taking Patient Symptoms: Supplemental Education for Chapter 2 (pages 37 to 46).

Health History Form

PATIENT HEALTH HISTORY

IDENTIFICATION DATA   Please print the following information.

Today's date _____   File no. _____

Name _____

____ Male ____ Female _____ Race   Date of Birth _____

Address _____

____ Married ____ Separated ____ Divorced ____ Widowed ____ Single

Zip Code _____

Insurance provider _____

Telephone _____   _____
Home number   Work number

Policy number _____

Occupation _____

Social Security or Medicare No. _____

A

FAMILY HISTORY

For each member of your family, follow the purple or blue line across the page and check boxes for:
1. Their present state of health
2. Any illnesses they have had

If deceased, write in age and cause of death. Include fatal accidents and suicides.

	Good health	Poor health	Deceased	If deceased...	Allergies or asthma	Anemia	Bleed easily	Diabetes	Cancer or tumor	Epilepsy	Glaucoma	Genetic disease	Alcoholism	Kidney or bladder trouble	Stomach/duodenal ulcer	Nervous breakdown	Rheumatism or arthritis	High blood pressure	Heart trouble	Gout
Father:																				
Mother:																				
Brothers/Sisters:																				
Spouse:																				
Child:																				
Child:																				
Child:																				
Child:																				
Paternal relatives (in each box, write how many affected with) ——→																				
Maternal relatives (in each box, write how many affected with) ——→																				

B

PAST HISTORY (begin here with illnesses) ——→

ADDITIONAL ILLNESSES OR PROBLEMS: mark an X in the box next to any of the following that you have now or have ever had:

☐ Eye infections	☐ Pneumonia	☐ Neuralgia or neuritis	☐ Scarlet fever	☐ Mononucleosis
☐ Thyroid disease	☐ Pancreatitis	☐ Tension/anxiety	☐ Measles	☐ Venereal disease
☐ Eczema	☐ Liver disease	☐ Depression	☐ Mumps	☐ Yellow jaundice
☐ Hive or rashes	☐ Diverticulosis	☐ Childhood hyperactivity	☐ Polio	☐ Tuberculosis
☐ Bronchitis	☐ Hernia	☐ Chicken Pox	☐ Rheumatic fever	☐ _____
☐ Emphysema	☐ Hemorrhoids	☐ German measles	☐ Malaria	☐ _____

Have you ever been turned down for life insurance, military service or employment because of health problems?   ☐ Yes   ☐ No

MAJOR HOSPITALIZATIONS: If you have ever been hospitalized for any major medical illness or operation, write in your most recent hospitalizations below. Check this box ☐ if you have had more than four such hospitalizations. (Do not include normal pregnancies.)

	Year	Operation or illness	Name of hospital	City and state
1st Hospitalization				
2nd Hospitalization				
3rd Hospitalization				
4th Hospitalization				

TESTS AND IMMUNIZATIONS: Mark an X next to those that you have had. Enter the year when you least were given the tests or "shots".

Year		Year	
☐ 19___ chest x-ray		☐ 19___ smallpox "shots"	
☐ 19___ kidney x-ray		☐ 19___ tetanus "shots"	
☐ 19___ G.I. series		☐ 19___ polio series	
☐ 19___ colon x-ray		☐ 19___ typhoid "shots"	
☐ 19___ gallbladder x-ray		☐ 19___ flu injections	
☐ 19___ electrocardiogram		☐ 19___ mumps "shots"	
☐ 19___ TB test		☐ 19___ measles "shots"	
☐ 19___ sigmoidoscopy		☐ 19___ _____	

MEDICINES: Mark an X in the box next to any medicines that you are now taking, or that you are sensitive or allergic to:

Taking	Allergic to:	Taking	Allergic to:
☐	☐ antibiotics	☐	☐ aspirin
☐	☐ penicillin	☐	☐ diet pills
☐	☐ sulfa	☐	☐ antacids
☐	☐ opiates/codeine	☐	☐ laxatives
☐	☐ diuretics/water pills	☐	☐ cold tablets
☐	☐ sedatives	☐	☐ _____
☐	☐ stimulants/caffeine	☐	☐ _____
☐	☐ Demarol	☐	☐ _____
☐	☐ Blood pressure medicine		

C

Health History Form

SOCIAL HISTORY

EDUCATION

_____ Years elementary   _____ Years high school   _____ Years college, technical, business, etc.

Occupation _____   Years _____

Previous occupation _____   Years _____

Military services _____

Overseas? _____

Have you ever been exposed to any of the following in your work environment?

☐ Excess dust (coal, lime, rock)   ☐ Cleaning fluids/solvents   ☐ Radiation   ☐ Other toxic materials

☐ Sand   ☐ Hair spray   ☐ Insecticides

☐ Chemicals   ☐ Smoke or auto exhaust fumes   ☐ Paints

Please answer the following questions by placing an X in the box in front of the word Yes or No, except where your are asked for specific information. If a question doesn't apply, skip it and go on to the next one. This information is obviously highly confidential and will be released to other health professionals or insurance carriers ONLY with your signed consent.

DIET HISTORY/EXERCISE

1. Do you eat a good breakfast? ☐ Yes ☐ No
2. Do you snack between meals (soft drinks, chips, candy bars)? ☐ Yes ☐ No
3. Do you eat fresh fruits and vegetables each day? ☐ Yes ☐ No
4. Do you eat whole grain breads and cereals? ☐ Yes ☐ No
5. Is your diet high in fat content? ☐ Yes ☐ No
6. Is your diet high in cholesterol content? ☐ Yes ☐ No
7. Is your diet high in salt content? ☐ Yes ☐ No
8. Do you habitually use laxatives? ☐ Yes ☐ No

9. Do you exercise on a regular basis? ☐ Yes ☐ No
10. Does your job require strenuous, sustained, physical work? ☐ Yes ☐ No
11. Are you allergic to any foods? ☐ Yes ☐ No
12. How many glasses of milk do you drink each day? ☐ Yes ☐ No
13. How many glasses of water do you drink each day? ☐ Yes ☐ No
14. How would you describe your overall eating habits?
☐ Excellent
☐ Good
☐ Fair
☐ Poor

SOCIAL HISTORY/EXERCISE

15. Are you very nervous around strangers? ☐ Yes ☐ No
16. Do you find it hard to make decisions? ☐ Yes ☐ No
17. Do you find it hard to concentrate or remember? ☐ Yes ☐ No
18. Do you usually feel lonely or depressed? ☐ Yes ☐ No
19. Do you often cry? ☐ Yes ☐ No
20. Would you say you have a hopeless outlook? ☐ Yes ☐ No
21. Do you have difficulty relaxing? ☐ Yes ☐ No
21. Do you have a tendency to worry a lot? ☐ Yes ☐ No
23. Are you troubled by frightening dreams or thoughts? ☐ Yes ☐ No
24. Do you have a tendency to be shy or sensitive? ☐ Yes ☐ No
25. Do you have a strong dislike for criticism? ☐ Yes ☐ No
26. Do you lose your temper often? ☐ Yes ☐ No
27. Do little things often annoy you? ☐ Yes ☐ No
28. Are you disturbed by any work or family problems? ☐ Yes ☐ No
29. Are you having sexual difficulties? ☐ Yes ☐ No
30. Have you ever considered committing suicide? ☐ Yes ☐ No
31. Have you ever desired or sought psychiatric help? ☐ Yes ☐ No
32 Have you gained or lost much weight recently? ☐ Yes ☐ No
33. Do you have a tendency to be too hot or too cold? ☐ Yes ☐ No
34. Have you lost your interest in eating lately? ☐ Yes ☐ No
35. Do you always seem to be hungry? ☐ Yes ☐ No

36. Are you more thirsty than usual lately? ☐ Yes ☐ No
37. Are there any swellings in your armpits or groin? ☐ Yes ☐ No
38. Do you seem to feel exhausted or fatigued most of the time? ☐ Yes ☐ No
39. Do you have difficulty either falling asleep or staying asleep? ☐ Yes ☐ No
40. Do you participate in physical activity or exercise less than three times a week? ☐ Yes ☐ No
41. How much do you smoke per day?
☐ Cigarettes
☐ Cigars/pipes
☐ Don't smoke
42. Do you take two or more alcoholic drinks per day? ☐ Yes ☐ No
43. Do you drink six or more cups of coffee or tea per day? ☐ Yes ☐ No
44. Are you a regular user of sleeping pills, marijuana, tranquilizers, pain killers, etc.? ☐ Yes ☐ No
45. Have you ever used heroin, cocaine, LSD, PCP, etc? ☐ Yes ☐ No
46. Do you drive a motor vehicle more than 25,000 miles a year? ☐ Yes ☐ No
47. How often do you use seat belts when riding in cars?
☐ Never
☐ Sometimes
☐ Always
48. List any country outside the USA you have visited in the past six months? _____
49. Do you live in: (A) an apartment (B) a house (C) a trailer (D) other _____
50. When did you have your last physical examination? _____

Health History Form

Name _____   Date _____

Doctor's notes _____

_____

_____

REVIEW OF SYSTEMS

HEAD AND NECK
92. ____ frequent headaches
93. ____ neck and pains
94. ____ neck lumps or sweating

EYES
95. ____ wears glasses
96. ____ blurry vision
97. ____ eyesight worsening
98. ____ sees double
99. ____ sees halo
100. ____ eye pains or itching
101. ____ watering eyes
102. ____ eye trouble

EARS
103. ____ hearing difficulties
104. ____ earaches
105. ____ running ears
106. ____ buzzing in ears
107. ____ motion sickness

MOUTH
108. ____ dental problems
109. ____ swellings on gums or jaws
110. ____ sore tongue
111. ____ taste changes

NOSE AND THROAT
112. ____ congested nose
113. ____ running nose
114. ____ sneezing spells
115. ____ headcolds
116. ____ nose bleeds
117. ____ sore throat
118. ____ enlarged tonsils
119. ____ hoarse voice

RESPIRATORY
120. ____ wheezed or gasps
121. ____ coughing spells
122. ____ coughs up phlegm
123. ____ coughed up blood
124. ____ chest colds
125. ____ excessive seating, night sweats

CARDIOVASCULAR
126. ____ high blood pressure
127. ____ racing heart
128. ____ chest pains
129. ____ dizzy spells
130. ____ shortness of breath
131. ____ shortness of breath at night
132. ____ more pillows to breathe
133. ____ swollen feet or ankles
134. ____ leg cramps
135. ____ heart murmur

DIGESTIVE
heartburn ____ 49.
bloated stomach ____ 50.
belching ____ 51.
stomach pains ____ 52.
nausea ____ 53.
vomited blood ____ 54.
difficulty swallowing ____ 55.
constipation ____ 56.
loose bowels ____ 57.
black stools ____ 58.
grey stools ____ 59.
pain in rectum ____ 60.
rectal bleeding ____ 61.

URINARY
night frequency ____ 62.
day frequency ____ 63.
wets pants or bed ____ 64.
burning on urination ____ 65.
brown, black or bloody urine ____ 66.
difficulty staring urine ____ 67.
urgency ____ 68.

MALE GENITAL
weak urine stream ____ 69.
prostate trouble ____ 70.
burning or discharge ____ 71.
lumps on testicles ____ 72.
painful testicles ____ 73.

FEMALE GENITAL
last menstrual period __/__/__ 74.
post-menopausal or hysterectomy ____ 75.
noticed vaginal bleeding ____ 76.
lumps on testicles ____ 72.
painful testicles ____ 73.
abnormal LMP ____ 77.
heavy bleeding during periods ____ 78.
bleeding between periods ____ 79.
bleeding after intercourse ____ 80.
recent vaginal itching/discharge ____ 81.
no monthly breast exam ____ 82.
lump or pain in breasts ____ 83.
complications with birth control ____ 84.
last Pap test __/__/__ 85.

OBSTETRIC HISTORY
gravida ____ 86.
para ____ 87.
pre-term ____ 88.
miscarriages ____ 89.
still births ____ 90.
has had an abortion ____ 91.

MUSCULOSKELETAL
1. ____ aching muscles
2. ____ swollen joints
3. ____ back or shoulder pains
4. ____ painful feet
5. ____ handicapped

SKIN
6. ____ skin problems
7. ____ itching or burning skin
8. ____ bleeds easily
9. ____ bruises easily

NEUROLOGICAL
10. ____ faintness
11. ____ numbness
12. ____ convulsions
13. ____ change in handwriting
14. ____ trembles

MOOD
15. ____ nervous with strangers
16. ____ difficulty in making decisions
17. ____ lack of concentration or memory
18. ____ lonely or depressed
19. ____ cries often
20. ____ hopeless outlook
21. ____ difficulty relaxing
22. ____ worries a lot
23. ____ frightening dreams or thoughts
24. ____ shy or sensitive
25. ____ dislikes criticism
26. ____ loses temper
27. ____ annoyed by little things
28. ____ work or family problems
29. ____ sexual difficulties
30. ____ considered suicide
31. ____ desired psychiatric help

GENERAL
32. ____ weight changes
33. ____ tends to be hot or cold
34. ____ loss of interest in eating
35. ____ always hungry
36. ____ more thirsty lately
37. ____ armpits or groin swelling
38. ____ fatigue
39. ____ sleeping difficulties
40. ____ exercises less than 3 times per week
41. ____ cigarettes ____ cigars/pipes ____ don't smoke
42. ____ two or more alcoholic drinks per day
43. ____ over 6 cups of coffee/tea per day
44. ____ uses sleeping pill, marijuana, tranquilizers
45. ____ has used hard drugs
46. ____ drives vehicle over 25,000 miles per year
47. ____ never ____ sometimes ____
         ____ always uses seat belts
48. _____ visited in the last 6 months

Special problems or symptoms _____

_____

_____

_____

PATIENT'S SIGNATURE _____

Health History Form

Name _____ Age _____

Occupation _____ Social Security Number _____

	BLOOD PRESSURE	VISION	DIAGNOSTIC TESTS	RESULTS
Height _____	Sitting R / :L /	Without glasses Far R20/ :L20 / Near R / :L /		
Weight _____				
Build _____	Standing R / :L /	With glasses Far R20/ :L20 / Near R / :L /		
(Sm. Med. Lg. Obese)				
Pulse _____		Tonometry R___ L___		
Resp. _____	Lying R / :L /	Colorvision _____ (Ishihara plates missed)		
Temp. _____		Peripheral fields R___ L___		

	250	500	1000	2000	4000	8000
AUDIOMETRIC TESTING	R__	R__	R__	R__	R__	R__
	L__	L__	L__	L__	L__	L__

Gross hearing _____

PULMONARY FUNCTIONS

F

CHIEF COMPLAINT AND PRESENT ILLNESS _____

Employment status _____ Physician's signature _____

Date _____

G

Consent to Treatment Form

(attach label or complete blanks)

First name: _____ Last name: _____

Date of Birth: _____ Month _____ Day _____ Year

Account Number: _____

Procedure Consent Form

I, _____ ,hereby consent to have

Dr. _____ , perform _____ .

I have been fully informed of the following by my physician:

1. The nature of my condition.
2. The nature and purpose of the procedure.
3. An explanation of risks involved with the procedure.
4. Alternative treatments or procedures available.
5. The likely results of the procedure.
6. The risks involved with declining or delaying the procedure.

My physician has offered to answer all questions concerning the proposed procedure.

I am aware that the practice of medicine and surgery is not an exact science, and I acknowledge that no guarantees have been made to me about the results of the procedure.

Patient _____   Date _____
              (or guardian and relationship)

Witnessed _____   Date _____

Release of Medical Information Form

CONSENT TO RELEASE MEDICAL INFORMATION

MEDICAL RECORD REQUEST

I hereby request to inspect and/or photocopy information contained in the medical record of

_____ compiled during

Print resident name

his/her stay at _____
Facility name

from _____ through _____ . The specific information requested shall include the

following items:_____

_____

The reason(s) for this request is:_____

_____

Print name of person requesting information | Signature of person requesting information | Date

Organization represented | Phone number

Address | City | State | Zip

RESIDENT REQUEST

I hereby grant authorization to _____
Facility

to release the information listed to _____
Name/Organization indicated above

above. In addition, I waive any and all privileges relating to the disclosure hereby authorized.

This consent will expire on _____ or six months after the date shown below. I reserve the right to revoke this consent at any time and further understand that the facility named above is not liable for any records sent prior to such revocation.

X _____
Resident or appropriate resident's representative | Date

If resident's representative signed, complete the following:

Print name | Relationship to resident

(1) Witness | Date

(2) Witness (Second witness signature required if acknowledged by resident "mark".) | Date

MEDICAL RECORDS OFFICE

Information as requested released: Date _____ Time: _____ AM/PM

Explanation of information released:_____

Signature of person accepting information X _____

Signature of person releasing information X _____ Date

NAME-Last | First | Middle | Attending Physician | Chart No.

Evaluation of Competency

PROCEDURE 2-1: COMPLETION OF A CONSENT TO TREATMENT FORM

Name _____   Date _____

Evaluated By _____   Score_____

Performance Objective

Outcome:	Complete a consent to treatment form.
Conditions:	Given a consent to treatment form.
Standards:	Time: 10 minutes.
	Accuracy: Satisfactory score on the Performance Evaluation Checklist.

Performance Evaluation Checklist

Trial 1	Trial 2	Point Value	*Performance Standards*
		●	Typed required information on the consent to treatment form.
		●	Made sure that the physician had an informed consent discussion with the patient.
		▷	Is able to state why the physician must have the discussion before the form is signed.
		●	Greeted and identified the patient.
		●	Introduced yourself and explained the purpose of the form.
		●	Gave the consent form to the patient to read.
		●	Asked if the patient had any questions.
		●	Asked the patient to sign the form.
		●	Witnessed the patient's signature.
		▷	Is able to state what witnessing the form means and what it does not mean.
		●	Provided the patient with a copy of the completed form.
		●	Filed the original form in the patient's medical record.
		▷	Is able to state why the form must be filed in the medical record.
		★	Completed the procedure within 10 minutes.

Evaluation of Student Performance

EVALUATION CRITERIA			COMMENTS
Symbol	**Category**	**Point Value**	
★	Critical Step	16 points	
●	Essential Step	6 points	
▷	Theory Question	2 points	
Score calculation: 100 points			
− points missed			
Score			
Satisfactory score: 85 or above			

AAMA/CAAHEP Competency Achieved:

☐ Respond to and initiate written communications.

Evaluation of Competency

PROCEDURE 2-2: RELEASE OF MEDICAL INFORMATION

Name _____ Date _____

Evaluation _____ Score_____

Performance Objective

Outcome: Assist a patient in the completion of a consent to release medical information form.

Conditions: Given a consent to release information form.

Standards: Time: 10 minutes.
Accuracy: Satisfactory score on the Performance Evaluation Checklist.

Performance Evaluation Checklist

Trial 1	Trial 2	Point Value	Performance Standards
		●	Greeted and identified the patient.
		●	Introduced yourself and explain the purpose of the form.
		●	Provided the patient with consent form.
		●	Asked the patient to complete the form.
		●	Asked the patient to complete the information section on the form.
		●	Offered to answer questions.
		●	Checked to make sure all information was completed.
		●	Asked the patient to sign the form.
		●	Witnessed the patient's signature.
		●	Provided the patient with a copy of the completed form.
		●	Made a copy of the completed form.
		●	Included a copy of the completed form with the medical information.
		●	Documented what information was released along with the date.
		●	Signed the document with your name and credentials.
		●	Filed the release document and the consent form in the patient's medical record.
		▷	Is able to state the reason for filing the form.
		●	Sent the medical information according to the medical office policy.
		★	Completed the procedure within 10 minutes.

Evaluation of Student Performance

EVALUATION CRITERIA			COMMENTS
Symbol	**Category**	**Point Value**	
★	Critical Step	16 points	
●	Essential Step	6 points	
▷	Theory Question	2 points	

Score calculation: 100 points

− _____ points missed

_____ Score

Satisfactory score: 85 or above

AAMA/CAAHEP Competencies Achieved:

☐ Identify and respond to issues of confidentiality.

☐ Perform within legal and ethical boundaries.

Evaluation of Competency

PROCEDURE 2-3: PREPARING A MEDICAL RECORD

Name _____   Date _____

Evaluated By _____   Score_____

Performance Objective

Outcome:	Prepare a medical record.
Conditions:	Given the following: file folder, metal fasteners, name labels, alphabetic labels, miscellaneous chart labels, chart dividers, preprinted forms, and a two-hole punch.
Standards:	Time: 10 minutes
	Accuracy: Satisfactory score on the Performance Evaluation Checklist.

Performance Evaluation Checklist

Trial 1	Trial 2	Point Value	Performance Standards
		●	Greeted and identified the patient.
		●	Introduced yourself and verified that the patient was a new patient.
		●	Asked the patient to complete a patient registration form.
		●	Offered to answer questions.
		●	Checked the form for accuracy and legibility.
		●	Copied the patient's insurance card.
		▷	Is able to state the purpose of copying the card.
		●	Entered the data on the completed registration form into the computer.
		●	Assembled supplies needed to prepare the medical record.
			Typed the patient's full name on the name label
		●	The patient's name was in transposed order.
		●	The name was typed using correct spacing.
		●	The patient's name was spelled correctly.
		●	Attached appropriate color-coded labels to the side tab.
		●	The labels were attached using the indentations on the tab.
		●	Attached the name label immediately above alphabetical label.
		●	Attached additional labels to the folder as required.
		●	Inserted chart divider onto the metal fasteners.

Trial 1	Trial 2	Point Value	Performance Standards
		●	Placed the original registration form in front of medical record.
		●	Placed the insurance card in the appropriate section of the record.
		●	Labeled preprinted forms with required information.
		●	Punched holes into the form if required.
		●	Inserted each form under its proper chart divider.
		●	Rechecked the medical record to make sure it was prepared properly.
		★	Completed the procedure within 10 minutes.

Evaluation of Student Performance

EVALUATION CRITERIA			COMMENTS
Symbol	Category	Point Value	
★	Critical Step	16 points	
●	Essential Step	6 points	
▷	Theory Question	2 points	

Score calculation: 100 points
− _____ points missed
_____ Score
Satisfactory score: 85 or above

AAMA/CAAHEP Competencies Achieved:
☐ Maintain medication and immunization records.
☐ Establish and maintain the medical record.
☐ Utilize computer software to maintain office systems.

Evaluation of Competency

PROCEDURE 2-4: OBTAINING AND RECORDING PATIENT SYMPTOMS

Name _____   Date _____

Evaluation _____   Score_____

Performance Objective

Outcome:	Obtain and record patient symptoms.
Conditions:	Given the following: medical record of the patient to be interviewed and a dark blue or black pen.
Standards:	Time: 10 minutes
	Accuracy: Satisfactory score on the Performance Evaluation Checklist.

Performance Evaluation Checklist

Trial 1	Trial 2	Point Value	*Performance Standards*
		●	Assembled equipment.
		●	Made sure the correct patient record was obtained.
		●	Went to the waiting room and asked the patient to come back.
		●	Escorted the patient to a quiet room.
		●	Greeted and identified the patient.
		●	Introduced yourself using a calm and friendly manner.
		●	Asked the patient to be seated.
		●	Seated yourself facing the patient at a distance of 3 to 4 feet.
		▷	Is able to state the purpose of this seating arrangement.
			Used good communication skills
		●	Used the patient's name of choice.
		●	Demonstrated genuine interest and concern for the patient.
		●	Maintained appropriate eye contact.
		●	Used terminology the patient could understand.
		●	Listened carefully and attentively to the patient.
		●	Payed attention to the patient's nonverbal messages.
		●	Avoided judgmental comments.
		●	Avoided rushing the patient.

Trial 1	Trial 2	Point Value	Performance Standards
		●	Located the progress note sheet.
		●	Charted the chief complaint correctly.
		●	Obtained additional information regarding the chief complaint.
		●	Thanked the patient and proceeded to the next step in the patient work-up.
		●	Informed the patient the physician will be in soon.
		●	Placed the medical record in the appropriate location.
		★	Completed the procedure within 10 minutes.

CHART	
Date	

Evaluation of Student Performance

EVALUATION CRITERIA			COMMENTS
Symbol	Category	Point Value	
★	Critical Step	16 points	
●	Essential Step	6 points	
▷	Theory Question	2 points	

Score calculation: 100 points

—_____ points missed

_____ Score

Satisfactory score: 85 or above

AAMA/CAAHEP Competencies Achieved:

☐ Perform telephone and in-person screening.
☐ Obtain and record patient history.
☐ Recognize and respond to verbal communications.
☐ Recognize and respond to nonverbal communications.
☐ Document appropriately.

Taking Patient Symptoms: Supplemental Education for Chapter 2

Taking patient symptoms is a frequent and important responsibility of the medical assistant. Because of this, the medical assistant must have a thorough knowledge of symptoms and related terminology. A **symptom** is defined as any change in the body or its functioning that indicates the presence of disease. The medical assistant will be able to observe **objective** symptoms presented by the patient, such as coughing, a rash, and swelling. On the other hand, the medical assistant must rely on information relayed by the patient in order to obtain data on **subjective** symptoms. Examples of subjective symptoms include pain, pruritus, and vertigo.

This section is designed as supplemental education for Chapter 2 (The Medical Record) in your textbook. Completion of the exercises in this section will assist you in taking patient symptoms effectively and thoroughly, which is essential to an accurate diagnosis by the physician.

Learning Objectives

After completing this chapter, you should be able to:

1. Explain the purpose of analyzing a symptom.

2. State the seven basic types of information that must be obtained to analyze a symptom.

3. Analyze a symptom by using direct questions.

Analysis of a Symptom

Before a symptom can be analyzed, the chief complaint must first be identified. The **chief complaint** (CC) is the patient's reason for seeking care, or the symptom causing the patient the most trouble. An open-ended question should be used to elicit the chief complaint from the patient, and it should be charted following the charting guidelines presented in your textbook (pages 66 and 68). The next step is to analyze the chief complaint in detail from the time of its onset. The purpose of this is to provide a complete description of the current status of the chief complaint.

Analyzing the chief complaint requires a combination of good listening and writing skills. The medical assistant must also acquire a knowledge of the basic information required for each symptom as well as examples of direct and detailed questions to ask the patient to obtain this information. A list and explanation of the information required for each symptom, along with examples of direct questions to ask the patient to obtain it, are presented below.

Type of Information Required

The following information is needed for each symptom to provide a full description of the current status of the chief complaint:

1. **Location of the Symptom.** This refers to the specific area of the body where the symptom is located. Locating the symptom is the first step in determining the cause of the patient's disease. The patient may refer to the location in general terms—for example, the head, arm, stomach, or back. It is important that the medical assistant be more specific than this, however, and determine the exact location such as "occurs in the lower back" or "occurs under the sternum." Questions that assist in accomplishing this are as follows:

   Where exactly does it hurt?
   Can you show me where it hurts?
   Do you feel it anywhere else?

2. **Quality of the Symptom.** The quality of the symptom includes a complete and concise description of the symptom. The medical assistant should use informative terms to describe the character of each symptom. For example, if the patient complains of pain, the character of the pain must be included. Terms that can be used to describe pain include burning, aching, sharp, dull, throbbing, cramplike, and squeezing. If the patient has vomited, the medical assistant will need to indicate the color, odor, and consistency of the vomitus. If the patient has a cough, the medical assistant will need to indicate if it is productive or nonproductive and whether or not blood is present. Refer to the table of terms on page 46 of this manual, which will assist you in describing symptoms. Specific examples of questions that are helpful in determining the quality of the symptom are as follows:

   Describe it (the symptom) to me as fully as possible.
   What is it (the symptom) like?

3. **Severity of the Symptom.** The severity refers to the quantitative aspect of the symptom. It includes the intensity of the symptom (e.g., mild, moderate, severe), the number (e.g., of convulsions, of nosebleeds), the volume (e.g., of vomitus, of blood, of mucus), and the size or extent (e.g., of the rash, edema, lumps or masses). This information assists the physician in determining the extensiveness or seriousness of the illness. Questions to determine severity are often specific to that symptom. For example, if the patient has a productive cough, the medical assistant will need to determine how much phlegm is being coughed up (e.g., a teaspoon, half a cup). At first, this area may appear difficult. As you practice taking symptoms, however, you will learn what questions to ask the patient and eventually it will become automatic. The examples at the end of this section as well as the student practice problems provide guidance in developing skill in this area. Some examples of general questions that can be used to determine the severity of a symptom are as follows:

   How bad is it (the symptom)?
   Does it (the symptom) limit your normal activities?

4. **Chronology and Timing of the Symptom.** Chronology and timing include a sequential account of the symptom up to the time the patient came to the medical office for treatment. This information is important in determining the duration of the symptom and change in it since it first occurred. Chronology and timing includes the following four areas:

    a. **Date of Onset:** The date of the onset of the symptom should be indicated, if possible, as a calendar date and clock time. Because of this, the patient may need some time to recall this information. Examples of the questions to obtain this information are as follows:

    When did you experience this (the symptom) for the first time?
    Exactly when did this begin?

    b. **Duration:** The duration of the symptom refers to how long the symptom lasts after it occurs, for example: 10 minutes, 2 hours, continuously. Examples of questions to obtain this information are as follows:

    How long does it last after occurring?
    For what length of time do you experience this symptom?

    c. **Frequency:** The frequency of the symptom refers to how often the symptom occurs, for example: twice a day, a single attack, every 2 weeks. Examples of questions to obtain this information are as follows:

    How often does it occur?
    How often has the symptom recurred?

    d. **Change Over Time:** This area refers to any change in the symptom since it first occurred. A change in a symptom reflects the nature of the underlying disease, which, in turn, assists the physician in making a diagnosis. Examples of questions to obtain this information are as follows:

    Has the symptom changed since it first occurred?
    Is it (the symptom) getting better, worse, or staying the same?

5. **Manner of Onset.** The manner of onset refers to what the patient was doing when the symptom first occurred and exactly what was experienced by the patient when the symptom began. These data help provide information on the pathologic process responsible for the symptom. For example, the patient may have been lifting a heavy object before experiencing low back pain. As is evident, this information helps the physician in making an accurate diagnosis. Examples of questions that are helpful in determining the manner of onset are as follows:

What exactly did you experience when it (the symptom) first occurred?
What was the first thing you noticed?
Did it (the symptom) come on suddenly or gradually?
What were you doing when it (the symptom) began?
Where were you when this happened?
How were you feeling before it (the symptom) began?

6. **Modifying Factors.** Symptoms are often influenced by activities or physiologic processes such as physical exercise, change in weather, bodily functions (e.g., bowel movements, eating, coughing), pregnancy, emotional states, and fatigue. Some activities may aggravate the symptom while others may alleviate it. These influences may help to determine what is causing the problem. For example, pain that becomes

worse after the patient eats but is relieved after taking an antacid assists the physician in focusing on gastrointestinal disorders. Questions to assist in determining modifying factors are as follows:

Does anything make it (the symptom) better?
Does anything make it worse?
What have you done to make it better?
What did you do to help it?
Are you taking any medication for it? Did it help?

7. **Associated Symptoms.** There is usually more than one symptom present with a disease process. Determining these additional symptoms gives the physician a complete picture of the illness. Examples of questions that help to identify the presence of additional symptoms are as follows:

Are you having any other symptoms?
What other problems have you noticed since you became ill?

EXAMPLES

The following examples illustrate how to analyze a symptom. The chief complaint is listed first, followed by seven basic categories of required information and examples of direct and detailed questions to ask the patient.

Example

> Chief Complaint: Headaches that began 2 months ago.

1. *Location:* With your finger, point to the location of the headache.

2. *Quality:* Describe the pain. Is it sharp, dull, throbbing?

3. *Severity:* Are you able to carry on normal activities when you have a headache? Is it more severe sometimes than at other times?

4. *Chronology and Timing:*

    a. *Date of Onset:* When exactly did your headaches begin?

    b. *Duration:* How long does your headache last when it occurs?

    c. *Frequency:* How often do you get a headache?

    d. *Change Over Time:* Since your headaches began, have they gotten better, worse, or stayed the same?

5. *Manner of Onset:* What were you doing the first time you experienced a headache? How was your health before your headaches began?

6. *Modifying Factors:* Do you get a headache before, during, or after a particular activity such as reading or watching TV? Does anything make your headache better? Are you taking any medication for your headache? Does it help?

7. *Associated Symptoms:* Have you had any other problems since your headaches began, such as nausea, vomiting, dizziness, or not seeing clearly?

Example

> Chief Complaint: The patient has been coughing for the past 3 days.

1. *Location:* Does it hurt when you cough? Where? Show me with one finger.

2. *Quality:* What is the cough like? Can you cough for me? Do you bring up any phlegm when you cough? What color is it? Is blood present? Describe the pain. Is it sharp, dull, squeezing?

3. *Severity:* Do you become exhausted when you cough? How much phlegm do you bring up? A teaspoon? Half a cup? How much blood is present in the phlegm?

4. *Chronology and Timing*

    a. *Date of Onset:* When did your cough first begin?

    b. *Duration:* Does it seem like an attack? How long does the attack last?

    c. *Frequency:* How often do you get a coughing attack?

    d. *Change Over Time:* Does your cough seem to be getting better or worse?

5. *Manner of Onset:* What was the first thing you noticed when you became ill? How were you feeling before your symptoms began?

6. *Modifying Factors:* Is there anything that makes your cough better? Is there anything that makes your cough worse? Do you cough more at night or during the day? Are you taking any medication for it? Does it help?

7. *Associated Symptoms:* Are you having any other problems?

PRACTICE PROBLEMS

In the space provided, indicate examples of direct questions to ask the patient to obtain the necessary information for the symptom(s) presented in the chief complaint. To assist you with this practice session, some of the categories have already been completed.

Problem 1

> Chief Complaint: Earache and fever for the past 2 days.

1. *Location:* Which ear hurts?

2. *Quality:* _____
   _____

3. *Severity:* Does the pain wake you at night? How high has your fever been?

4. *Chronology and Timing*

    a. *Date of Onset:* _____

    b. *Duration:* _____

    c. *Frequency:* _____

    d. *Change Over Time:* _____

5. *Manner of Onset:* What was the first thing you noticed when you became ill? Did the pain start suddenly or gradually? How were you feeling before your earache began?

6. *Modifying Factors:* _____

_____

_____

_____

7. *Associated Symptoms:* Have you had any other problems, such as an ear discharge, difficulty in hearing, or dizziness?

Problem 2

Chief Complaint: Rash with itching which began 3 days ago.

1. *Location:* Where did you first notice the rash? And then where? Please show me the rash.

2. *Quality:* _____

_____

_____

3. *Severity:* _____

_____

_____

4. *Chronology and Timing*

   a. *Date of Onset:* _____

   b. *Duration:* _____

   c. *Frequency:* _____

   d. *Change Over Time:* _____

5. *Manner of Onset:* What were you doing before the rash began? What was the first thing you noticed? How were you feeling before the rash began?

6. *Modifying Factors:* Does anything make the rash worse? What have you done to try to help it?

7. *Associated Symptoms:* _____

_____

_____

Problem 3

> Chief Complaint: Pain during urination that began yesterday.

1. *Location:* _____
   _____
   _____

2. *Quality:* Describe the pain. Is it burning, sharp, dull, aching? Do you have any difficulty in beginning to urinate? What color is your urine? Is there any blood present?

3. *Severity:* _____
   _____
   _____

4. *Chronology and Timing*
   a. *Date of Onset:* When did the pain first begin?
   b. *Duration:* How long does the burning sensation last?
   c. *Frequency:* Do you have burning each time you urinate?
   d. *Change Over Time:* Does it seem to be getting better or worse?

5. *Manner of Onset:* _____
   _____
   _____

6. *Modifying Factors:* _____
   _____
   _____

7. *Associated Symptoms:* Have you had any other symptoms such as lower back pain, abdominal cramps, or fever? _____
   _____
   _____

Problem 4

> Chief Complaint: Low back pain for the past 3 months.

1. *Location:* Can you show me where it hurts?

2. *Quality:* _____
   _____
   _____

3. *Severity:* _____

_____

_____

4. *Chronology and Timing*

  a. *Date of Onset:* _____

  b. *Duration:* _____

  c. *Frequency:* _____

  d. *Change Over Time:* _____

5. *Manner of Onset:* What were you doing just before you started having low back pain? What was the first thing you noticed? How was your health before you started having back pain?

6. *Modifying Factors:* Does anything make it better such as lying down or applying heat? What makes it worse? Are you taking any medication for it? Does it help?

7. *Associated Symptoms:* _____

_____

_____

Note: To assess your progress in analyzing symptoms, complete all seven categories in the remaining practice problems.

Problem 5

Chief Complaint: Sore throat and fever for the past 24 hours.

1. *Location:* _____

_____

_____

2. *Quality:* _____

_____

_____

3. *Severity:* _____

_____

_____

4. *Chronology and Timing*

  a. *Date of Onset:* _____

  b. *Duration:* _____

  c. *Frequency:* _____

  d. *Change Over Time:* _____

5. *Manner of Onset:* _____

_____

_____

6. *Modifying Factors:*_____

_____

_____

7. *Associated Symptoms:* _____

_____

_____

Problem 6

Chief Complaint: Chest pain that occurred this morning.

1. *Location:* _____

_____

_____

2. *Quality:* _____

_____

_____

3. *Severity:* _____

_____

_____

4. *Chronology and Timing*
   a. *Date of Onset:* _____
   b. *Duration:* _____
   c. *Frequency:* _____
   d. *Change Over Time:* _____

5. *Manner of Onset:* _____

_____

_____

6. *Modifying Factors:* _____

_____

_____

7. *Associated Symptoms:* _____

_____

_____

Terms for Describing Symptoms

PAIN
Burning, aching, sharp, dull, throbbing, cramping, squeezing
Radiating, transient, constant
Localized, superficial, deep

RESPIRATIONS
Rapid, irregular, shallow, deep, labored, gasping, noisy, wheezing
Apnea, dyspnea, orthopnea
Discomfort, pain, cyanosis, cough

COUGH
Nonproductive, productive
Persistent, dry, hacking, barking, spasmodic
Phlegm: color, consistency, presence or absence of blood
Exhausting or painful

CARDIOVASCULAR
Pain, palpitations
Sharp, radiating
Dyspnea, orthopnea
Cyanosis

GASTROINTESTINAL
Abdomen: flaccid, rigid, distended
Appetite: anorexia, intolerance to foods
Heartburn, pain after eating, belching, nausea, vomiting, flatulence, change in bowel habits, constipation, diarrhea, black stools

URINE/STOOL
Abnormality: color, odor, consistency, frequency
Contents: sediment, mucus, blood
Elimination: urgency, nocturia, pain, burning

SKIN
Rash: pruritus, red, swelling, distribution
Lesions: color, character, distribution
Pallor, flushing, jaundice, warm, dry, cold, clammy
Ecchymosis, petechiae, cyanosis, edema
Pruritus, sweating, change in color, bruises easily

EARS
Pain, loss of hearing, tinnitus, vertigo
Discharge, infection

EYES
Itching, burning, blurry vision, seeing double, photophobia
Discharge, watering, infection

Vital Signs

Temperature

NAME _____

Key Terminology Assessment

Directions: Match each medical term with its definition.

_____ 1. afebrile
_____ 2. antipyretic
_____ 3. axilla
_____ 4. Centigrade thermometer
_____ 5. conduction
_____ 6. convection
_____ 7. crisis
_____ 8. disinfectant
_____ 9. Fahrenheit thermometer
_____ 10. febrile
_____ 11. frenulum linguae
_____ 12. hyperpyrexia
_____ 13. hypothermia
_____ 14. lysis
_____ 15. radiation

A. An extremely high fever.
B. A substance that kills disease-producing organisms.
C. A body temperature that is below normal.
D. The armpit.
E. The transfer of energy, such as heat, in the form of currents.
F. The gradual return of the body temperature to normal.
G. An agent that reduces fever.
H. A thermometer on which the freezing point of water is 32° and the boiling point of water is 212°.
I. The transfer of energy, such as heat, in the form of waves.
J. A thermometer on which the freezing point of water is 0° and the boiling point is 100°.
K. The midline fold that connects the undersurface of the tongue with the floor of the mouth.
L. Pertaining to fever.
M. The transfer of energy, such as heat, from one object to another.
N. The sudden falling of an elevated body temperature to normal.
O. Without fever; the body temperature is normal.

Self-Evaluation

Directions: Fill in each blank with correct answer.

1. Define a vital sign.

   _____

   _____

   _____

2. What are the four vital signs?

   _____

   _____

   _____

   _____

3. What general guidelines should be followed when measuring vital signs?

   _____

   _____

   _____

4. List four ways in which heat is produced in the body.

   _____

   _____

   _____

   _____

5. List four ways in which heat is lost from the body.

   _____

   _____

   _____

   _____

6. What is the normal body temperature range?

   _____

7. What is a fever?

   _____

   _____

8. How do diurnal variations affect body temperature?

   _____

   _____

9. How does vigorous physical exercise affect body temperature?

_____

_____

10. How do emotional states affect the body temperature?

_____

_____

11. What symptoms occur with a fever?

_____

_____

12. Describe the following fever patterns:
    a.   continuous fever

          _____

          _____

    b.   intermittent fever

          _____

          _____

    c.   remittent fever

          _____

          _____

13. What is the subsiding stage of a fever?

_____

14. What four sites are used for taking body temperature?

_____

_____

15. Why is the rectal method for taking body temperature considered the most accurate method?

_____

_____

_____

16. List three instances in which the axillary site for taking body temperature would be preferred over the oral site.

_____

_____

_____

17. How does a temperature taken through the rectal and axillary method compare (in terms of degrees) with a temperature taken through the oral method?

_____

_____

18. List and describe the four types of thermometers available for taking body temperature.

_____

_____

_____

_____

19. What is the purpose of using a probe cover with an electronic thermometer?

_____

20. Describe the advantages of a tympanic membrane thermometer.

_____

_____

21. Explain how a tympanic membrane thermometer measures body temperature.

_____

_____

_____

22. Explain how to clean the lens of a tympanic membrane thermometer.

_____

_____

23. Where should a chemical thermometer be stored? Explain why.

_____

_____

24. Why is the bulb of an oral mercury glass thermometer long and slender?

_____

_____

25. What is the purpose of temperature sheaths?

_____

_____

Critical Thinking Skills

1. For each of the following situations involving the measurement of body temperature using a tympanic membrane thermometer, write **C** if the technique is correct and **I** if the technique is incorrect. If the situation is correct, state the principle underlying the technique. If the situation is incorrect, explain what might happen if the technique were performed in the incorrect manner.

   _____ a. A tympanic membrane thermometer is used to take the temperature of a patient with impacted cerumen.

   _____ b. A thermometer with a dirty probe lens is used to take the patient's temperature.

   _____ c. The ear canal is straightened before taking a patient's aural temperature.

   _____ d. The medical assistant does not seal the opening of the ear canal with the probe when taking aural temperature.

   _____ e. The probe is positioned toward the opposite temple when taking aural temperature.

   _____ f. The medical assistant waits 30 seconds before taking the patient's temperature in the same ear.

2. Using the principles outlined in the Procedures for Measuring Body Temperature, tell what might happen if any of the following occurred during the procedure:

   _____ a. The mercury level is not below 96°F before inserting a glass thermometer in the patient's mouth.

   _____ b. The rectal thermometer is not lubricated before being inserted into the rectum.

   _____ c. The medical assistant walks into the examining room to take a patient's oral temperature and finds him drinking a cold liquid.

   _____ d. The patient talks while having his oral temperature measured.

   _____ e. A _rectal_ temperature reading is recorded as follows: 99.8°F.

   _____ f. The mercury glass thermometer is left in the patient's axilla for 3 minutes.

3. Record the following temperature readings in the spaces provided. For each oral temperature recording (g through n), indicate whether the reading is normal, sub-normal, or above normal (pyrexia).

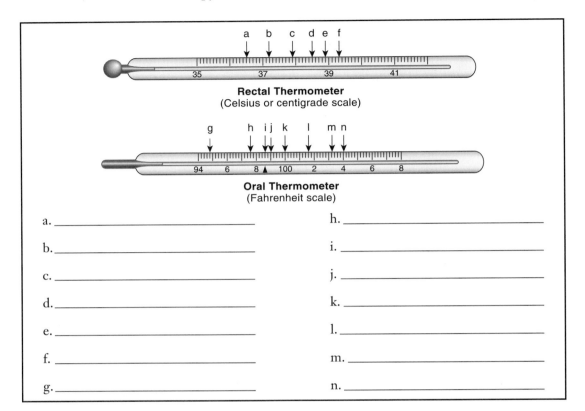

a. _____

b. _____

c. _____

d. _____

e. _____

f. _____

g. _____

h. _____

i. _____

j. _____

k. _____

l. _____

m. _____

n. _____

Pulse

Key Terminology Assessment

Directions: Match each medical term with its definition.

_____ 1. antecubital space
_____ 2. aorta
_____ 3. arrhythmia
_____ 4. bounding pulse
_____ 5. bradycardia
_____ 6. intercostal
_____ 7. pulse rhythm
_____ 8. pulse volume
_____ 9. tachycardia
_____10. thready pulse

A. Between the ribs.
B. A pulse with an increased volume that feels very strong and full.
C. The strength of the heart beat.
D. The space located at the front of the elbow.
E. An abnormally fast heart rate (over 100 beats per minute).
F. The major trunk of the arterial system of the body.
G. The time interval between heart beats.
H. A pulse with a decreased volume that feels weak and thin.
I. An irregular rhythm.
J. An abnormally slow heart rate (below 60 beats per minute).

Self-Evaluation

Directions: Fill in each blank with the correct answer.

1. What causes the pulse to occur?

2. What measurement unit is used in checking the pulse rate?

3. How does physical activity affect the pulse rate?

4. What is the most common site for taking the pulse?

5. When is the brachial artery used as a pulse site?

6. When is the carotid artery used as a pulse site?

_____

7. When is the femoral artery used as a pulse site?

_____

8. List two reasons for taking the pulse at the apical pulse site.

_____

_____

9. List two reasons for measuring the pulse rate.

_____

_____

10. State the normal range for a pulse rate for an adult.

_____

11. Which of the following individuals would have the faster pulse rate, a 30-year-old adult or a 5-year-old child?

_____

_____

12. If the rhythm and volume of a patient's pulse are normal, the medical assistant would record it as

_____

Critical Thinking Skills

Complete the following exercises:

1. Take the radial pulse rate of three children. Determine the rhythm and volume of each. Record the pulse rate, rhythm, and volume below:

    a. _____

    b. _____

    c. _____

2. Locate the pulse at the following sites and record the pulse rates below:

    a. Brachial pulse

    _____

    b. Temporal pulse

c. Carotid pulse

_____

d. Femoral pulse

_____

e. Popliteal pulse

_____

f. Dorsalis pedis

_____

3. Take the radial pulse rate of a person before and after vigorous exercise. Record results below:

a. Before vigorous exercise

_____

b. After vigorous exercise

_____

c. Compare the results and explain how exercise affects the pulse rate.

_____

Respiration

Key Terminology Assessment

Direction: Match each medical term with its definition.

_____ 1. alveolus
_____ 2. apnea
_____ 3. bradypnea
_____ 4. cyanosis
_____ 5. dyspnea
_____ 6. eupnea
_____ 7. exhalation
_____ 8. hyperventilation
_____ 9. hypopnea
_____ 10. hypoxia
_____ 11. inhalation
_____ 12. orthopnea
_____ 13. tachypnea

A. The act of breathing out.
B. A reduction in the oxygen supply to the tissues of the body.
C. The temporary cessation of breathing.
D. An abnormal increase in the respiratory rate of more than 20 respirations per minute.
E. An abnormal decrease in the rate and depth of respiration.
ß. A thin-walled air sac of the lungs in which the exchange of oxygen and carbon dioxide takes place.
G. The act of breathing in.
H. A bluish discoloration of the skin and mucous membranes.
I. The condition in which breathing is easier when an individual is in a standing or sitting position.
J. Labored or difficult breathing.
K. Normal respiration.
L. An abnormally fast and deep type of breathing usually associated with acute anxiety or emotional tension.
M. An abnormal decrease in the respiratory rate of less than 10 respirations per minute.

Self-Evaluation

Directions: Fill in each blank with the correct answer.

1. What is the purpose of respiration?

   _____

   _____

2. What is the purpose of inhalation?

   _____

   _____

3. What is the purpose of exhalation?

   _____

   _____

4. What is included in one complete respiration?

_____

_____

5. The exchange of oxygen and carbon dioxide between the body cells and blood is known as

_____

6. What is the name of the control center for involuntary respiration?

_____

7. Why must respiration be taken without the patient's awareness?

_____

_____

8. What is the normal respiratory rate (range) for a normal adult?

_____

_____

9. An abnormal decrease in the respiratory rate is known as

_____

_____

10. List two factors that will increase the respiratory rate.

_____

_____

11. Describe a normal rhythm for respiration.

_____

_____

12. Where is cyanosis first observed?

_____

_____

13. What are two conditions in which dyspnea may occur?

_____

_____

14. Describe the character of normal breath sounds.

_____

_____

15. Describe the character of the following abnormal breath sounds:

    a. stertor

_____

_____

    b. crackles

_____

_____

    c. gurgles

_____

_____

    d. wheezes

_____

_____

Critical Thinking Skills

1. Mrs. Allen is upset over the constant temper tantrums of her three-year-old son, during which he holds his breath until he turns blue. What can you tell her about breathholding that may help to reduce her anxiety?

_____

_____

_____

2. a. Take a person's respiratory rate before and after vigorous exercise. Record results below:

Before vigorous exercise

_____

After vigorous exercise

_____

    b. Compare the results and explain how vigorous exercise affects the respiratory rate.

_____

_____

_____

3. Mr. Bateman has difficulty breathing and tells you it is easier for him to breathe while in a sitting position. How would you record his condition?

_____

_____

4. Mr. Gilbert's respiratory rate is 16. What would you expect his pulse to be?

_____

5. Using a reference source, define the following chronic obstructive pulmonary diseases (COPD) and list the symptoms of each:

   a. emphysema

   _____
   _____
   _____
   _____

   b. asthma

   _____
   _____
   _____
   _____

   c. chronic bronchitis

   _____
   _____
   _____
   _____

Blood Pressure

Key Terminology Assessment

Directions: Match each medical term with its definition.

_____ 1. diastole
_____ 2. diastolic pressure
_____ 3. hypertension
_____ 4. hypotension
_____ 5. meniscus
_____ 6. pulse pressure
_____ 7. sphygmomanometer
_____ 8. stethoscope
_____ 9. systole
_____ 10. systolic pressure

A. The curved surface on a column of liquid in a tube.
B. High blood pressure.
C. The point of maximum pressure on the arterial walls.
D. The phase in the cardiac cycle in which the heart relaxes between contractions.
E. An instrument for measuring arterial blood pressure.
F. The point of lesser pressure on the arterial walls.
G. Low blood pressure.

H. The phase in the cardiac cycle in which the ventricles contract, sending blood out of the heart and into the aorta and pulmonary aorta.
I. An instrument for amplifying and hearing sounds produced by the body.
J. The difference between the systolic and diastolic pressures.

Self-Evaluation

Directions: Fill in each blank with the correct answer.

1. What does blood pressure measure?

   _____
   _____

2. Why is the diastolic pressure lower than the systolic pressure?

   _____
   _____
   _____

3. What is the normal range for blood pressure for an adult?

   _____

4. Why should blood pressure readings always be interpreted using the patient's baseline blood pressure?

   _____
   _____
   _____

5. How does age affect blood pressure?

   _____
   _____

6. How do diurnal variations affect the blood pressure?

   _____
   _____

7. What are the parts of a sphygmomanometer?

   _____
   _____

8. List the two types of sphygmomanometers.

_____

_____

9. List the three different cuff sizes and give examples of when each would be employed.

_____

_____

_____

10. List the five phases included in the Korotkoff sounds and what type of sound is heard during each phase.

_____

_____

_____

_____

_____

_____

Critical Thinking Skills

1. What would you tell patients who are having their blood pressure taken for the first time to help them understand the purpose and procedure for taking blood pressure?

_____

_____

_____

_____

2. Using the principles outlined in the Procedure for Measuring Blood Pressure, tell what happens under the following circumstances:

   a. The blood pressure is taken on a patient who has just undergone vigorous physical exercise.

   _____

   _____

   b. The blood pressure is taken on a patient with tight sleeves.

   _____

   _____

   c. An adult cuff is used to measure blood pressure on a young child.

   _____

   _____

d. The rubber bladder is not centered over the brachial artery.

_____

_____

e. The cuff is placed 1/2 inch above the bend in the elbows.

_____

_____

f. The manometer is viewed from a distance of 4 feet.

_____

_____

3. Read and record the following blood pressure measurements in the space provided.

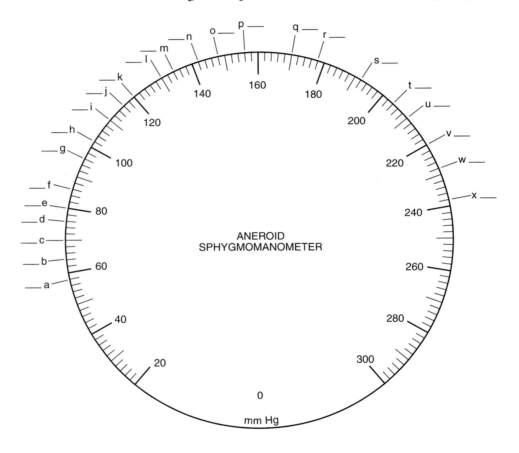

4. What should the medical assistant do if she enters the room to take blood pressure and discovers that the patient is in a very fearful and apprehensive state? Explain your answer.

_____

_____

_____

_____

Practice for Competency

BODY TEMPERATURE

Assignment

Measure body temperature with each of the following types of thermometers and record in the chart provided.

1. Electronic thermometer
2. Tympanic membrane thermometer
3. Mercury glass thermometer
4. Chemical thermometer

CHART	
Date	

CHART	
Date	

Evaluation of Competency

PROCEDURE 3-1: MEASURING BODY TEMPERATURE—ELECTRONIC THERMOMETER

Name _____   Date _____

Evaluated By _____   Score_____

Performance Objective

Outcome:	Measure oral body temperature.
Conditions:	Given the following: electronic thermometer and oral probe, oral probe cover, and a biohazard waste container.
Standards:	Time: 5 minutes
	Accuracy: Satisfactory score on the Performance Evaluation Checklist.

Performance Evaluation Checklist

Trial 1	Trial 2	Point Value	Performance Standards
		●	Washed hands.
		●	Assembled equipment.
		●	Attached oral temperature probe to thermometer unit.
		●	Inserted probe into the face of thermometer.
		●	Greeted and identified the patient.
		●	Introduced yourself and explained the procedure.
		●	Removed thermometer unit from its rechargeable base.
		●	Grasped probe by the collar and removed it from the face of the thermometer.
		▷	Is able to state what occurs when probe is removed from the face of the thermometer.
		●	Attached disposable probe cover to probe.
		▷	Is able to state the purpose of probe cover.
		●	Correctly inserted the oral probe in patient's mouth.
		●	Held probe in place until the audible tone was heard.
		●	Noted patient's temperature reading on the digital display screen.
		●	Removed probe from patient's mouth.

Trial 1	Trial 2	Point Value	Performance Standards
		●	Discarded probe cover in a biohazard waste container.
		●	Did not allow fingers to come in contact with cover.
		●	Returned probe to its stored position in the thermometer unit.
		▷	Is able to state what occurs when probe is returned to face of the thermometer.
		●	Washed hands.
		●	Charted the results correctly.
		★	The temperature recording was identical to the reading on the display screen.
		●	Stored thermometer unit in its base.
		▷	Is able to state why thermometer unit must be stored in its base.
		★	Completed the procedure within 5 minutes.

CHART	
Date	

Evaluation of Student Performance

EVALUATION CRITERIA			COMMENTS
Symbol	**Category**	**Point Value**	
★	Critical Step	16 points	
●	Essential Step	6 points	
▷	Theory Question	2 points	
Score calculation: 100 points			
− _____ points missed			
_____ Score			
Satisfactory score: 85 or above			

AAMA/CAAHEP Competency Achieved:
☐ Obtain vital signs.

Evaluation of Competency

PROCEDURE 3-2: MEASURING AURAL BODY TEMPERATURE— TYMPANIC MEMBRANE THERMOMETER

Name _____   Date _____

Evaluated By _____   Score_____

Performance Objective

Outcome:	Measure aural body temperature.
Conditions:	Given the following: tympanic membrane thermometer, probe cover, and a biohazard waste container.
Standards:	Time: 5 minutes
	Accuracy: Satisfactory score on the Performance Evaluation Checklist.

Performance Evaluation Checklist

Trial 1	Trial 2	Point Value	Performance Standards
		●	Washed hands.
		●	Assembled equipment.
		●	Greeted and identified the patient.
		●	Introduced yourself and explained the procedure.
		●	Removed the thermometer from its base.
		●	Checked to make sure the probe lens was clean and intact.
		▷	Is able to state what would occur if the lens was dirty.
		●	Checked the display screen to make sure the thermometer is set on the proper mode for the patient's age.
		●	Placed a cover on the probe.
		▷	Is able to state the purpose of the probe cover.
		●	Pulled the probe straight up and observed the screen until the word READY appeared.
		●	Held the thermometer in the dominant hand.
		●	Straightened the patient's ear canal with the nondominant hand.
		▷	Is able to state the purpose of straightening the ear canal.

Trial 1	Trial 2	Point Value	Performance Standards
		●	Inserted the probe into the patient's ear canal and sealed the opening without causing the patient discomfort.
		●	Pointed the tip of the probe toward the opposite temple.
		▷	Is able to state the reason for pointing the probe toward the opposite temple.
		●	Asked the patient to remain still.
		●	Held the thermometer steady and depressed the activation button for 1 full second.
		●	Read the patient's temperature on the display screen.
		▷	Is able to state what should be done if the temperature seems too low.
		●	Disposed of the probe cover in a biohazard waste container.
		●	Replaced the thermometer in its base.
		▷	Is able to state the reason for storing the thermometer in its base.
		●	Washed hands.
		●	Charted the results correctly.
		★	The temperature recording was identical to the reading on the display screen.
		★	Completed the procedure within 5 minutes.

CHART	
Date	

Evaluation of Student Performance

EVALUATION CRITERIA			COMMENTS
Symbol	Category	Point Value	
★	Critical Step	16 points	
●	Essential Step	6 points	
▷	Theory Question	2 points	

Score calculation: 100 points

−_____ points missed

_____ Score

Satisfactory score: 85 or above

AAMA/CAAHEP Competency Achieved:
☐ Obtain vital signs.

Evaluation of Competency

PROCEDURE 3-3: MEASURING BODY TEMPERATURE—ORAL/MERCURY GLASS THERMOMETER

Name _____   Date _____

Evaluated By _____   Score_____

Performance Objective

Outcome:	Measure oral body temperature.
Conditions:	Given the following: oral mercury glass thermometer, oral temperature sheath, disposable gloves, and a biohazard waste container.
	Using a watch with a sweep second hand.
Standards:	Time: 5 minutes
	Accuracy: Satisfactory score on the Performance Evaluation Checklist.

Performance Evaluation Checklist

Trial 1	Trial 2	Point Value	*Performance Standards*
		●	Washed hands.
		●	Assembled equipment.
		●	Greeted and identified the patient.
		●	Introduced yourself and explained the procedure.
		▷	Is able to state what should be done if patient is drinking a hot liquid.
		●	Checked the level of mercury in thermometer.
		●	Shook mercury level to 96°F or below, if necessary using a snapping wrist movement.
		▷	Is able to state why mercury level does not fall on its own.
		●	Applied gloves.
		●	Applied the temperature sheath.
		▷	Is able to state the purpose of the temperature sheath.
		●	Correctly placed thermometer in patient's mouth.
		▷	Is able to state why the mouth is used as a site to take body temperature.

Trial 1	Trial 2	Point Value	Performance Standards
		●	Instructed patient to keep the mouth closed and to hold thermometer in place with the lips.
		▷	Is able to state why the mouth must be kept closed.
		●	Left thermometer in place for 2 to 3 minutes.
		●	Removed thermometer from the patient's mouth.
		●	Removed the thermometer sheath and disposed of it in a biohazard waste container.
		●	Held thermometer horizontally at eye level.
		●	Read thermometer accurately.
		★	The reading was identical to evaluator's reading.
		●	Placed the thermometer in the designated container for cleansing and disinfecting.
		●	Removed gloves and washed hands.
		●	Charted the results correctly.
		★	Completed the procedure within 5 minutes.

CHART	
Date	

Evaluation of Student Performance

EVALUATION CRITERIA			COMMENTS
Symbol	Category	Point Value	
★	Critical Step	16 points	
●	Essential Step	6 points	
▷	Theory Question	2 points	

Score calculation: 100 points

— _____ points missed

_____ Score

Satisfactory score: 85 or above

AAMA/CAAHEP Competency Achieved:
☐ Obtain vital signs.

Evaluation of Competency

PROCEDURE 3-4: MEASURING BODY TEMPERATURE— RECTAL/MERCURY THERMOMETER

Name _____   Date _____

Evaluated By _____   Score_____

Performance Objective

Outcome:	Measure rectal body temperature.
Conditions:	Given the following: rectal mercury glass thermometer, rectal temperature sheath, disposable gloves, soft tissues, and a biohazard waste container.
	Using a watch with a sweep second hand.
Standards:	Time: 5 minutes
	Accuracy: Satisfactory score on the Performance Evaluation Checklist.

Performance Evaluation Checklist

Trial 1	Trial 2	Point Value	Performance Standards
		●	Washed hands.
		●	Assembled equipment.
		●	Greeted and identified the patient.
		●	Introduced yourself and explained the procedure.
		●	Positioned the patient.
		●	Checked the level of mercury in the thermometer.
		●	Shook mercury level to 96°F or below, if necessary using a snapping wrist movement.
		●	Applied gloves.
		●	Applied a prelubricated temperature sheath to the thermometer.
		▷	Is able to state why the temperature sheath is lubricated.
		●	Spread buttocks and properly inserted the thermometer into the rectum.

Trial 1	Trial 2	Point Value	Performance Standards
		▷	Is able to state how far the thermometer should be inserted for adults, children, and infants.
		●	Instructed patient to remain still.
		●	Held the thermometer in place for 2 to 3 minutes.
		●	Removed thermometer in the same manner as it was inserted.
		●	Removed the temperature sheath and disposed of it in a biohazard waste container.
		●	Held thermometer horizontally at eye level.
		●	Read thermometer accurately.
		★	The reading was identical to the evaluator's reading.
		▷	Is able to state how the rectal temperature reading compares to the oral temperature reading.
		●	Placed thermometer in the designated container for cleansing and disinfecting.
		●	Wiped the anal area with tissues.
		●	Removed gloves and washed hands.
		●	Charted the results correctly.
		★	Completed the procedure within 5 minutes.

CHART	
Date	

Evaluation of Student Performance

EVALUATION CRITERIA			COMMENTS
Symbol	Category	Point Value	
★	Critical Step	16 points	
●	Essential Step	6 points	
▷	Theory Question	2 points	

Score calculation: 100 points

$-$ _____ points missed

_____ Score

Satisfactory score: 85 or above

AAMA/CAAHEP Competency Achieved:
☐ Obtain vital signs.

Evaluation of Competency

PROCEDURE 3-5: MEASURING BODY TEMPERATURE— AXILLARY/MERCURY GLASS THERMOMETER

Name _____   Date _____

Evaluated By _____   Score_____

Performance Objective

Outcome: Measure axillary body temperature.

Conditions: Given the following: axillary mercury glass thermometer, oral temperature sheath, and a biohazard waste container.

Using a watch with a sweep second hand.

Standards: Time: 12 minutes.

Accuracy: Satisfactory score on the Performance Evaluation Checklist.

Performance Evaluation Checklist

Trial 1	Trial 2	Point Value	Performance Standards
		●	Washed hands.
		●	Assembled equipment.
		●	Greeted and identified the patient.
		●	Introduced yourself and explained the procedure.
		●	Checked the level of mercury in thermometer.
		●	Shook mercury level to 96°F or below, if necessary using a snapping wrist movement.
		●	Removed clothing from patient's shoulder and arm.
		●	Made sure the axilla was dry.
		●	Applied the temperature sheath to the thermometer.
		●	Placed bulb of thermometer in the center of the axilla.
		●	Instructed patient to hold arm close to the body with the forearm across the chest.
		▷	Is able to explain why arm must be held tightly against chest.
		●	Left thermometer in place for 5 to 10 minutes.

Trial 1	Trial 2	Point Value	*Performance Standards*
		●	Removed thermometer from the patient's axilla.
		●	Removed the temperature sheath and disposed of it in a biohazard waste container.
		●	Held thermometer horizontally at eye level.
		●	Read thermometer accurately.
		★	The reading was identical to the evaluator's reading.
		▷	Is able to state how the axillary temperature reading compares to the oral temperature reading.
		●	Placed thermometer in the designated container for cleansing and disinfecting.
		●	Washed hands.
		●	Charted the results correctly.
		★	Completed the procedure within 12 minutes.

CHART	
Date	

Evaluation of Student Performance

EVALUATION CRITERIA			COMMENTS
Symbol	**Category**	**Point Value**	
★	Critical Step	16 points	
●	Essential Step	6 points	
▷	Theory Question	2 points	
Score calculation: 100 points			
<div align="right">− points missed</div>			
<div align="right"> Score</div>			
Satisfactory score: 85 or above			

AAMA/CAAHEP Competency Achieved:
☐ Obtain vital signs.

Practice for Competency

PULSE

Assignment:

Radial Pulse. Measure the radial pulse. Describe the rhythm and volume of the pulse. Record the results in the chart provided.

Apical Pulse. Measure apical pulse. Describe the rhythm and volume of the pulse. Record the results in the chart provided.

CHART	
Date	

CHART	
Date	

Evaluation of Competency

PROCEDURE 3-6: MEASURING RADIAL PULSE

Name _____ Date _____

Evaluated By _____ Score_____

Performance Objective

Outcome:	Measure radial pulse.
Conditions:	Using a watch with a sweep second hand.
Standards:	Time: 3 minutes.
	Accuracy: Satisfactory score on the Performance Evaluation Checklist.

Performance Evaluation Checklist

Trial 1	Trial 2	Point Value	Performance Standards
		●	Washed hands.
		●	Greeted and identified the patient.
		●	Introduced yourself and explained the procedure.
		●	Observed patient for any signs that might influence the pulse rate.
		▷	Is able to state two factors that would increase the pulse rate.
		●	Positioned patient, making sure that the arm rests alongside the body with the palm facing downward.
		●	Placed three middle fingertips over the radial pulse site.
		▷	Is able to state why the pulse should not be taken with the thumb.
		●	Applied moderate, gentle pressure until the pulse was felt.
		▷	Is able to state what will occur if too much pressure is applied over the radial artery.
		●	Counted the pulse for 30 seconds and multiplied by 2.
		★	The reading was within ±2 beats of the evaluator's reading.
		●	Determined the rhythm and volume of the pulse.
		▷	Is able to state when the pulse should be measured for a full minute.
		●	Charted the results correctly.
		★	Completed the procedure within 3 minutes.

CHART

Date	

Evaluation of Student Performance

EVALUATION CRITERIA			COMMENTS
Symbol	**Category**	**Point Value**	
★	Critical Step	16 points	
●	Essential Step	6 points	
▷	Theory Question	2 points	

Score calculation: 100 points

−_____ points missed

_____ Score

Satisfactory score: 85 or above

AAMA/CAAHEP Competency Achieved:
☐ Obtain vital signs.

Evaluation of Competency

PROCEDURE 3-7: MEASURING APICAL PULSE

Name _____   Date _____

Evaluated By _____   Score_____

Performance Objective

Outcome:	Measure apical pulse
Conditions:	Given the following: stethoscope and antiseptic wipe.
	Using a watch with a sweep second hand.
Standards:	Time: 5 minutes
	Accuracy: Satisfactory score on the Performance Evaluation Checklist.

Performance Evaluation Checklist

Trial 1	Trial 2	Point Value	*Performance Standards*
		●	Washed hands.
		●	Greeted and identified the patient.
		●	Introduced yourself and explained the procedure.
		●	Assembled equipment.
		●	Cleaned earpieces of stethoscope with antiseptic wipe.
		▷	Is able to state the reason for cleaning earpieces with an antiseptic.
		●	Positioned patient.
		●	Warmed chestpiece of the stethoscope.
		▷	Is able to state the reason for warming chestpiece.
		●	Inserted earpieces of stethoscope correctly in the ears.
		▷	Is able to state why the earpieces must be inserted correctly.
		●	Correctly placed the chestpiece over the apex of the heart.
		●	Counted the number of heart beats for 30 seconds and multiplied by 2.
		★	The reading was within ±2 beats of the evaluator's reading.
		●	Charted the results correctly.
		●	Cleaned earpieces of stethoscope with an antiseptic wipe.
		★	Completed the procedure within 5 minutes.

CHART	
Date	

Evaluation of Student Performance

EVALUATION CRITERIA			COMMENTS
Symbol	**Category**	**Point Value**	
★	Critical Step	16 points	
●	Essential Step	6 points	
▷	Theory Question	2 points	
Score calculation: 100 points			
− _____ points missed			
_____ Score			
Satisfactory score: 85 or above			

AAMA/CAAHEP Competency Achieved:
☐ Obtain vital signs.

Practice for Competency

RESPIRATION

Assignment

Measure respiratory rate and describe the rhythm and depth of the respirations. Record results in the chart provided.

CHART	
Date	

CHART	
Date	

Evaluation of Competency

PROCEDURE 3-8: MEASURING RESPIRATION

Name _____ Date _____

Evaluated By _____ Score_____

Performance Objective

Outcome: Measure respirations.
Conditions: Using a watch with a sweep second hand.
Standards: Time: 3 minutes.
Accuracy: Satisfactory score on the Performance Evaluation Checklist.

Performance Evaluation Checklist

Trial 1	Trial 2	Point Value	*Performance Standards*
		●	Took respirations without patient's awareness.
		▷	Is able to state why respirations should be taken without patient's awareness.
		●	Observed the rise and fall of patient's chest.
		●	Counted the number of respirations for 30 seconds and multiplied by 2.
		★	The measurement was within ±1 respiration of the evaluator's measurement.
		▷	Is able to state what makes up one respiration.
		●	Determined the rhythm and depth of the respirations.
		●	Charted the results correctly.
		★	Completed the procedure within 3 minutes.

CHART	
Date	

Evaluation of Student Performance

EVALUATION CRITERIA			COMMENTS
Symbol	**Category**	**Point Value**	
★	Critical Step	16 points	
●	Essential Step	6 points	
▷	Theory Question	2 points	
Score calculation: 100 points			
− _____ points missed			
_____ Score			
Satisfactory score: 85 or above			

AAMA/CAAHEP Competency Achieved:

☐ Obtain vital signs.

Practice for Competency

BLOOD PRESSURE

Assignment

Measure blood pressure. Record results in the chart provided.

CHART	
Date	

CHART	
Date	

Evaluation of Competency

PROCEDURE 3-9: MEASURING BLOOD PRESSURE

Name _____ Date _____

Evaluated By _____ Score_____

Performance Objective

Outcome: Measure blood pressure.

Conditions: Give the following: stethoscope, sphygmomanometer, and an antiseptic wipe.

Standards: Time: 5 minutes

Accuracy: Satisfactory score on the Performance Evaluation Checklist.

Performance Evaluation Checklist

Trial 1	Trial 2	Point Value	*Performance Standards*
		●	Washed hands.
		●	Assembled equipment, making sure to choose proper cuff size.
		●	Cleaned earpieces of stethoscope.
		●	Greeted and identified the patient.
		●	Introduced yourself and explained the procedure.
		●	Observed patient for any signs that might influence the blood pressure reading.
		▷	Is able to list signs that would influence the blood pressure reading.
		●	Positioned patient in a sitting position.
		●	Made sure that the patient's arm was uncovered.
		●	Correctly positioned patient's arm.
		●	Placed cuff on patient's arm 1 inch above bend in elbow.
		●	Centered rubber bladder over the brachial artery.
		●	Wrapped cuff smoothly and snugly around patient's arm and secured the end of cuff.
		●	Positioned self and/or manometer for direct viewing and at a distance of no more than 3 feet.
		●	Inserted earpieces of stethoscope correctly in the ears.
		●	Located the brachial pulse with fingertips.

Trial 1	Trial 2	Point Value	Performance Standards
		▷	Is able to state the purpose for locating the brachial pulse.
		●	Placed chestpiece of the stethoscope over the brachial artery.
		●	Made sure chestpiece was not touching cuff.
		▷	Is able to state why the chestpiece should not touch the cuff.
		●	Closed valve on bulb and pumped air into cuff up to level of 20 to 30 mm of mercury above the palpated or previously measured systolic pressure.
		●	Released pressure at a moderate, steady rate.
		●	Heard and noted the first clear tapping sound (systolic pressure).
		●	Heard and noted the onset of the muffled sound (diastolic pressure).
		●	Heard and noted the point on scale at which the sounds ceased (if Phase V is to be recorded).
		●	Quickly and completely deflated cuff to zero and removed earpieces of stethoscope from ears.
		▷	Is able to state how long one should wait before taking the blood pressure again on the same arm.
		●	Carefully removed cuff from patient's arm.
		●	Charted the results correctly.
		★	The reading was within ± 2 mm of mercury of the evaluator's reading.
		●	Cleaned earpieces with an antiseptic wipe.
		★	Completed the procedure within 5 minutes.

CHART	
Date	

Evaluation of Student Performance

EVALUATION CRITERIA			COMMENTS
Symbol	Category	Point Value	
★	Critical Step	16 points	
●	Essential Step	6 points	
▷	Theory Question	2 points	

Score calculation: 100 points

− _____ points missed

_____ Score

Satisfactory score: 85 or above

AAMA/CAAHEP Competency Achieved:

☐ Obtain vital signs.

The Physical Examination

## CHAPTER 4

NAME _____

Key Terminology Assessment

Directions: Match each medical term with its definition.

_____ 1. audiometer	A. An instrument for examining the interior of the eye.
_____ 2. auscultation	
_____ 3. charting	B. A tentative diagnosis obtained through the evaluation of the health history and the physical examination, without the benefit of laboratory or diagnostic tests.
_____ 4. clinical diagnosis	
_____ 5. conjunctiva	
_____ 6. diagnosis	
_____ 7. differential diagnosis	C. An instrument for opening a body orifice or cavity for viewing.
_____ 8. inspection	
_____ 9. medical record	D. A written record of the important aspects regarding a patient, his/her care, and the progress of his/her illness.
_____10. mensuration	
_____11. ophthalmoscope	
_____12. otoscope	E. An instrument used to measure hearing.
_____13. palpation	F. The process of measuring the patient.
_____14. percussion	G. The scientific method for determining and identifying a disease.
_____15. percussion hammer	
_____16. prognosis	H. The process of tapping the body to detect signs of disease.
_____17. retina	
_____18. speculum	I. The mucous membrane that lines the eyelids and covers the eyeball, except for the cornea.
_____19. symptom	
_____20. tympanic membrane	

J. The process of observing a patient to detect any signs of disease.

K. The process of making written entries about a patient in the medical record.

L. Any change in the body or its functioning that indicates that a disease is present.

M. The process of listening to the sounds produced within the body to detect any signs of disease.

N. A determination of which of two or more diseases with similar symptoms is producing the patient's symptoms.

O. An instrument for examining the external ear canal and tympanic membrane.

P. A thin, semitransparent membrane located between the external ear canal and middle ear that receives and transmits sound waves.

Q. The process of feeling with the hands to detect signs of disease.

R. The interior structure of the eye, which picks up and transmits light impulses to the optic nerve.

S. An instrument with a rubber head, used for testing reflexes.

T. The probable course and outcome of a disease and the prospects of patient recovery.

Self-Evaluation

Directions: Fill in each blank with the correct answer.

1. What are the three parts of a complete patient examination?

_____

_____

2. List two functions of the patient examination.

_____

_____

3. What is the purpose for establishing a final diagnosis?

_____

_____

4. Why is there a space for indicating the clinical diagnosis on the laboratory request form?

_____

_____

5. What is a risk factor?

_____

_____

6. What is an acute illness? List two examples of acute illnesses.

_____

_____

7. What is a chronic illness? List two examples of chronic illnesses.

_____

_____

8. What is the difference between a therapeutic procedure and a diagnostic procedure?

_____

_____

_____

9. How can patient apprehension be reduced during a physical examination?

_____

_____

10. Why is it recommended that the patient's medical record be placed outside the examining room?

_____

_____

11. What is the purpose for measuring weight?

_____

_____

_____

12. What is the purpose of positioning and draping?

_____

_____

_____

13. Indicate three types of examinations for which the supine position is used.

_____

_____

14. Indicate two types of examinations for which the lithotomy position is used.

_____

_____

15. Indicate one type of examination for which the knee-chest position is used.

_____

_____

16. List four types of assessments that can be made through inspection.

_____

_____

17. List four types of assessments that can be made through palpation.

_____

_____

18. Explain what can be assessed through the use of percussion.

_____

_____

19. What type of assessments can be made using auscultation?

_____

_____

20. What type of stethoscope chestpiece should be used to assess the heart?

_____

_____

Critical Thinking Skills

1. The diagram below is an illustration of a portion of the calibration bar of an upright balance beam scale. In the spaces provided record the weight measurements indicated on the calibration bar. In **all** cases, assume that the lower weight is resting in the 100 pound notched groove.

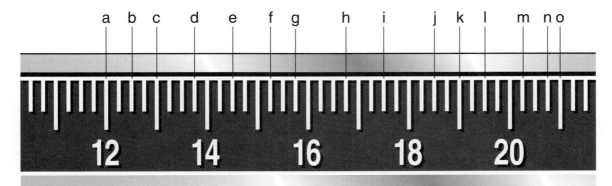

a. _____

b. _____

c. _____

d. _____

e. _____

f. _____

g. _____

h. _____

i. _____

j. _____

k. _____

l. _____

m. _____

n. _____

o. _____

94   THE PHYSICAL EXAMINATION

2. The diagram below is an illustration of a portion of the calibration rod of an upright balance beam scale. In the spaces provided, indicate the height measurement in feet and inches indicated on the calibration rod.

a. _____
b. _____
c. _____
d. _____
e. _____
f. _____
g. _____
h. _____
i. _____
j. _____
k. _____

3. a. Using the Highlight on Interpreting Body Weight box on pages 132 and 133 of your textbook, calculate and interpret your BMI and record results below.

_____

b. List the diseases that an individual with an above normal BMI has an increased chance of developing.

_____
_____
_____
_____

4. In which position would you place the patient for the following examinations or procedures?

a. Measurement of rectal temperature of an adult _____
b. Examination of the back _____
c. Measurement of vital signs _____
d. Pelvic examination _____
e. Examination of the upper extremities _____

f. Examination of the eyes, ears, nose, and throat _____

g. Examination of the breasts _____

h. Flexible sigmoidoscopy _____

i. Administration of an enema _____

j. To examine the upper body of a patient with emphysema _____

5. List the examination technique (inspection, palpation, percussion, auscultation) that is used in each of the following situations:

a. A patient with a stutter _____

b. Taking the radial pulse _____

c. Finding the location of the apical pulse _____

d. Taking the apical pulse _____

e. Taking respiration (may be two answers, depending on method)_____

f. A patient with cracked lips _____

g. Checking for lumps in the breast_____

h. Checking reflexes_____

i. Obtaining the fetal heart rate_____

j. A patient with a fever (may be several methods) _____

6. Obtain an otoscope and an ophthalmoscope. Following the manufacturer's instructions, perform the following. Place a check mark next to each after performing it.

_____ a. Turn the otoscope and ophthalmoscope on and off.

_____ b. Change the bulbs in the otoscope and ophthalmoscope.

_____ c. Change the batteries or recharge the otoscope and ophthalmoscope.

_____ d. Change the speculum of the otoscope.

Notes

Practice for Competency

WEIGHT AND HEIGHT

Assignment

Take weight and height measurements. Record results in the chart provided below.

CHART	
Date	

CHART	
Date	

Practice for Competency

POSITIONING AND DRAPING

Assignment

Position and drape an individual in each of the following positions: sitting, supine, prone, dorsal recumbent, lithotomy, Sims, and knee-chest. In the space provided below, list the name of each position and the number of times you practiced it.

POSITION   **NUMBER OF PRACTICES**

Practice for Competency

ASSISTING WITH THE PHYSICAL EXAMINATION

Assignment

1. Complete the health history form on the following pages using yourself as the patient.
2. Prepare the patient and assist with a physical examination. In the chart provided below, record the results of the procedures you performed while assisting with the examination (e.g., vital signs, height and weight, visual acuity).

CHART	
Date	

Evaluation of Competency

PROCEDURE 4-1: MEASURING WEIGHT AND HEIGHT

Name _____   Date _____

Evaluated By _____   Score_____

Performance Objective

Outcome:	Measure weight and height.
Conditions:	Given a paper towel.
	Using an upright balance scale.
Standards:	Time: 5 minutes.
	Accuracy: Satisfactory score on the Performance Evaluation Checklist.

Performance Evaluation Checklist

Trial 1	Trial 2	Point Value	*Performance Standards*
			WEIGHT
		●	Washed hands.
			Checked the balance scale for accuracy
		●	Made sure the upper and lower weights were on zero.
		●	Looked at the indicator point to make sure the scale is balanced.
		▷	Is able to state what will be observed if the scale is balanced.
		▷	Is able to state what to do if the indicator point rests below the center.
		▷	Is able to state what to do if the indicator point rests above the center.
		▷	Is able to state what occurs if the scale is not balanced.
		●	Greeted and identified the patient.
		●	Introduced yourself and explained the procedure.
		●	Instructed patient to remove shoes and heavy outer clothing.
		●	Placed paper towel on the scale.
		●	Assisted patient onto the scale.
		●	Instructed patient not to move.

Trial 1	Trial 2	Point Value	Performance Standards
			Balanced the scale
		●	Moved the lower weight to the groove that did not cause the indicator point to drop to the bottom of the balance area.
		▷	Is able to state why the lower weight should be seated firmly in its groove.
		●	Slid the upper weight slowly until the indicator point came to a rest at the center of the balance area.
		●	Read the results to the nearest quarter pound.
		★	The reading was identical to the evaluator's reading.
		●	Assisted the patient off of the scale platform.
			HEIGHT
		●	Slid the calibration rod until it is above the patient's height.
		●	Opened the measuring bar to its horizontal position.
		●	Instructed the patient to step onto the scale platform with the back to the scale.
		●	Instructed patient to stand erect and to look straight ahead.
		●	Carefully lowered the measuring bar until it rested gently on top of the patient's head.
		●	The bar was in a horizontal position.
		●	Instructed the patient to step down and put on his/her shoes.
		●	Read the marking to the nearest quarter inch.
		★	The reading was identical to the evaluator's reading.
		●	Returned the bar to the resting position.
		●	Charted the weight and height correctly.
		●	Returned the weights to zero.
		●	Returned the measuring bar to its vertical position.
		●	Slid the calibration rod to its lowest position.
		★	Completed the procedure within 5 minutes.
			CHART
	Date		

Evaluation of Student Performance

EVALUATION CRITERIA			COMMENTS
Symbol	**Category**	**Point Value**	
★	Critical Step	16 points	
●	Essential Step	6 points	
▷	Theory Question	2 points	

Score calculation: 100 points
− _____ points missed
_____ Score

Satisfactory score: 85 or above

AAMA/CAAHEP Competency Achieved:
☐ Prepare patient for and assist with routine and specialty examinations.

Notes

Evaluation of Competency

PROCEDURE 4-2: SITTING POSITION

Name _____   Date _____

Evaluated By _____   Score_____

Performance Objective

Outcome:	Position and drape an individual in the sitting position.
Conditions:	Using an examining table.
	Given the following: a patient gown and a drape.
Standards:	Time: 5 minutes
	Accuracy: Satisfactory score on the Performance Evaluation Checklist.

Performance Evaluation Checklist

Trial 1	Trial 2	Point Value	Performance Standards
		●	Washed hands.
		●	Greeted and identified the patient.
		●	Introduced yourself.
		●	Explained what type of examination will be performed.
		●	Provided patient with a patient gown.
		●	Instructed patient to remove clothing and to put on a patient gown with the opening in front.
		▷	Is able to state what qualities the disrobing facility should have.
		●	Pulled out the footrest and assisted the patient into a sitting position.
		●	The patient's buttocks and thighs were firmly supported on the edge of the table.
		●	Placed a drape over the patient's thighs and legs.
		●	After the exam, assisted the patient down from the table.
		●	Instructed the patient to get dressed.
		●	Returned the footrest to its normal position.
		▷	Is able to state one use of the sitting position.
		★	Completed the procedure within 5 minutes.

Evaluation of Student Performance

EVALUATION CRITERIA			COMMENTS
Symbol	**Category**	**Point Value**	
★	Critical Step	16 points	
●	Essential Step	6 points	
▷	Theory Question	2 points	

Score calculation: 100 points

− _____ points missed

_____ Score

Satisfactory score: 85 or above

AAMA/CAAHEP Competency Achieved:

☐ Prepare patient for and assist with routine and specialty examinations.

Evaluation of Competency

PROCEDURE 4-3: SUPINE POSITION

Name _____   Date _____

Evaluated By _____   Score_____

Performance Objective

Outcome:	Position and drape an individual in the supine position.
Conditions:	Using an examining table.
	Given the following: a patient gown and a drape.
Standards:	Time: 5 minutes
	Accuracy: Satisfactory score on the Performance Evaluation Checklist.

Performance Evaluation Checklist

Trial 1	Trial 2	Point Value	*Performance Standards*
		●	Washed hands.
		●	Greeted and identified the patient.
		●	Introduced yourself.
		●	Explained what type of examination will be performed.
		●	Provided patient with a patient gown.
		●	Instructed patient to remove clothing and to put on a patient gown with the opening in front.
		●	Pulled out the footrest and assisted the patient into a sitting position.
		●	Asked the patient to move back on the table.
		●	Pulled out the table extension while supporting the patient's lower legs.
		●	Asked the patient to lie down on the back with the legs together.
		●	The arms were placed above the head or alongside the body.
		●	Placed a drape over the patient.
		▷	Is able to state the purpose of the drape.
		●	Moved the drape according to the body parts being examined.
		●	After the exam, assisted the patient back into a sitting position.
		●	Slid the table extension back into place while supporting the patient's lower legs.

Trial 1	Trial 2	Point Value	Performance Standards
		●	Assisted the patient from the examining table.
		●	Instructed the patient to get dressed.
		●	Returned the footrest to its normal position.
		▷	Is able to state one use of the supine position.
		★	Completed the procedure within 5 minutes.

Evaluation of Student Performance

EVALUATION CRITERIA			COMMENTS
Symbol	Category	Point Value	
★	Critical Step	16 points	
●	Essential Step	6 points	
▷	Theory Question	2 points	
Score calculation: 100 points			
— _____ points missed			
_____ Score			
Satisfactory score: 85 or above			

AAMA/CAAHEP Competency Achieved:

☐ Prepare patient for and assist with routine and specialty examinations.

Evaluation of Competency

PROCEDURE 4-4: PRONE POSITION

Name _____   Date _____

Evaluated By _____   Score _____

Performance Objective

Outcome:	Position and drape an individual in the prone position.
Conditions:	Using an examining table.
	Given the following: a patient gown and a drape.
Standards:	Time: 5 minutes
	Accuracy: Satisfactory score on the Performance Evaluation Checklist

Performance Evaluation Checklist

Trial 1	Trial 2	Point Value	Performance Standards
		●	Washed hands.
		●	Greeted and identified the patient.
		●	Introduced yourself.
		●	Explained what type of examination will be performed.
		●	Provided patient with a patient gown.
		●	Instructed patient to remove clothing and to put on a patient gown with the opening in back.
		●	Pulled out the footrest and assisted the patient into a sitting position.
		●	Asked the patient to move back on the table.
		●	Pulled out the table extension while supporting the patient's lower legs.
		●	Asked the patient to lie down on the back.
		●	Asked the patient to turn his/her body over and lie on the abdomen with the legs together and the head turned to one side.
		●	Provided assistance.
		▷	Is able to state the reason for providing assistance.
		●	The arms were placed above the head or alongside the body.
		●	Placed a drape over the patient.
		●	Moved the drape according to the body parts being examined.

Trial 1	Trial 2	Point Value	Performance Standards
		●	After the exam, assisted the patient back into a supine position and then into a sitting position.
		●	Slid the table extension back into place while supporting the patient's lower legs.
		●	Assisted the patient from the examining table.
		●	Instructed the patient to get dressed.
		●	Returned the footrest to its normal position.
		▷	Is able to state one use of the prone position.
		★	Completed the procedure within 5 minutes.

Evaluation of Student Performance

EVALUATION CRITERIA			COMMENTS
Symbol	Category	Point Value	
★	Critical Step	16 points	
●	Essential Step	6 points	
▷	Theory Question	2 points	
Score calculation: 100 points			
− _____ points missed			
_____ Score			
Satisfactory score: 85 or above			

AAMA/CAAHEP Competency Achieved:
☐ Prepare patient for and assist with routine and specialty examinations.

Evaluation of Competency

PROCEDURE 4-5: DORSAL RECUMBENT POSITION

Name _____ Date _____

Evaluated By _____ Score_____

Performance Objective

Outcome:	Position and drape an individual in the dorsal recumbent position.
Conditions:	Using an examining table.
	Given the following: a patient gown and a drape.
Standards:	Time: 5 minutes
	Accuracy: Satisfactory score on the Performance Evaluation Checklist.

Performance Evaluation Checklist

Trial 1	Trial 2	Point Value	Performance Standards
		●	Washed hands.
		●	Greeted and identified the patient.
		●	Introduced yourself.
		●	Explained what type of examination will be performed.
		●	Provided patient with a patient gown.
		●	Instructed patient to remove clothing and to put on a patient gown with the opening in front.
		●	Pulled out the footrest and assisted the patient into a sitting position.
		●	Asked the patient to move back on the table.
		●	Pulled out the table extension while supporting the patient's lower legs.
		●	Asked the patient to lie down on the back.
		●	The arms were placed above the head or alongside the body.
		●	Placed a drape over the patient in a diagonal position.
		●	Asked the patient to bend the knees and place each foot at the edge of the table with the soles of the feet flat on the table.
		●	Provided assistance.
		●	Pushed in the table extension and the footrest.

Trial 1	Trial 2	Point Value		Performance Standards
		●		Folded back the center corner of the drape when the physician was ready to examine the patient.
		●		After the exam, pulled out the footrest and the table extension.
		●		Assisted the patient back into a supine position and then into a sitting position.
		●		Slid the table extension back into place while supporting the patient's lower legs.
		●		Assisted the patient from the examining table.
		●		Instructed the patient to get dressed.
		●		Returned the footrest to its normal position.
		▷		Is able to state one use of the dorsal recumbent position.
		★		Completed the procedure within 5 minutes.

Evaluation of Student Performance

EVALUATION CRITERIA			COMMENTS
Symbol	Category	Point Value	
★	Critical Step	16 points	
●	Essential Step	6 points	
▷	Theory Question	2 points	
Score calculation: 100 points			
— points missed			
_____Score			
Satisfactory score: 85 or above			

AAMA/CAAHEP Competency Achieved:
☐ Prepare patient for and assist with routine and specialty examinations.

Evaluation of Competency

PROCEDURE 4-6: LITHOTOMY POSITION

Name _____ Date _____

Evaluated By _____ Score_____

Performance Objective

Outcome:	Position and drape an individual in the lithotomy position.
Conditions:	Using an examining table.
	Given the following: a patient gown and a drape.
Standards:	Time: 5 minutes
	Accuracy: Satisfactory score on the Performance Evaluation Checklist.

Performance Evaluation Checklist

Trial 1	Trial 2	Point Value	Performance Standards
		●	Washed hands.
		●	Greeted and identified the patient.
		●	Introduced yourself.
		●	Explained what type of examination will be performed.
		●	Provided patient with a patient gown.
		●	Instructed patient to remove clothing and to put on a patient gown with the opening in front.
		●	Pulled out the footrest and assisted the patient into a sitting position.
		●	Asked the patient to move back on the table.
		●	Pulled out the table extension while supporting the patient's lower legs.
		●	Asked the patient to lie down on the back.
		●	The arms were placed above the head or alongside the body.
		●	Placed a drape over the patient in a diagonal position.
		●	Asked the patient to bend the knees and place each foot at the edge of the table with the soles of the feet flat on the table.
		●	Provided assistance.
		●	Pushed in the table extension and the footrest.
		●	Positioned the stirrups so that they are level with the examining table and pulled out approximately 1 foot from the edge of the table.

Trial 1	Trial 2	Point Value	Performance Standards
		●	Asked the patient to move the feet into the stirrups.
		●	Provided assistance.
		●	Instructed the patient to slide the buttocks to the edge of the table and to rotate the thighs outward as far as is comfortable.
		●	Folded back the center corner of the drape when the physician was ready to examine the genital area.
		●	After the exam, asked the patient to slide the buttocks back from the end of the table.
		●	Pulled out the footrest and the table extension.
		●	Lifted the patient's legs out of the stirrups at the same time and placed them on the table extension.
		▷	Is able to state why both legs should be lifted at the same time.
		●	Returned stirrups to the normal position.
		●	Assisted the patient into a sitting position.
		●	Slid the table extension back into place while supporting the patient's lower legs.
		●	Assisted the patient from the examining table.
		●	Instructed the patient to get dressed.
		●	Returned the footrest to its normal position.
		▷	Is able to state one use of the lithotomy position.
		★	Completed the procedure within 5 minutes.

Evaluation of Student Performance

EVALUATION CRITERIA			COMMENTS
Symbol	**Category**	**Point Value**	
★	Critical Step	16 points	
●	Essential Step	6 points	
▷	Theory Question	2 points	

Score calculation: 100 points

−   points missed

_____ Score

Satisfactory score: 85 or above

AAMA/CAAHEP Competency Achieved:

☐ Prepare patient for and assist with routine and specialty examinations.

Evaluation of Competency

PROCEDURE 4-7: SIMS POSITION

Name _____ Date _____

Evaluated By _____ Score_____

Performance Objective

Outcome:	Position and drape an individual in the Sims position.
Conditions:	Using an examining table.
	Given the following: a patient gown and a drape.
Standards:	Time: 5 minutes
	Accuracy: Satisfactory score on the Performance Evaluation Checklist.

Performance Evaluation Checklist

Trial 1	Trial 2	Point Value	Performance Standards
		●	Washed hands.
		●	Greeted and identified the patient.
		●	Introduced yourself.
		●	Explained what type of examination will be performed.
		●	Provided patient with a patient gown.
		●	Instructed patient to remove clothing from the waist down and to put on a patient gown with the opening in back.
		●	Pulled out the footrest and assisted the patient into a sitting position.
		●	Asked the patient to move back on the table.
		●	Pulled out the table extension while supporting the patient's lower legs.
		●	Asked the patient to lie down on the back.
		●	Placed a drape over the patient.
		●	Asked the patient to turn on the left side.
		●	Provided assistance.
		●	Positioned the left arm behind the body and the right arm forward with the elbow bent.
		●	Assisted the patient in flexing the legs with the right leg flexed sharply and the left leg flexed slightly.

Trial 1	Trial 2	Point Value	Performance Standards
		●	Adjusted the drape by folding back the drape to expose the anal area when the physician was ready to examine the patient.
		●	After the exam, assisted the patient into a supine position and then into a sitting position.
		●	Slid the table extension back into place while supporting the patient's lower legs.
		●	Assisted the patient from the examining table.
		●	Instructed the patient to get dressed.
		●	Returned the footrest to its normal position.
		▷	Is able to state one use of the Sims position.
		★	Completed the procedure within 5 minutes.

Evaluation of Student Performance

EVALUATION CRITERIA			COMMENTS
Symbol	**Category**	**Point Value**	
★	Critical Step	16 points	
●	Essential Step	6 points	
▷	Theory Question	2 points	
Score calculation: 100 points			
− _____ points missed			
_____ Score			
Satisfactory score: 85 or above			

AAMA/CAAHEP Competency Achieved:

☐ Prepare patient for and assist with routine and specialty examinations.

Evaluation of Competency

PROCEDURE 4-8: KNEE-CHEST POSITION

Name _____ Date _____

Evaluated By _____ Score_____

Performance Objective

Outcome:	Position and drape an individual in the knee-chest position.
Conditions:	Using an examining table.
	Given the following: a patient gown and a drape.
Standards:	Time: 5 minutes
	Accuracy: Satisfactory score on the Performance Evaluation Checklist.

Performance Evaluation Checklist

Trial 1	Trial 2	Point Value	Performance Standards
		●	Washed hands.
		●	Greeted and identified the patient.
		●	Introduced yourself.
		●	Explained what type of examination will be performed.
		●	Provided patient with a patient gown.
		●	Instructed patient to remove clothing from the waist down and to put on a patient gown with the opening in back.
		●	Pulled out the footrest and assisted the patient into a sitting position.
		●	Asked the patient to move back on the table.
		●	Pulled out the table extension while supporting the patient's lower legs.
		●	Assisted the patient into the supine position and then into the prone position.
		●	Placed a drape over the patient.
		●	Asked the patient to bend the arms at the elbows and rest them alongside the head.
		●	Asked the patient to elevate the buttocks while keeping the back straight.
		●	The patient's head was turned to one side, and the weight of the body was supported by the chest.

Trial 1	Trial 2	Point Value	Performance Standards
		●	A pillow was used for additional support, if needed.
		●	Separated the knees and lower legs approximately 12 inches.
		●	Positioned the drape diagonally.
		●	Folded back a small portion of the drape to expose the anal area when the physician was ready to examine the patient.
		●	After the exam, assisted the patient into a prone position and then into a supine position.
		●	Allowed the patient to rest in a supine position before sitting up.
			Is able to state why the patient should be allowed to rest.
		●	Assisted the patient into a sitting position.
		●	Slid the table extension back into place while supporting the patient's lower legs.
		●	Assisted the patient from the examining table.
		●	Instructed the patient to get dressed.
		●	Returned the footrest to its normal position.
		▷	Is able to state one use of the knee-chest position.
		★	Completed the procedure within 5 minutes.

Evaluation of Student Performance

EVALUATION CRITERIA			COMMENTS
Symbol	Category	Point Value	
★	Critical Step	16 points	
●	Essential Step	6 points	
▷	Theory Question	2 points	

Score calculation: 100 points

_____ − points missed

_____ Score

Satisfactory score: 85 or above

AAMA/CAAHEP Competency Achieved:
☐ Prepare patient for and assist with routine and specialty examinations.

Evaluation of Competency

PROCEDURE 4-9: FOWLER'S POSITION

Name _____   Date _____

Evaluated By _____   Score_____

Performance Objective

Outcome:	Position and drape an individual in the Fowler's position.
Conditions:	Using an examining table.
	Given the following: a patient gown and a drape.
Standards:	Time: 5 minutes
	Accuracy: Satisfactory score on the Performance Evaluation Checklist.

Performance Evaluation Checklist

Trial 1	Trial 2	Point Value	*Performance Standards*
		●	Washed hands.
		●	Greeted and identified the patient.
		●	Introduced yourself.
		●	Explained what type of examination or procedure will be performed.
		●	Provided patient with a patient gown.
		●	Instructed patient to remove clothing and to put on a patient gown with the opening in front.
		●	Positioned the head of the table at a 45-degree angle for a semi-Fowler's position or at a 90-degree angle for a full Fowler's position.
		●	Pulled out the footrest and assisted the patient into a sitting position.
		●	Pulled out the table extension while supporting the patient's lower legs.
		●	Asked the patient to lean back against the table head.
		●	Provided assistance.
		●	Placed a drape over the patient.
		●	Moved the drape according to the body parts being examined.
		●	After the exam, assisted the patient into a sitting position.
		●	Slid the table extension back into place while supporting the patient's lower legs.
		●	Assisted the patient from the examining table.

Trial 1	Trial 2	Point Value	Performance Standards
		●	Instructed the patient to get dressed.
		●	Returned the footrest to its normal position.
		▷	Is able to state one use of Fowler's position.
		★	Completed the procedure within 5 minutes.

Evaluation of Student Performance

EVALUATION CRITERIA			COMMENTS
Symbol	**Category**	**Point Value**	
★	Critical Step	16 points	
●	Essential Step	6 points	
▷	Theory Question	2 points	

Score calculation: 100 points

− _____ points missed

_____ Score

Satisfactory score: 85 or above

AAMA/CAAHEP Competency Achieved:

☐ Prepare patient for and assist with routine and specialty examinations.

Evaluation of Competency

PROCEDURE 4-10: ASSISTING WITH THE PHYSICAL EXAMINATION

Name _____   Date _____

Evaluated By _____   Score_____

Performance Objective

Outcome:	Prepare the patient and assist with a physical examination.
Conditions:	Using an examining table.
	Given the following: equipment for the type of examination to be performed, patient examination gown, and drapes.
Standards:	Time: 20 minutes
	Accuracy: Satisfactory score on the Performance Evaluation Checklist.

Performance Evaluation Checklist

Trial 1	Trial 2	Point Value	Performance Standards
		●	Prepared examining room.
		●	Washed hands.
		●	Assembled all necessary equipment.
		●	Arranged istruments in a neat and orderly manner.
		●	Obtained the patient's medical record.
		●	Went to the waiting room and asked the patient to come back.
		●	Escorted the patient to the examining room.
		●	Asked the patient to be seated.
		●	Greeted and identified the patient.
		●	Introduced yourself.
		▷	Is able to state why a calm and friendly manner should be used.
		●	Seated yourself facing the patient at a distance of 3 to 4 feet.
		●	Obtained and recorded patient symptoms.
		●	Measured vital signs and charted results.
		●	Measured weight and height and charted results.
		●	Asked patient is he or she needs to void.
		▷	Is able to state why the patient should be asked to void.

Trial 1	Trial 2	Point Value	Performance Standards
		●	Instructed patient to remove all clothing and put on an examining gown.
		●	Asked the patient to have a seat.
		●	Informed the patient that the physician will be in soon.
		●	Informed physician that the patient is ready.
		●	Made patient's medical record available.
		●	Assisted the patient onto examining table and into a sitting position.
		●	Handed the ophthalmoscope to examiner when requested.
		●	Dimmed the lights when the physician was ready to use the ophthalmoscope.
		▷	Is able to state why the lights are dimmed.
		▷	Is able to state the proper use of the ophthalmoscope.
		●	Handed the otoscope to the examiner when requested.
		▷	Is able to state the proper use of the otoscope.
		▷	Is able to change the speculum and bulb in the otoscope.
		●	Handed the tongue depressor to the examiner when requested.
		●	Offered reassurance to patient as needed.
		●	Positioned patient as required for examination of the remaining body systems.
			Assisted and instructed patient
		●	Assisted patient off the examining table.
		●	Instructed patient to get dressed.
		●	Provided patient with any necessary instructions.
		▷	Is able to state what type of instructions may need to be relayed to the patient.
		●	Charted any instructions given to the patient.
		●	Escorted the patient to the reception area.
			Cleaned the examining room
		●	Discarded paper on the examining table and unrolled a fresh length.
		●	Discarded all disposable supplies into an appropriate waste container.
		●	Checked to make sure ample supplies are available
		●	Removed reusable equipment for sanitization, sterilization, or disinfection.
		★	Completed the procedure within 20 minutes.

CHART

Date	

Evaluation of Student Performance

EVALUATION CRITERIA			COMMENTS
Symbol	**Category**	**Point Value**	
★	Critical Step	16 points	
●	Essential Step	6 points	
▷	Theory Question	2 points	

Score calculation: 100 points

_____ − points missed

_____ Score

Satisfactory score: 85 or above

AAMA/CAAHEP Competencies Achieved:

☐ Prepare and maintain examination and treatment areas.
☐ Prepare patient for and assist with routine and specialty examinations.
☐ Dispose of biohazardous materials.
☐ Explain general office policies.
☐ Instruct individuals according to their needs.
☐ Instruct and demonstrate the use and care of patient equipment.
☐ Provide instruction for health maintenance and disease prevention.
☐ Identify community resources.
☐ Perform an inventory of supplies and equipment.
☐ Perform routine maintenance of administrative and clinical equipment.

Notes

Sterilization and Disinfection

CHAPTER 5

NAME _____

Key Terminology Assessment

Directions: Match each medical term with its definition.

_____ 1. antiseptic
_____ 2. autoclave
_____ 3. contaminate
_____ 4. critical item
_____ 5. detergent
_____ 6. disinfectant
_____ 7. incubate
_____ 8. load
_____ 9. material data safety sheet
_____ 10. noncritical item
_____ 11. sanitization
_____ 12. semi-critical item
_____ 13. spore
_____ 14. sterilization
_____ 15. thermolabile

A. To provide proper conditions for growth and development.
B. To soil, stain, or pollute; to make impure.
C. Easily affected or changed by heat.
D. A substance that inhibits disease-producing microorganisms but not their spores (usually applied to living tissues).
E. An item that comes in contact with intact skin but not mucous membranes.
F. A hard, thick-walled capsule formed by some bacteria that contains only the essential parts of the protoplasm of the bacterial cell.
G. An item that comes in contact with sterile tissue or the vascular system.
H. An apparatus for the sterilization of materials, using steam under pressure.
I. An agent that cleanses by emulsifying dirt and oil.

J. An item that comes in contact with intact mucous membranes.

K. The articles that are being sterilized.

L. A substance used to destroy disease-producing microorganisms but not necessarily their spores (usually applied to inanimate objects).

M. A sheet that provides information regarding a chemical, its hazards, and measures to take to avoid injury and illness when handling the chemical.

N. A cleaning process to reduce the number of microorganisms to a safe level as determined by public health requirements.

O. The process of destroying all forms of microbial life, including bacterial spores.

Self-Evaluation

Directions: Fill in each blank with correct answer.

1. How does one determine what type of physical or chemical agent to use to destroy microorganisms on an article?

_____

_____

_____

2. List two diseases that are caused by bacteria that produce spores.

_____

_____

3. What is the purpose of the Hazard Communications Standard?

_____

_____

4. List four examples of hazardous chemicals that may be used in the medical office.

_____

_____

5. What information must be included on a hazardous chemical label as required by the Hazard Communications Standard?

_____

_____

6. List and describe the information that must be included in a Material Data Safety Sheet.

_____

_____

_____

_____

_____

_____

_____

_____

7. What is the purpose of sanitizing an article?

_____

_____

8. List the general steps in the sanitization procedure.

_____

_____

_____

_____

9. What is the advantage of using the ultrasound method to clean instruments?

_____

_____

10. What is the definition of high-level disinfection.

_____

_____

11. List two examples of items that require high-level disinfection.

_____

12. List two examples of items that can be disinfected through intermediate-level disinfection. List one example of an intermediate-level disinfectant.

_____

_____

13. List two examples of items that are disinfected by low-level disinfection.

_____

14. What disinfectant does OSHA recommend for the decontamination of blood spills?

_____

15. Why should an article be dry before it is placed in a chemical disinfectant?

_____

_____

128 STERILIZATION AND DISINFECTION

16. Explain the difference between shelf life and use life.

_____

_____

_____

17. What is the purpose of the pressure used in the autoclaving process?

_____

_____

18. Why is it important that all air be removed from the autoclave during the sterilization process?

_____

_____

19. What is the most common temperature and pressure used to sterilize materials with the autoclave?

_____

_____

20. What information does the CDC recommend be recorded in an autoclave log regarding each cycle?

_____

_____

_____

21. What is the function of a sterilization indicator?

_____

_____

22. What is the purpose of wrapping articles to be autoclaved?

_____

_____

23. List two properties of a good wrapper for use in autoclaving.

_____

_____

24. List three examples of wrapping material used for autoclave and identify an advantage of each type.

_____

_____

_____

25. Why is more time needed to autoclave a large minor office surgery pack?

_____

_____

26. How long is an article wrapped in sterilization paper considered sterile after it has been autoclaved?

_____

27. Describe the care an autoclave should receive on a daily basis.

_____

_____

_____

28. Why is a longer exposure period needed to ensure sterilization when using the dry heat oven?

_____

_____

29. What effect does moist heat have on instruments with sharp points or cutting edges?

_____

30. How does the medical manufacturing industry use ethylene oxide gas sterilization?

_____

_____

_____

Critical Thinking Skills

1. Refer to the Material Safety Data Sheet (Figure 5-2) and answer the following questions.
   a. What is the hazard rating of glutaraldehyde?

   _____

   b. Can glutaraldehyde enter the body through the skin?

   _____

   c. What type of symptoms occur if glutaraldehyde is inhaled?

   _____

   d. What is the emergency and first aid procedures if glutaraldehyde gets on the skin?

   _____

   e. What should be done if there is a small spill of glutaraldehyde?

   _____

   f. What is the disposal method for a glutaraldehyde solution?

   _____

   g. What eye and skin protection should be taken with glutaraldehyde?

   _____

2. You are responsible for disinfecting articles and surfaces in your medical office. Using Table 5-1, indicate the disinfectant that should be used for each of the following: (Note: There may be more than one answer for some of the items listed below).

    a. Mercury glass thermometers

_____

    b. Percussion hammer

_____

    c. Laboratory work surface

_____

    d. Stethoscope

_____

    e. Otoscope speculum

_____

    f. Rubber stopper of a multiple-dose medication vial

_____

    g. Decontamination of a blood spill

_____

    h. Flexible fiberoptic sigmoidoscope

_____

3. Refer to the instruction manual that comes with your autoclave and describe the basic procedure for operating it.

_____

_____

_____

_____

_____

_____

_____

4. For each of the following situations involving sanitization and sterilization, write **C** if the technique is correct and **I** if the technique is incorrect. If the situation is correct, state the principle underlying the technique. If the situation is incorrect, explain what might happen if the technique was performed in the incorrect manner.

_____ a. A contaminated surgical instrument is left in the examination room.

_____

_____

_____ b. The medical assistant wears gloves during the entire sanitization process.

_____

_____

_____ c. The medical assistant piles instruments in a heap while preparing them for sanitization.

_____

_____

_____ d. The medical assistant follows all personal safety precautions listed on the label of the instrument cleaner.

_____

_____

_____ e. The medical assistant uses laundry detergent to sanitize surgical instruments.

_____

_____

_____ f. Dried blood is not completely cleansed from hemostatic forceps before they are sterilized in the autoclave.

_____

_____

_____ g. The medical assistant checks all instruments for proper working condition before sterilizing them.

_____

_____

_____ h. The medical assistant lubricates hemostatic forceps before sterilizing them with a steam penetrable lubricant.

_____

_____

_____ i. The medical assistant opens all hinged instruments before sterilizing them.

_____

_____

_____ j. Tap water is used to fill the water reservoir of the autoclave.

_____

_____

_____ k. When loading the autoclave, the medical assistant places glass jars in an upright position.

_____

_____

_____ l.   The medical assistant places sterilization pouches on their sides in the autoclave.

_____

_____

_____ m. The medical assistant places small packs to be sterilized approximately 1 to 3 inches apart in the autoclave.

_____

_____

_____ n.   Spore strips are placed in the autoclave where steam will penetrate them most easily.

_____

_____

_____ o.   The medical assistant begins timing the load in the autoclave after the proper temperature of 250°F has been reached.

_____

_____

_____ p.   The medical assistant removes the load from the autoclave while it is still wet.

_____

_____

_____ q.   The medical assistant notices a tear in one of the wrappers while removing articles from the autoclave. She rewraps and resterilizes the article.

_____

_____

_____ r.   The medical assistant resterilizes an article wrapped in a sterilization pouch after 4 weeks.

_____

_____

Practice for Competency

Assignment

Sanitizing Instruments. Sanitize instruments. In space provided, indicate the name of each instrument you sanitized.

Chemical Disinfection of Articles. Chemically disinfect contaminated articles. In the space provided, indicate the articles you disinfected.

Wrapping Articles for the Autoclave. Wrap articles for autoclaving. In the space provided, list the information you indicated on the label of each pack.

Sterilizing Articles in the Autoclave. Sterilize articles in the autoclave. In the space provided, indicate the articles you sterilized.

Names of Instruments Sanitized

Names of Articles Disinfected

Information Indicated on the Label of the Wrapped Article

Names of Articles Sterilized

Notes

Evaluation of Competency

PROCEDURE 5-1: SANITIZING INSTRUMENTS

Name _____ Date _____

Evaluated By _____ Score_____

Performance Objective

Outcome:	Sanitize instruments
Conditions:	Given the following: disposable gloves, utility gloves, contaminated instruments, instrument container, cleaning solution, paper towels, lubricant, nylon brush, wire brush, and an ultrasonic cleaner.
Standards:	Time: 10 minutes
	Accuracy: Satisfactory score on the Performance Evaluation

Performance Evaluation Checklist

Trial 1	Trial 2	Point Value	Performance Standards
		●	Applied gloves.
		●	Removed the contaminated instruments to the cleaning area.
		●	Applied heavy-duty utility gloves over the disposable gloves.
		▷	Is able to state the purpose of the utility gloves.
		●	Separated sharp instruments and delicate instruments from other instruments.
		▷	Is able to state why instruments should be separated.
		●	Immediately rinsed the instruments thoroughly under warm to hot running water.
		▷	Is able to state why the instruments should be rinsed immediately.
			Cleaned the Instruments-Manual Method
		●	Checked the expiration date of the cleaning agent.
		▷	Is able to state the reason for checking the expiration date.
		●	Followed the manufacturer's label for proper use and mixing of the cleaning agent.
		●	Observed all personal safety precautions listed on the label.
		●	Cleaned the surface of the instruments with a nylon brush.
		●	Cleaned grooves, crevices, or serrations with a wire brush.

Trial 1	Trial 2	Point Value	Performance Standards
		●	Removed stains using commercial stain remover.
		●	Scrubbed the instruments until they were visibly clean.
		▷	Is able to state why all organic matter must be removed.
		●	Disposed of the cleaning solution according to the manufacturer's instructions.
			Cleaned the Instruments-Ultrasound Method
		●	Prepared the cleaning solution in the ultrasonic cleaner.
		●	Separated instruments of dissimilar metals.
		●	Properly placed the instruments in the ultrasonic cleaner.
		●	Hinged instruments were in an open position.
		▷	Is able to state why hinged instruments must be in an open position.
		●	Sharp instruments did not touch other instruments.
		●	All instruments were fully submerged.
		●	Placed the lid on the ultrasonic cleaner.
		●	Turned on the ultrasonic cleaner.
		●	Cleaned the instruments for the length of time recommended by the manufacturer.
		●	Removed the instruments from the machine.
		●	Changed the cleaning solution as recommended by the manufacturer.
		●	Rinsed each instrument thoroughly with warm to hot water.
		▷	Is able to state why instruments should be rinsed thoroughly.
		●	Dried each instrument with a paper towel.
		●	Placed instrument on a towel for additional drying.
		▷	Is able to state the reason for drying the instruments.
		●	Checked each instrument for defects and proper working condition.
		●	Lubricated hinged instruments.
		▷	Is able to state the reason for lubricating instruments.
		●	Removed both sets of gloves.
		●	Washed hands.
		●	Wrapped the instruments.
		●	Sterilized the instruments in the autoclave.
		★	Completed the procedure within 10 minutes.

Evaluation of Student Performance

EVALUATION CRITERIA			COMMENTS
Symbol	**Category**	**Point Value**	
★	Critical Step	16 points	
●	Essential Step	6 points	
▷	Theory Question	2 points	

Score calculation: 100 points

− _____ points missed

_____ Score

Satisfactory score: 85 or above

AAMA/CAAHEP Competency Achieved:

☐ Perform sterilization techniques.

Notes

Evaluation of Competency

PROCEDURE 5-2: CHEMICAL DISINFECTION OF ARTICLES

Name _____   Date _____

Evaluated By _____   Score_____

Performance Objective

Outcome:	Chemically disinfect articles.
Conditions:	Given the following: disposable gloves, utility gloves, contaminated articles, chemical disinfectant, MSDS, container to hold the disinfectant, and paper towels.
Standards:	Time: 10 minutes
	Accuracy: Satisfactory score on the Performance Evaluation Checklist.

Performance Evaluation Checklist

Trial 1	Trial 2	Point Value	*Performance Standards*
		●	Reviewed the MSDS.
		▷	Is able to state what information is included on an MSDS.
		●	Applied gloves.
		●	Removed contaminated articles to a separate work area.
		●	Applied utility gloves.
		●	Rinsed the articles.
		●	Cleaned the articles.
		▷	Is able to state why all organic matter must be removed.
		●	Thoroughly rinsed articles again.
		▷	Is able to state why articles must be rinsed thoroughly.
		●	Dried articles completely.
		▷	Is able to state the reason for drying articles.
		●	Checked the expiration date of the disinfectant.
		●	Followed the directions on the manufacturer's label for proper use and mixing of the disinfectant.
		●	Observed all personal safety precautions listed on the label.
		●	Completely immersed articles in the chemical disinfectant.

Trial 1	Trial 2	Point Value	Performance Standards
		●	Covered disinfectant container.
		▷	Is able to state the reason for covering container.
		●	Disinfected articles for the proper length of time as indicated on the label of the container.
		●	Rinsed the articles thoroughly.
		▷	Is able to state the reason for rinsing the articles.
		●	Dried the articles.
		●	Properly disposed of the disinfectant.
		▷	Is able to state the purpose of proper disposal.
		●	Removed both sets of gloves.
		●	Washed hands.
		●	Properly stored the articles.
		★	Completed the procedure within 10 minutes.

Evaluation of Student Performance

EVALUATION CRITERIA			COMMENTS
Symbol	Category	Point Value	
★	Critical Step	16 points	
●	Essential Step	6 points	
▷	Theory Question	2 points	

Score calculation: 100   points

−　_____   points missed

_____   Score

Satisfactory score: 85 or above

AAMA/CAAHEP Competency Achieved:
☐ Perform sterilization techniques.

Evaluation of Competency

PROCEDURE 5-3: WRAPPING INSTRUMENTS FOR THE AUTOCLAVE USING STERILIZATION PAPER OR MUSLIN

Name _____ Date _____

Evaluated By _____ Score_____

Performance Objective

Outcome:	Wrap an instrument for autoclaving.
Conditions:	Given the following: sanitized instrument, wrapping material, sterilization indicator strip, autoclave tape, and a permanent marker.
Standards:	Time: 5 minutes
	Accuracy: Satisfactory score on the Performance Evaluation Checklist.

Performance Evaluation Checklist

Trial 1	Trial 2	Point Value	Performance Standards
		●	Washed the hands.
		●	Assembled the equipment.
		●	Selected the appropriate-sized wrapping material.
		●	Checked the expiration date on the sterilization indicator box.
		▷	Is able to state why outdated strips should not be used.
		●	Placed wrapping material on clean, flat surface.
		●	Turned the wrap in a diagonal position.
		●	Placed instrument in the center of wrapping material.
		●	Placed an instrument with a movable joint in an open position.
		▷	Is able to state why instruments with movable joints must be placed in an open position.
		●	Placed a sterilization indicator in the center of the pack.
		●	Folded wrapping material up from the bottom and doubled back a small corner.
		●	Folded over the right edge of wrapping material and doubled back the corner.
		●	Folded over the left edge of wrapping material and doubled back the corner.

Trial 1	Trial 2	Point Value	Performance Standards
		●	Folded the pack up from the bottom and secured with autoclave tape.
		●	Dated and labeled the pack according to its contents.
		▷	Is able to state the purpose for dating the pack.
		●	The pack was firm enough for handling, but loose enough to permit proper circulation of steam.
		▷	Is able to state why instruments are wrapped for autoclaving.
		★	Completed the procedure within 5 minutes.

Evaluation of Student Performance

EVALUATION CRITERIA			COMMENTS
Symbol	**Category**	**Point Value**	
★	Critical Step	16 points	
●	Essential Step	6 points	
▷	Theory Question	2 points	
Score calculation: 100 points			
− _____ points missed			
_____ Score			
Satisfactory score: 85 or above			

AAMA/CAAHEP Competency Achieved:

☐ Wrap items for autoclaving.

Evaluation of Competency

PROCEDURE 5-4: WRAPPING INSTRUMENTS FOR THE AUTOCLAVE USING A STERILIZATION POUCH

Name _____ Date _____

Evaluated By _____ Score_____

Performance Objective

Outcome:	Wrap an instruments for autoclaving.
Conditions:	Given the following: sanitized instrument, sterilization pouch, and a permanent marker.
Standards:	Time: 5 minutes
	Accuracy: Satisfactory score on the Performance Evaluation Checklist.

Performance Evaluation Checklist

Trial 1	Trial 2	Point Value	Performance Standards
		●	Washed hands.
		●	Assembled equipment.
		●	Selected the appropriate-sized pouch.
		●	Placed the sterilization pouch on a clean, flat surface.
		●	Labeled the pack according to its contents.
		●	Dated the pack.
		▷	Is able to state the reason for dating the pack.
		●	Inserted the instrument into the open end of the pouch.
		●	Sealed the pouch.
		●	Sterilized the pack in the autoclave.
		★	Completed the procedure within 5 minutes.

Evaluation of Student Performance

EVALUATION CRITERIA			COMMENTS
Symbol	Category	Point Value	
★	Critical Step	16 points	
●	Essential Step	6 points	
▷	Theory Question	2 points	
Score calculation: 100 points			
−_____ points missed			
_____ Score			
Satisfactory score: 85 or above			

AAMA/CAAHEP Competency Achieved:

☐ Perform sterilization techniques.

Evaluation of Competency

PROCEDURE 5-5: STERILIZING ARTICLES IN THE AUTOCLAVE

Name _____ Date _____

Evaluated By _____ Score_____

Performance Objective

Outcome:	Sterilize a load of contaminated articles in the auto-clave.
Conditions:	Using an autoclave.
	Given the following: autoclave instruction manual, distilled water, wrapped articles, and heat-resistant gloves.
Standards:	Time: 10 minutes
	Accuracy: Satisfactory score on the Performance Evaluation Checklist.

Performance Evaluation Checklist

Trial 1	Trial 2	Point Value	Performance Standards
		●	Assembled equipment.
		●	Checked the water level in the autoclave.
		●	Properly loaded the autoclave.
			Manually Operated the Autoclave
		●	Determined the sterilizing time for the type of articles being autoclaved.
		●	Turned on the autoclave.
		●	Filled the chamber with water.
		●	Closed and latched the door.
		●	Set the timing control.
		▷	Is able to state when the timer should be set.
		●	Vented the chamber of steam.
		●	Dried the load.
		▷	Is able to state the reason for drying the load.

Trial 1	Trial 2	Point Value	Performance Standards
			Automatically Operated the Autoclave
		●	Closed and latched the door.
		●	Turned on the autoclave.
		●	Determined the sterilization program.
		●	Pressed the appropriate program button.
		●	Pressed the start button.
		▷	Is able to state the purpose of each indicator.
		●	Turned off the autoclave.
		●	Removed the load with heat-resistant gloves.
		▷	Is able to state the reason for using heat-resistant gloves.
		●	Inspected the packs as they were removed for damage.
		▷	Is able to state what should be done if a pack is torn.
		●	Checked the sterilization indicators on the outside of the packs.
		●	Recorded monitoring information in the autoclave log.
		●	Stored the articles in a clean dustproof area.
		●	Maintained appropriate daily care of the autoclave.
		▷	Is able to state what care the autoclave should receive each day.
		★	Completed the procedure within 10 minutes.

Evaluation of Student Performance

EVALUATION CRITERIA			COMMENTS
Symbol	Category	Point Value	
★	Critical Step	16 points	
●	Essential Step	6 points	
▷	Theory Question	2 points	

Score calculation: 100 points

− _____ points missed

_____ Score

Satisfactory score: 85 or above

AAMA/CAAHEP Competency Achieved:

☐ Perform sterilization techniques.

Minor Office Surgery

NAME _____

Key Terminology Assessment

Directions: Match each medical term with its definition.

_____ 1. abrasion
_____ 2. abscess
_____ 3. absorbable suture
_____ 4. approximation
_____ 5. bandage
_____ 6. biopsy
_____ 7. capillary action
_____ 8. colposcope
_____ 9. colposcopy
_____ 10. contaminate
_____ 11. contusion
_____ 12. cryosurgery
_____ 13. fibroblast
_____ 14. forceps
_____ 15. furuncle
_____ 16. hemostasis
_____ 17. incision
_____ 18. infection
_____ 19. inflammation
_____ 20. laceration
_____ 21. nonabsorbable suture
_____ 22. puncture
_____ 23. sterile
_____ 24. surgical asepsis
_____ 25. wound

A. A protective response of the body to trauma and the entrance of foreign matter.
B. To cause a sterile object or surface to become unsterile.
C. A wound made by a sharp, pointed object piercing the skin.
D. The condition in which the body or part of it is invaded by a pathogen.
E. A collection of pus in a cavity surrounded by inflamed tissue.
F. The arrest of bleeding by natural or artificial means.
G. Free from all living microorganisms and bacterial spores.
H. A wound in which the tissues are torn apart, leaving ragged and irregular edges.
I. A lighted instrument with a binocular magnifying lens used for the examination of the vagina and cervix.
J. A localized staphylococcal infection that originates deep within a follicle; also known as a boil.
K. An injury to the tissues under the skin, causing blood vessels to rupture and allowing blood to seep into tissues.

L. The surgical removal and examination of tissue from the living body.

M. A wound in which the outer layers of the skin are damaged.

N. That action that causes liquid to rise along a wick, a tube, or a gauze dressing.

O. A two-pronged instrument for grasping and squeezing.

P. Those practices that keep objects and areas sterile or free from microorganisms.

Q. A break in the continuity of an external or internal surface caused by physical means.

R. The therapeutic use of freezing temperatures to destroy abnormal tissue.

S. The visual examination of the vagina and cervix using a colposcope.

T. Suture material that is gradually digested by tissue enzymes and absorbed by the body.

U. The process of bringing two parts, such as tissue, together, through the use of sutures or other means.

V. A strip of woven material used to wrap or cover a part of the body.

W. A clean cut caused by a cutting instrument.

X. Suture material that is not absorbed by the body.

Y. An immature cell from which connective tissue can develop.

Self-Evaluation

Directions: Fill in each blank with the correct answer.

1. List the responsibilities of the medical assistant during a minor surgical operation.

_____

_____

_____

_____

2. What is the function of the speculum?

_____

_____

3. List five guidelines that should be followed in caring for instruments.

_____

_____

_____

_____

4. What is the difference between a closed and open wound?

_____

_____

5. Why might a tetanus booster be required with a puncture wound?

_____

_____

6. Explain the purpose of inflammation.

_____

_____

7. List the four local signs that occur during inflammation.

_____

_____

8. Describe what occurs during the inflammatory phase of wound healing.

_____

_____

9. Describe what occurs during the granulation phase of wound healing.

_____

_____

10. Describe what occurs during the maturation phase of wound healing.

_____

_____

11. What is an exudate?

_____

_____

12. Define the following types of exudates.

    a.   serous _____

    b.   sanguineous _____

    c.   purulent _____

13. List two functions of a sterile dressing.

_____

_____

14. Listed below are the names and sizes of sutures. In each of the following, circle the suture that has the smaller diameter.
    a. 4-0 surgical silk
        00 surgical silk

    b. 0 chromic gut
        3-0 chromic gut

    c. 2-0 polypropylene
        2 polypropylene

15. List five examples of materials used for nonabsorbable sutures.

_____

_____

16. What is a swaged needle? List advantages of using a swaged needle.

_____

_____

17. Why are sutures inserted in the head and neck generally removed sooner than other sutures?

_____

_____

18. List two advantages of using surgical skin staples to approximate a wound.

_____

_____

19. List three advantages of adhesive skin closures.

_____

_____

_____

20. What is the purpose of preparing the patient's skin before minor office surgery?

_____

21. What is the purpose of a fenestrated drape?

_____

_____

22. List the names of two local anesthetics commonly used in the medical office during minor office surgery.

_____

23. Explain how an instrument should be handed to the physician during minor office surgery.

_____

_____

24. What is a sebaceous cyst, and what causes it to form?

_____

_____

25. What is the purpose of using a rubber Penrose drain after incising a localized infection?

_____

_____

_____

26. What is the purpose of a needle biopsy?

_____

_____

27. What is an ingrown toenail?

_____

_____

28. List three causes of an ingrown toenail.

_____

_____

_____

29. List three reasons for performing colposcopy.

_____

_____

30. What is the purpose of performing a cervical punch biopsy?

_____

31. List the postoperative instructions that must be relayed to the patient following a cervical punch biopsy.

_____

_____

_____

32. List two uses of cryosurgery.

_____

_____

33. List the postoperative instructions that must be relayed to the patient following cervical cryosurgery.

_____

_____

_____

34. List three functions of a bandage.

_____

_____

_____

35. List four guidelines to follow when applying a bandage.

_____

_____

_____

_____

36. List four signs that may indicate a bandage is too tight.

_____

_____

37. Why should the medical assistant be careful when applying an elastic bandage?

_____

_____

38. What is the purpose of reversing the spiral during a spiral-reverse turn?

_____

_____

39. List two uses of the figure-eight bandage turn.

_____

_____

40. What type of bandage turn is used to anchor a bandage?

_____

41. List four examples of body parts to which a tubular bandage can be applied.

_____

_____

42. List two advantages for using a tubular bandage (as compared with roller bandage).

_____

_____

43. Explain why a tubular bandage cannot be used over an open wound.

_____

_____

Critical Thinking Skills

1.   a. Refer to Chapter 1 and describe the difference between medical asepsis and surgical asepsis.

_____

_____

_____

    b. Which technique (medical asepsis or surgical asepsis) would be employed during the following procedures? In those procedures requiring surgical asepsis, indicate which of the following reasons necessitate the use of surgical asepsis: caring for broken skin, the penetration of a skin surface, or entering a body cavity that is normally sterile.

      1. Administering oral medication _____

_____

      2. Inserting sutures _____

_____

      3. Measuring oral temperature _____

_____

      4. Applying a bandage to the forearm_____

_____

      5. Performing a needle biopsy _____

_____

      6. Removing a sebaceous cyst _____

_____

7. Obtaining a Pap smear _____

_____

8. Inserting a urinary catheter _____

_____

9. Incision and drainage of an abscess_____

_____

10. Applying a dressing to an open wound_____

_____

2. In the situations that follow, the principles of surgical asepsis have been violated. In the space provided, explain why the techniques should not be performed in this manner.

a. Not checking the expiration date on a sterile package before opening it

_____

_____

b. Wearing rings during the application of sterile gloves

_____

_____

c. Laughing or talking over a sterile field

_____

_____

d. Reaching over a sterile field

_____

_____

e. Holding articles below waist level

_____

_____

f. Not palming the label when pouring an antiseptic solution

_____

_____

g. Spilling an antiseptic on the sterile field

_____

_____

h. A soiled dressing is passed over the sterile field.

_____

_____

i.   Sutures are removed from an infected incision.

_____

_____

j.   A vial of Xylocaine is placed on the sterile field.

_____

_____

k.   The bare hands are used to arrange articles on the sterile field.

_____

_____

3.   In the space provided, state the name and use of each of the following types of surgical instruments. Identify any of the following parts present on each instrument by labeling the instrument: box lock, spring handle, ratchets, serrations, cutting edge, and teeth.

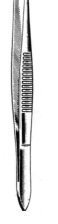

a. Name _____   b. Name _____   c. Name _____

Use _____   Use _____   Use _____

_____   _____   _____

(Courtesy of Elmed Incorporated, Addison, Illinois.)

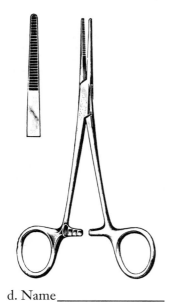

d. Name_____

Use _____

_____

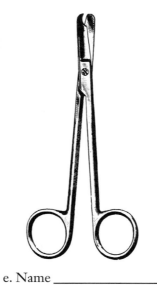

e. Name _____

Use _____

_____

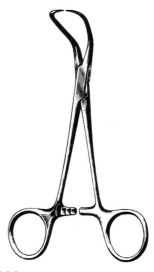

f. Name _____

Use _____

_____

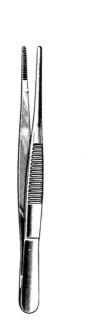

g. Name_____

Use _____

_____

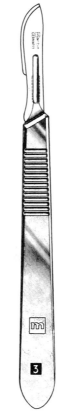

h. Name_____

Use _____

_____

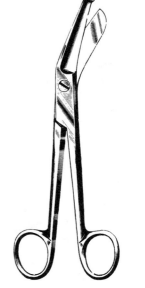

i. Name _____

Use _____

_____

(Courtesy of Elmed Incorporated, Addison, Illinois.)

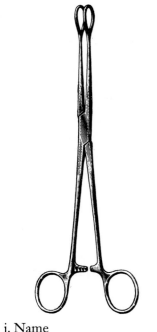

j. Name _____

Use _____

_____

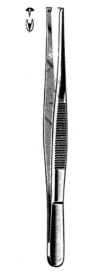

k. Name _____

Use _____

_____

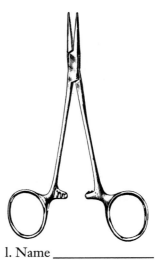

l. Name _____

Use _____

_____

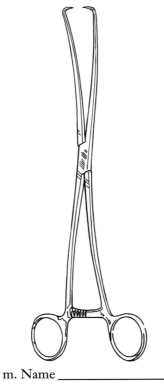

m. Name _____

Use _____

_____

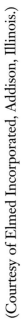

4. Prepare an index card for each minor surgical operation performed in your medical office. File the cards in alphabetical order and use them as reference cards when you prepare for a surgical procedure. Include the following information on each:

   a. The instruments and supplies needed to prepare the surgical tray. If a prepackaged setup is used, make a list of the articles already contained in the set-up and another list of the articles that need to be added. Be able to identify the surgical instruments needed for each procedure. Also list those articles that are to be set up off to the side on an adjacent table or stand.

   b. The type of patient preparation required. Include any type of preoperative patient instruction, skin preparation, or positioning and draping of the patient that may be needed.

   c. The type of medical assistance needed by the physician.

   d. Any postoperative care and instructions that may be required.

5. Obtain a reference source and, in the space provided, describe the contributions the following men made to medicine, especially regarding surgical asepsis.

   a. Ignaz Semmelweis

   _____
   _____
   _____

   b. Louis Pasteur

   _____
   _____
   _____

   c. Joseph Lister

   _____
   _____
   _____

6. Using a reference source, look up **inflammation** and answer the following questions:

   a. What specific physiologic changes take place in the body during inflammation?

   _____
   _____

   b. How do the changes listed in the previous answer aid in repairing injured tissue?

   _____
   _____
   _____
   _____

c. Try to determine how these physiologic changes cause the local symptoms of inflammation (redness, swelling, pain, and warmth).

_____

_____

_____

7. Which type of wound, closed or open, would be more prone to developing an infection? Explain your answer.

_____

_____

_____

Notes

Practice for Competency

Assignment

Applying and Removing Sterile Gloves. Apply and remove sterile gloves.

Opening a Sterile Package. Open a sterile package.

Using Commercially Prepared Sterile Packages. Add a sterile article to a sterile field using a peel-apart package. Practice each of the methods used to transfer articles to a sterile field as shown in Figure 6-3 of your textbook.

Pouring a Sterile Solution. Pour a sterile solution into a container on a sterile field.

Practice for Competency

BANDAGE TURNS

Assignment

Practice the following bandage turns:

a. circular turn

b. spiral turn

c. spiral-reverse turn

d. figure-eight turn

e. recurrent turn

TUBULAR GAUZE BANDAGE

Assignment

Apply a tubular gauze bandage. Practice the procedure for applying a tubular gauze bandage.

Practice for Competency

Assignment

Changing a Sterile Dressing. Change a sterile dressing and record the procedure in the chart provided.

Suture and Removal. Practice the procedure for removing sutures and staples and record the procedure in the chart provided.

Application and Removal of Adhesive Skin Closures. Practice the procedure for applying and removing adhesive skin closures and record the procedure in the chart provided.

Assisting with Minor Office Surgery. Set up a surgical tray for the procedures listed below and assist with minor office surgery. In the chart provided, record the instructions relayed to the patient following the surgery.

1. Suture insertion
2. Sebaceous cyst removal
3. Incision and drainage of a localized infection
4. Needle biopsy
5. Ingrown toenail removal
6. Colposcopy
7. Cervical punch biopsy
8. Cervical cryosurgery

CHART	
Date	

CHART	
Date	

Evaluation of Competency

PROCEDURES 6-1 AND 6-2: APPLYING AND REMOVING STERILE GLOVES

Name _____   Date _____

Evaluated By _____   Score_____

Performance Objective

Outcome:	Apply and remove sterile gloves.
Conditions:	Given the appropriate sized sterile gloves.
	Using a clean flat surface.
Standards:	Time: 5 minutes
	Accuracy: Satisfactory score on the Performance Evaluation Checklist.

Performance Evaluation Checklist

Trial 1	Trial 2	Point Value	*Performance Standards*
			APPLICATION OF GLOVES
		●	Removed rings and washed hands.
		▷	Is able to state why hands should be washed.
		●	Placed the glove package on a clean flat surface.
		●	Opened the sterile glove package without touching the inside of wrapper.
		▷	Is able to state why the inside of wrapper should not be touched.
		●	Picked up the first glove on the inside of cuff without contaminating.
		▷	Is able to state why the inside of the cuff can be touched with the bare hand.
		●	Did not touch the outside of the glove with the bare hand.
		●	Pulled on glove and allowed the cuff to remain turned back on itself.
		●	Picked up the second glove by slipping sterile gloved fingers under the cuff of second glove without contaminating.
		▷	Is able to state how the above step prevents contamination.
		●	Pulled the glove on and turned back the cuff.
		●	Turned back the cuff of first glove.
		●	Adjusted the gloves to a comfortable position.

Trial 1	Trial 2	Point Value	Performance Standards
		●	Inspected the gloves for tears.
		▷	Is able to state what should be done if a glove is torn.
			REMOVAL OF GLOVES
		●	Grasped the outside of the right glove 1 to 2 inches from the top with the gloved left hand.
		●	Slowly pulled right glove off the hand.
		●	Pulled the right glove free and scrunched it into a ball with the gloved left hand.
		●	Placed index and middle fingers of the right hand on the inside of left glove.
		●	Did not allow the clean hand to touch the outside of glove.
		●	Pulled the glove off the left hand enclosing the balled-up right glove.
		●	Discarded both gloves in an appropriate waste container.
		●	Washed hands.
		★	Completed the procedure within 5 minutes.

Evaluation of Student Performance

EVALUATION CRITERIA			COMMENTS
Symbol	Category	Point Value	
★	Critical Step	16 points	
●	Essential Step	6 points	
▷	Theory Question	2 points	
Score calculation: 100 points			
− _____ points missed			
_____ Score			
Satisfactory score: 85 or above			

AAMA/CAAHEP Competency Achieved:

☐ Prepare patient for and assist with procedures, treatments, and minor office surgery.

Evaluation of Competency

PROCEDURE 6-3: OPENING A STERILE PACKAGE

Name _____ Date _____

Evaluated By _____ Score_____

Performance Objective

Outcome: Open a sterile package.
Conditions: Given a sterile package.
Using a clean flat surface.
Standards: Time: 5 minutes.
Accuracy: Satisfactory score on the Performance Evaluation Checklist.

Performance Evaluation Checklist

Trial 1	Trial 2	Point Value	Performance Standards
		●	Washed hands.
		●	Assembled equipment.
		●	Checked the sterilization indicator and expiration date on the package.
		▷	Is able to state why the indicator and date must be checked.
		●	Placed the wrapped package so that the top flap of wrapper will open away from the body.
		●	Removed the fastener on wrapped package and discarded it.
		●	Opened the first flap away from the body.
		●	Opened the left and right flaps without contaminating.
		●	Opened the flap closest to the body.
		●	In all cases, only touched the outside of wrapper.
		●	In all cases, did not reach over the sterile contents of package.
		▷	Is able to state why the medical assistant should not reach over the contents of package.
		●	Utilized package as a sterile set-up or transferred the contents of package to the sterile field, according to medical office procedure.
		★	Completed the procedure within 5 minutes.

Evaluation of Student Performance

EVALUATION CRITERIA			COMMENTS
Symbol	Category	Point Value	
★	Critical Step	16 points	
●	Essential Step	6 points	
▷	Theory Question	2 points	
Score calculation: 100 points			
− _____ points missed			
_____ Score			
Satisfactory score: 85 or above			

AAMA/CAAHEP Competency Achieved:
☐ Prepare patient for and assist with procedures, treatments, and minor office surgery.

Evaluation of Competency

USING COMMERCIALLY PREPARED STERILE PACKAGES

Name _____   Date _____

Evaluated By _____   Score_____

Performance Objective

Outcome:	Add a sterile article to a sterile field from a peel-apart package by ejecting its contents onto the field.
Conditions:	Given the following: peel-apart package and a sterile field.
Standards:	Time: 3 minutes
	Accuracy: Satisfactory score on the Performance Evaluation Checklist.

Performance Evaluation Checklist

Trial 1	Trial 2	Point Value	Performance Standards
		●	Washed hands.
		●	Grasped the two unsterile flaps of the peel-pack between thumbs.
		●	Pulled the package apart using a rolling-outward motion.
		▷	Is able to state what parts of the peel-pack must remain sterile.
		●	Stepped back slightly from the sterile field.
		▷	Is able to state the reason for stepping back.
		●	Gently ejected contents of the peel-pack onto the sterile field.
		★	Completed the procedure within 3 minutes.

Evaluation of Student Performance

EVALUATION CRITERIA			COMMENTS
Symbol	**Category**	**Point Value**	
★	Critical Step	16 points	
●	Essential Step	6 points	
▷	Theory Question	2 points	
Score calculation: 100 points			
− _____ points missed			
_____ Score			
Satisfactory score: 85 or above			

AAMA/CAAHEP Competency Achieved:

☐ Prepare patient for and assist with procedures, treatments, and minor office surgery.

Evaluation of Competency

PROCEDURE 6-4: POURING A STERILE SOLUTION

Name _____ Date _____

Evaluated By _____ Score_____

Performance Objective

Outcome:	Pour a sterile solution.
Conditions:	Given the following: sterile solution, sterile container, and a sterile towel.
Standards:	Time: 5 minutes
	Accuracy: Satisfactory score on the Performance Evaluation Checklist.

Performance Evaluation Checklist

Trial 1	Trial 2	Point Value	Performance Standards
		●	Read the label and checked expiration date on the solution.
		●	Palmed the label of bottle.
		▷	Is able to state why the label should be palmed.
		●	Removed cap and placed it on a flat surface with the open end facing up.
		▷	Is able to state why cap should be placed with the open end facing up.
		●	Rinsed the lip of bottle.
		▷	Is able to state why the lip of bottle should be rinsed.
		●	Poured the proper amount of solution into sterile container.
		●	Did not allow the neck of bottle to come in contact with container.
		●	Did not allow any of the solution to splash onto the sterile field.
		▷	Is able to state why the sterile solution should not be allowed to splash onto the sterile field.
		●	Replaced cap on container without contaminating.
		●	Read the label again.
		★	Completed the procedure within 5 minutes.

Evaluation of Student Performance

EVALUATION CRITERIA			COMMENTS
Symbol	**Category**	**Point Value**	
★	Critical Step	16 points	
●	Essential Step	6 points	
▷	Theory Question	2 points	

Score calculation: 100 points

− _____ points missed

_____ Score

Satisfactory score: 85 or above

AAMA/CAAHEP Competency Achieved:

☐ Prepare patient for and assist with procedures, treatments, and minor office surgery.

Evaluation of Competency

PROCEDURE 6-5: CHANGING A STERILE DRESSING

Name _____   Date _____

Evaluated By _____   Score_____

Performance Objective

Outcome:	Change a sterile dressing.
Conditions:	Given the following: clean disposable gloves, antiseptic swabs, sterile gloves, waterproof waste bag, adhesive tape and scissors, biohazard waste container, sterile dressing, and thumb forceps.
Standards:	Time: 10 minutes.
	Accuracy: Satisfactory score on the Performance Evaluation Checklist.

Performance Evaluation Checklist

Trial 1	Trial 2	Point Value	Performance Standards
		●	Washed hands.
		●	Assembled equipment.
		●	Prepared the sterile field using surgical asepsis.
		●	Positioned the waterproof waste bag in a convenient location.
		●	Greeted and identified the patient.
		●	Introduced yourself and explained the procedure.
		●	Instructed patient not to move during procedure or to talk, laugh, sneeze, or cough over the sterile field.
		●	Applied clean gloves.
		●	Loosened the tape and carefully removed soiled dressing.
		▷	Is able to state what should be done if the dressing is stuck to the wound.
		●	Placed soiled dressing in the waste bag without allowing it to pass over the sterile field.
		●	Inspected the wound.
		▷	Is able to state what type of inspection should be performed.
		●	Removed gloves and discarded them without contaminating.

Trial 1	Trial 2	Point Value	Performance Standards
		●	Opened the antiseptic swabs and placed the pouch in a convenient location.
		●	Opened sterile glove package and applied sterile gloves.
		●	Cleansed the wound using antiseptic swabs.
		●	Discarded contaminated swabs in the waste bag.
		●	Placed sterile dressing over the wound.
		▷	Is able to state why the dressing should be dropped onto the wound.
		●	Discarded gloves or forceps in the waste bag.
		●	Applied adhesive tape to hold sterile dressing in place.
		●	Instructed patient in wound care.
		▷	Is able to state the wound care that should be relayed to the patient.
		●	Provided the patient with written instructions.
		●	Asked patient to sign instruction sheet.
		●	Witnessed the patient's signature.
		●	Gave a signed copy to the patient.
		●	Filed a copy in the patient's medical record.
		●	Returned equipment.
		●	Disposed of contaminated articles in a biohazard waste container.
		●	Washed hands.
		●	Charted the procedure correctly.
		★	Completed the procedure within 10 minutes.

CHART	
Date	

Evaluation of Student Performance

EVALUATION CRITERIA			COMMENTS
Symbol	**Category**	**Point Value**	
★	Critical Step	16 points	
●	Essential Step	6 points	
▷	Theory Question	2 points	
Score calculation: 100 points			
− _____ points missed			
_____ Score			
Satisfactory score: 85 or above			

AAMA/CAAHEP Competency Achieved:

☐ Prepare patient for and assist with procedures, treatments, and minor office surgery.

Notes

Evaluation of Competency

PROCEDURE 6-6: SUTURE AND STAPLE REMOVAL

Name _____ Date _____

Evaluated By _____ Score_____

Performance Objective

Outcome:	Remove sutures and staples.
Conditions:	Given the following: antiseptic swabs, clean disposable gloves, sterile 4 x 4 gauze, surgical tape, biohazard waste container, suture removal kit, and staple removal kit.
Standards:	Time: 10 minutes.
	Accuracy: Satisfactory score on the Performance Evaluation Checklist.

Performance Evaluation Checklist

Trial 1	Trial 2	Point Value	Performance Standards
		●	Washed hands.
		●	Assembled equipment.
		●	Greeted and identified the patient.
		●	Introduced yourself and explained the procedure.
		●	Positioned the patient as required.
		●	Checked to make sure the sutures (or staples) were intact.
		●	Checked to make sure the incision line was approximated and free from infection.
		▷	Is able to state what to do if the incision line was not approximated.
		●	Opened the suture or staple removal kit.
		●	Applied clean gloves.
		●	Cleaned the incision line with an antiseptic swab.
		●	Allowed the skin to dry.
			Removed Sutures as Follows:
		●	Informed the patient that he/she would feel a pulling sensation.
		●	Picked up the knot of suture with thumb forceps.
		●	Placed curved tip of suture scissors under the suture.
		●	Cut suture below the knot on the side of suture closest to the skin.

Trial 1	Trial 2	Point Value	Performance Standards
		●	Gently pulled suture out through the outer skin orifice, using a smooth continuous motion.
		●	Did not allow any portion of suture previously on the outside to be pulled through the skin.
		●	Placed the suture on the gauze.
		●	Repeated above sequence until all sutures were removed.
			Removed Staples as Follows:
		●	Placed the jaws of the staple remover under the staple.
		●	Squeezed the staple handles until they were closed.
		●	Lifted the staple remover upward to remove the staple.
		●	Continued until all the staples were removed.
		●	Cleansed the site with antiseptic swab.
		●	Applied DSD, if directed to do so by physician.
		●	Properly disposed of all contaminated supplies in biohazard waste container.
		●	Removed gloves and washed hands.
		●	Charted the procedure correctly.
		★	Completed the procedure within 10 minutes.

CHART	
Date	

Evaluation of Student Performance

EVALUATION CRITERIA			COMMENTS
Symbol	Category	Point Value	
★	Critical Step	16 points	
●	Essential Step	6 points	
▷	Theory Question	2 points	

Score calculation: 100   points

−_____ points missed

_____ Score

Satisfactory score: 85 or above

AAMA/CAAHEP Competency Achieved:
☐ Prepare patient for and assist with procedures, treatments, and minor office surgery.

Evaluation of Competency

PROCEDURE 6-7: APPLICATION AND REMOVAL OF ADHESIVE SKIN CLOSURES

Name _____ Date _____

Evaluated By _____ Score_____

Performance Objective

Outcome:	Apply and remove adhesive skin closures.
Conditions:	Given the following: box of clean disposable gloves, sterile gloves, antiseptic solution, surgical scrub brush, antiseptic swabs, tincture of benzoin, sterile cotton-tipped applicator, adhesive skin closure strips, sterile 4 x 4 gauze pads, surgical tape, and a biohazard waste container.
Standards:	Time: 10 minutes
	Accuracy: Satisfactory score on the Performance Evaluation Checklist.

Performance Evaluation Checklist

Trial 1	Trial 2	Point Value	Performance Standards
			APPLICATION OF ADHESIVE SKIN CLOSURES
		●	Washed hands.
		●	Assembled equipment.
		●	Greeted and identified the patient.
		●	Introduced yourself and explained the procedure.
		●	Positioned the patient as required.
		●	Applied clean gloves.
		●	Inspected the wound.
		●	Scrubbed the wound with an antiseptic solution.
		●	Allowed the skin to dry or patted dry.
		●	Cleansed the site with an antiseptic swab.
		●	Allowed the skin to dry.
		●	Applied tincture of benzoin without letting it touch the wound.
		▷	Is able to state the purpose of tincture of benzoin.
		●	Allowed the skin to dry.

Trial 1	Trial 2	Point Value	Performance Standards
		●	Removed gloves and washed hands.
		●	Opened the package of adhesive strips.
		●	Applied sterile gloves.
		●	Peeled a strip of tape off the card.
		●	Checked to make sure the skin surface was dry.
		●	Secured one end of the strip to the skin by pressing down firmly.
		●	Stretched the strip across the incision until the edges of the wound were approximated.
		●	Secured the strip on the skin on the other side of the wound.
		●	Applied the next strip midway between the first strip and the end of the wound.
		●	Applied a third strip between the middle strip and the other end of the wound.
		●	Continued applying the strips at 1/8 inch intervals until the edges of the wound were approximated.
		▷	Is able to state why the strips should be spaced at 1/8 inch intervals.
		●	Applied two closures approximately 1/2 inch from the ends of the strips.
		▷	Is able to state the purpose of applying a strip along each edge.
		●	Applied a sterile dressing over the strips if indicated by the physician.
		●	Removed gloves and washed hands.
		●	Instructed the patient in wound care.
		●	Charted the procedure correctly.
			REMOVAL OF ADHESIVE SKIN CLOSURES
		●	Washed hands.
		●	Greeted and identified the patient.
		●	Introduced yourself and explained the procedure.
		●	Positioned the patient as required.
		●	Checked to make sure the incision line was approximated and free from infection.
		●	Positioned a 4 x 4 gauze pad in a convenient location.
		●	Applied clean gloves.
		●	Peeled off each half of the strip from the outside toward the wound margin.
		●	Lifted the strip away from the wound and placed on the gauze.
		●	Continued until all closures were removed.
		●	Cleansed the site with antiseptic swab.
		●	Applied a sterile dressing if indicated by the physician.
		●	Properly disposed of all contaminated supplies.

Trial 1	Trial 2	Point Value	Performance Standards
		●	Removed gloves and washed hands.
		●	Charted the procedure.
		★	Completed the procedure within 10 minutes.

CHART	
Date	

Evaluation of Student Performance

EVALUATION CRITERIA			COMMENTS
Symbol	Category	Point Value	
★	Critical Step	16 points	
●	Essential Step	6 points	
▷	Theory Question	2 points	

Score calculation: 100 points

−_____ points missed

_____ Score

Satisfactory score: 85 or above

AAMA/CAAHEP Competency Achieved:

☐ Prepare patient for and assist with procedures, treatments, and minor office surgery.

Notes

Evaluation of Competency

PROCEDURE 6-8: ASSISTING WITH MINOR OFFICE SURGERY

Name _____   Date _____

Evaluated By _____   Score _____

Performance Objective

Outcome:	Set up the surgical tray and assist with minor office surgery.
Conditions:	Given the instruments and supplies required for a specific minor office surgery as designed by the instructor.
Standards:	Time: 15 minutes
	Accuracy: Satisfactory score on the Performance Evaluation Checklist.

Performance Evaluation Checklist

Trial 1	Trial 2	Point Value	*Performance Standards*
		●	Determined the type of minor office surgery to be performed.
		●	Prepared examining room.
		●	Washed hands.
		●	Set up any medically aseptic articles required on a side stand or table.
		●	Washed hands.
		●	Set up the minor office surgery tray on a clean, dry, flat surface, using the principles of surgical asepsis.
			Prepackaged Sterile Set-Up
		●	Selected the appropriate package from supply shelf and placed it on a flat surface.
		●	Opened the set-up using the inside of wrapper as the sterile field.
		●	Added any additional articles required for the surgery.
			Transferring Articles to a Sterile Field
		●	Placed sterile towel on a flat surface by two corner ends, making sure not to contaminate it.
		●	Added sterile articles to the field, using peel-apart packages.
		●	Arranged articles neatly on the sterile field, using sterile gloves.
		●	Rechecked to make sure all articles were available on the sterile field.

Trial 1	Trial 2	Point Value	Performance Standards
		●	Covered the tray set-up with sterile towel without allowing arms to pass over the sterile field.
		●	Greeted and identified the patient.
		●	Introduced yourself and explained the procedure.
		●	Asked patient if he/she needs to void before the surgery.
		●	Instructed patient on clothing removal.
		●	Instructed patient not to move during procedure or to talk, laugh, sneeze, or cough over the sterile field.
		●	Positioned patient as required by the type of surgery to be performed.
		●	Adjusted the light so that it was focused on the operative site.
		●	Applied clean disposable gloves.
		●	Prepared patient's skin by shaving it (if required) and cleansing it with an antiseptic solution.
		●	Rinsed and dried the area.
		●	Cleansed the site using antiseptic swabs.
		●	Allowed the skin to dry.
		●	Removed gloves and washed hands.
		●	Checked to make sure that everything was ready and informed physician.
			Assisted the Physician
		●	Uncovered the tray set-up.
		●	Withdrew the local anesthetic into syringe and handed it to physician or held the vial while physician withdrew the anesthetic.
		●	Opened the outer glove wrapper for physician.
		●	Adjusted the light as required.
		●	Restrained patient.
		●	Relaxed and reassured patient.
		●	Handed instruments and supplies to physician. (Sterile gloves required.)
		●	Kept the sterile field neat and orderly. (Sterile gloves required.)
		●	Held basin for physician to deposit soiled instruments and supplies. (Sterile gloves required.)
		●	Retracted tissue. (Sterile gloves required.)
		●	Sponged blood from operative site. (Sterile gloves required.)
		●	Added additional instruments and supplies as necessary to the sterile field.
		●	Held specimen container to accept specimen. (Clean gloves required.)
		●	Labeled specimen container.
		●	Applied sterile dressing to the surgical wound if ordered by physician.

Trial 1	Trial 2	Point Value	Performance Standards
		●	Stayed with patient as a safety precaution.
		●	Assisted and instructed patient as required.
		▷	Is able to state the patient instructions that should be relayed for wound and suture care.
		●	Transferred any specimens collected to the laboratory with a completed biopsy request.
		●	Cleaned examining room.
		●	Discarded disposable contaminated articles in a biohazard waste container.
		●	Sanitized and sterilized instruments.
		★	Completed the procedure within 15 minutes.

CHART	
Date	

Evaluation of Student Performance

EVALUATION CRITERIA			COMMENTS
Symbol	Category	Point Value	
★	Critical Step	16 points	
●	Essential Step	6 points	
▷	Theory Question	2 points	

Score calculation: 100 points

− _____ points missed

_____ Score

Satisfactory score: 85 or above

AAMA/CAAHEP Competencies Achieved:
☐ Identify and respond to issues of confidentiality.
☐ Perform within legal and ethical boundaries.
☐ Prepare patient for and assist with procedures, treatments, and minor office surgery.

Notes

Evaluation of Competency

BANDAGE TURNS

Name _____ Date _____

Evaluated By _____ Score_____

Performance Objective

Outcome:	Apply the following bandage turns: circular, spiral, spiral-reverse, figure-eight, and recurrent.
Conditions:	Given the following: a roller bandage and an elastic bandage.
Standards:	Time: 15 minutes
	Accuracy: Satisfactory score on the Performance Evaluation Checklist.

Performance Evaluation Checklist

Trial 1	Trial 2	Point Value	Performance Standards
			Circular Turn
		●	Placed the end of a bandage on a slant.
		●	Encircled the body part while allowing the corner of the bandage to extend.
		●	Turned down corner of bandage.
		●	Made another circular turn around the body part.
		▷	Is able to state a use of the circular turn.
			Spiral Turn
		●	Anchored bandage using a circular turn.
		●	Encircled the body part while keeping bandage at a slant.
		●	Carried each spiral turn upward at a slight angle.
		●	Overlapped each previous turn by one-half to two-thirds the width of bandage.
		▷	Is able to state a use of the spiral turn.
			Spiral-Reverse Turn
		●	Anchored bandage using a circular turn.
		●	Encircled the body part while keeping bandage at a slant.
		●	Reversed the spiral turn using the thumb.
		●	Directed bandage downward and folded it on itself.

Trial 1	Trial 2	Point Value	Performance Standards
		●	Kept bandage parallel to the lower edge of the previous turn.
		●	Overlapped each previous turn by two-thirds the width of the bandage.
		▷	Is able to state a use of the spiral-reverse turn.
			Figure-Eight Turn
		●	Anchored bandage using a circular turn.
		●	Slanted bandage turns to alternately ascend and descend around the body part.
		●	Crossed the turns over one another in the middle to resemble a figure eight.
		●	Overlapped each previous turn by two-thirds the width of bandage.
		▷	Is able to state a use of the figure-eight turn.
			Recurrent Turn
		●	Anchored bandage using two circular turns.
		●	Passed bandage back and forth over the tip of the body part being bandaged.
		●	Overlapped each previous turn by two-thirds of the width of the bandage.
		▷	Is able to state a use of the recurrent turn.
		★	Completed the procedure within 15 minutes.

CHART	
Date	

Evaluation of Student Performance

EVALUATION CRITERIA			COMMENTS
Symbol	Category	Point Value	
★	Critical Step	16 points	
●	Essential Step	6 points	
▷	Theory Question	2 points	

Score calculation: 100 points

− _____ points missed

_____ Score

Satisfactory score: 85 or above

AAMA/CAAHEP Competency Achieved:

☐ Prepare patient for and assist with procedures, treatments, and minor office surgery.

Evaluation of Competency

PROCEDURE 6-9: APPLYING A TUBULAR GAUZE BANDAGE

Name _____   Date _____

Evaluated By _____   Score_____

Performance Objective

Outcome:	Apply a tubular gauze bandage.
Conditions:	Given the following: applicator, tubular gauze, and adhesive tape.
Standards:	Time: 5 minutes
	Accuracy: Satisfactory score on the Performance Evaluation Checklist.

Performance Evaluation Checklist

Trial 1	Trial 2	Point Value	Performance Standards
		●	Washed hands.
		●	Greeted and identified the patient.
		●	Introduced yourself and explained the procedure.
		●	Assembled equipment.
		●	Pulled a sufficient length of gauze from dispensing box roll.
		●	Spread apart the open end of gauze.
		●	Slid gauze over one end of applicator.
		●	Continuing loading applicator by gathering enough gauze on it to complete the bandage.
		●	Cut roll of gauze near the opening of box.
		●	Placed applicator over the proximal end of patient's finger.
		●	Moved applicator from the proximal to the distal end of patient's finger.
		●	Held bandage in place with the fingers.
		▷	Is able to state why bandage should be held in place.
		●	Pulled applicator 1 to 2 inches past the end of patient's finger.
		●	Rotated applicator one full turn to anchor bandage.
		●	Moved applicator forward toward the proximal end of patient's finger.
		●	Moved applicator forward approximately 1 inch past the original starting point of bandage.

Trial 1	Trial 2	Point Value	Performance Standards
		●	Anchored bandage using a rotating motion.
		●	Repeated procedure for the number of layers desired.
		●	Finished the last layer at the proximal end.
		●	Cut gauze from applicator.
		●	Removed applicator.
		●	Applied adhesive tape at the base of patient's finger.
		●	Washed hands.
		●	Charted the procedure correctly.
		★	Completed the procedure within 5 minutes.

CHART	
Date	

Evaluation of Student Performance

EVALUATION CRITERIA			COMMENTS
Symbol	Category	Point Value	
★	Critical Step	16 points	
●	Essential Step	6 points	
▷	Theory Question	2 points	

Score calculation: 100   points
−   _____ points missed
_____ Score
Satisfactory score: 85 or above

AAMA/CAAHEP Competency Achieved:
☐ Prepare patient for and assist with procedures, treatments, and minor office surgery.

Administration of Medication

NAME _____

Key Terminology Assessment

Directions: Match each medical term with its definition.

_____ 1. allergen
_____ 2. ampule
_____ 3. aspirate
_____ 4. dermis
_____ 5. dose
_____ 6. epidermis
_____ 7. induration
_____ 8. inhalation administration
_____ 9. intradermal injection
_____ 10. intramuscular injection
_____ 11. intravenous injection
_____ 12. oral administration
_____ 13. prescription
_____ 14. subcutaneous injection
_____ 15. sublingual administration
_____ 16. topical administration
_____ 17. vesiculation
_____ 18. vial
_____ 19. wheal

A. Applying a drug to a particular spot, usually for a local action.
B. Introducing medication into the dermal layer of the skin.
C. A small sealed glass container containing a single dose of medication.
D. Order for a drug or other therapy, written by a physician.
E. The outermost, nonvascular layer of the skin.
F. To remove by suction.
G. Introducing medication into the bloodstream directly through a vein.
H. A small raised area of the skin.
I. Introducing medication beneath the skin, into the fatty layer of the body.
J. An area of hardened tissue.
K. A closed glass container with a rubber stopper.

L. The administration of medication by way of air or other vapor being drawn into the lungs.
M. The true skin; the main thickness of the skin, with an active blood supply.
N. Administration of medication by mouth.
O. The formation of fluid-containing lesions of the skin.
P. Introducing medication into the muscular layer of the body.
Q. Administration of medication by placing it under the tongue.
R. The quantity of a drug to be administered at one time.
S. A substance that is capable of causing an allergic reaction.

Self-Evaluation

Directions: Fill in each blank with the correct answer.

1. The study of drugs is known as

   _____

2. What does the term *parenteral* mean?

   _____

   _____

3. What is the difference between administering, prescribing, and dispensing medication at the medical office?

   _____

   _____

   _____

   _____

4. Explain the difference between the generic name and the brand name of a drug.

   _____

   _____

   _____

   _____

5. When a drug is dissolved in a solution of sugar and water, with added flavoring to disguise its unpleasant taste, the preparation is called

   _____

6. What is a capsule?

_____

7. What is a tablet?

_____

8. Why must a suppository have a cylindrical or conical shape?

_____

9. How should a liniment be applied?

_____

10. What is the purpose of scoring a tablet?

_____

11. List two reasons for enterically coating a tablet.

_____

_____

12. What is the name given to the type of drug that relieves pain?

_____

13. What is the name given to the type of drug that neutralizes gastric acid?

_____

14. What is the name given to the type of drug that inhibits the growth of or kills susceptible bacteria?

_____

15. What is the name given to the type of drug that prevents nausea and vomiting?

_____

16. What is the name given to the type of drug that suppresses the cough reflex?

_____

17. What is the name given to the type of drug that increases urine output by the kidney?

_____

18. What is the name given to the type of drug that decreases the viscosity of bronchial secretions?

_____

19. What is the name given to the type of drug that reduces anxiety and promotes sleep?

_____

20. What is the name given to the type of drug that reduces blood pressure?

_____

21. Why is the metric system used most often to administer medication?

_____

_____

22. Define the term *volume*.

_____

_____

23. What is a cubic centimeter?

_____

_____

24. Describe the use of the household system of measurement.

_____

_____

25. When is conversion required?

_____

_____

26. What is a prescription?

_____

_____

_____

27. List three factors that affect the action of drugs in the body.

_____

_____

_____

28. List the six "rights" of preparing and administering medication.

_____

_____

_____

_____

29. List advantages and disadvantages of using the parenteral route of administration.

_____

_____

_____

_____

30. What is the purpose of using a filter needle when withdrawing medication from an ampule?

_____

31. What sites are used most frequently to administer a subcutaneous injection?

_____

_____

32. List three medications commonly administered through a subcutaneous injection.

_____

_____

_____

33. Why is medication absorbed faster through the intramuscular route than through the subcutaneous route?

_____

_____

_____

34. List the four intramuscular injection sites and explain why these sites must be used to administer an IM injection.

_____

_____

_____

35. What types of medication are given using the Z-track technique?

_____

_____

36. What sites are used most frequently to administer an intradermal injection?

_____

37. What is the most frequent use of an intradermal injection?

_____

38. Why is tuberculin skin testing performed as a screening measure?

_____

_____

39. What is induration and what causes it?

_____

_____

40. What will be done if the patient has a positive reaction to a tuberculin skin test?

_____

_____

41. What is an allergy?

_____

_____

42. What are the symptoms of an anaphylactic reaction?

_____

_____

_____

43. What are ten examples of common allergens?

_____

_____

_____

_____

44. Explain what is meant by each of the following intradermal skin test reactions.
   a.   ±1 _____
   b.   +2 _____
   c.   +3 _____

45. What are the advantages of RAST testing over direct skin testing?

_____

_____

_____

Critical Thinking Skills

1. Inspect the package labels of 10 drugs (or use other means) to assess the classification of each drug based on preparation and action. List the name of each drug along with its appropriate category in the spaces provided. Compare results. Example: *Drug:* Tylenol Elixir. *Classification based on preparation:* elixir. *Classification based on action:* analgesic, antipyretic.

	Drug	**Classification Based On:** Preparation	Action
a.	_____	_____	_____
b.	_____	_____	_____
c.	_____	_____	_____
d.	_____	_____	_____
e.	_____	_____	_____
f.	_____	_____	_____
g.	_____	_____	_____
h.	_____	_____	_____
i.	_____	_____	_____
j.	_____	_____	_____

2. Obtain a medicine cup that is graduated into the metric (milliliters), apothecary (drams and ounces), and household (teaspoons and tablespoons) systems. Complete the following:

   a. What is its capacity?   _____ ounce(s)

   _____ milliliter(s)

   _____ tablespoon(s)

   _____ dram(s)

   b. Practice pouring oral liquid medication by pouring the following amounts of water into the medicine cup. Place a check mark by each amount after it has been properly poured.

   20 ml   _____

   4 drams   _____

   1 ounce   _____

   10 ml   _____

   ½ ounce   _____

   1 tablespoon   _____

   2 drams   _____

3.   Obtain a needle and syringe. Locate the following parts of each and explain their function.

Needle   **Function**

   a.   hub _____

   b.   shaft, or cannula_____

   c.   lumen _____

   d.   point _____

   e.   bevel _____

   f.   What is the gauge of the needle?_____

   g.   What is the length of the needle? _____

Syringe   **Function**

   a.   barrel_____

   b.   flange_____

   c.   plunger _____

   d.   What is the capacity of the syringe? _____

4a. Obtain a 3 cc syringe that is divided into tenths of a cubic centimeter. Locate the fol-
     lowing calibrations on the syringe. Place a check mark in the blank next to each cali-
     bration after it has been correctly located.

**Calibration
(cc)**   **Correct Location**

   a.   0.5   _____

   b.   1.0   _____

   c.   1.2   _____

   d.   2.5   _____

   e.   2.7   _____

4b. Locate each calibration (listed in 4a) on the illustration of the hypodermic syringe by
     placing an arrow on the correct calibration line and labeling it with the calibration.

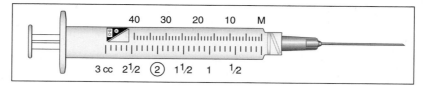

5a. Obtain a U-100 insulin syringe. Locate the following calibrations on the syringe.
     Place a check mark in the blank next to each calibration after it has been correctly
     located.

**Calibration
(units)**   **Correct Location**

   a.   10   _____

   b.   16   _____

c. 20 _____

d. 44 _____

e. 60 _____

f. 68 _____

g. 70 _____

h. 86 _____

i. 90 _____

j. 100 _____

5b. Locate each calibration (listed in 5a) on the illustration of the insulin syringe by placing an arrow on the correct calibration line and labeling it with the calibration.

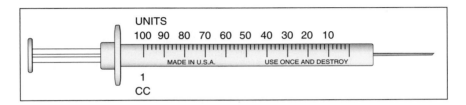

6a. Obtain a 1 cc tuberculin syringe that is divided into tenths and hundredths of a cubic
centimeter. Locate the following calibrations on the syringe. Place a check mark in
the blank next to each calibration after it has been correctly located.

**Calibration
(cc)**   **Correct Location**

a. 0.05 _____

b. 0.10 _____

c. 0.15 _____

d. 0.34 _____

e. 0.52 _____

f. 0.75 _____

g. 0.92 _____

6b. Locate each calibration (listed in 6a) on the illustration of the tuberculin syringe by
placing an arrow on the correct calibration line and labeling it with the calibration.

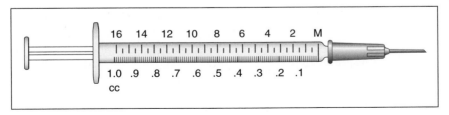

7. Refer to Figure 7-3 in your textbook. Indicate the following information for each syringe and needle: the syringe capacity and the gauge and length of the needle.

_____

_____

_____

_____

_____

8. In the diagram below, draw 3 lines indicating the angle of insertion into the correct body tissue for an intradermal, a subcutaneous, and an intramuscular injection. Label the lines.

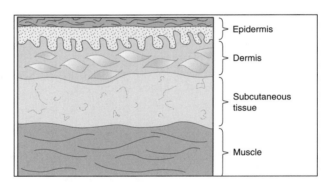

9. For each of the following situations involving the preparation and administration of medication, write **C** if the technique is correct and **I** if it is incorrect. If the technique is correct, state the principle underlying the technique. If the technique is incorrect, explain what might happen if it were performed.

_____ a. The expiration date of the bottle of medication is checked before administering the medication.

_____

_____

_____ b. The medical assistant is unfamiliar with the drug to be administered, so he or she looks it up in a drug reference.

_____

_____

_____ c. The medical assistant compares the medication label with the physician's instructions three times: as it is taken from the shelf, before pouring the medication, and before replacing the medication on the shelf.

_____

_____

_____ d. The medical assistant's fingers touch the inside of the bottle cap while pouring oral solid medication.

_____

_____

_____ e. The label on the liquid medication bottle is not palmed when pouring the medication.

_____

_____

_____ f. The medical assistant offers the patient water after administering Tylenol elixir.

_____

_____

_____ g. The rubber stopper of the multi-dose vial is cleansed with an antiseptic wipe before withdrawing the medication.

_____

_____

_____ h. Air is not injected into the multi-dose vial before withdrawing the medication.

_____

_____

_____ i. The medical assistant is careful to make sure the needle remains sterile during the procedure.

_____

_____

_____ j. Air bubbles are present in the medication in the syringe that has been withdrawn from an ampule.

_____

_____

_____ k. The injection sites are not rotated when repeated injections are given.

_____

_____ l. The antiseptic is not allowed to dry before administering an injection.

_____

_____

_____m. The medical assistant touches the injection site after cleansing it.

_____

_____

_____ n. The skin is stretched taut before an intramuscular injection is given.

_____

_____

_____ o. The needle is inserted slowly and steadily for an IM injection.

_____

_____

_____ p. An IM injection is given in the deltoid site to a patient who has a tight sleeve.

_____

_____

_____ q. An IM injection is given into the dorsogluteal site when the site is not fully exposed.

_____

_____

_____ r. The medical assistant does not aspirate when giving an intramuscular injection.

_____

_____

_____ s. The medication is injected quickly for an IM injection.

_____

_____

_____ t. The skin is pulled away laterally from the injection site before the needle is inserted for a Z-track injection.

_____

_____

_____ u. The needle is withdrawn at the same angle as for insertion.

_____

_____

_____ v. The intradermal needle is inserted with the bevel facing downward.

_____

_____

_____ w. The medical assistant does not aspirate when giving an intradermal injection.

_____

_____

_____ x. The injection site is gently massaged after an intradermal injection is given.

_____

_____

_____ y. The injection site is massaged after an IM injection has been given.

_____

_____

_____ z. The needle is recapped after administering an IM injection.

_____

_____

10. In the space provided, indicate whether the following Mantoux test results are positive, doubtful or negative:

    a. 12 mm of induration _____

    b. 7 mm of induration _____

    c. 5 mm (The patient is infected with HIV) _____

    d. 2 mm of induration _____

    e. Erythema, 6 mm wide _____

11. Table 7-1 in your textbook is a list of drugs frequently prescribed in the medical office. Using the Pharmacology Drug Sheets on the following pages, record the name (generic and brand) and drug classification for each of the drugs in Table 7-1. Obtain a drug reference book, and research indications and patient teaching for each drug. Record this information in the appropriate space on the Pharmacology Drug Sheets.

Pharmacology Drug Sheet

Name _____

Generic Name, Brand Name, Drug Classification	Indications	Patient Teaching

Pharmacology Drug Sheet

Name _____

Generic Name, Brand Name, Drug Classification	Indications	Patient Teaching

Pharmacology Drug Sheet

Name _____

Generic Name, Brand Name, Drug Classification	Indications	Patient Teaching

Pharmacology Drug Sheet

Name _____

Generic Name, Brand Name, Drug Classification	Indications	Patient Teaching

Pharmacology Drug Sheet

Name _____

Generic Name, Brand Name, Drug Classification	Indications	Patient Teaching

Pharmacology Drug Sheet

Name _____

Generic Name, Brand Name, Drug Classification	Indications	Patient Teaching

Pharmacology Drug Sheet

Name _____

Generic Name, Brand Name, Drug Classification	Indications	Patient Teaching

Pharmacology Drug Sheet

Name _____

Generic Name, Brand Name, Drug Classification	Indications	Patient Teaching

Pharmacology Drug Sheet

Name _____

Generic Name, Brand Name, Drug Classification	Indications	Patient Teaching

Pharmacology Drug Sheet

Name _____

Generic Name, Brand Name, Drug Classification	Indications	Patient Teaching

Pharmacology Drug Sheet

Name _____

Generic Name, Brand Name, Drug Classification	Indications	Patient Teaching

Practice for Competency

ADMINISTRATION OF MEDICATION

Assignment

Prerequisite. Complete *Supplemental Education for Chapter 7: Drug Dosage Calculation* (Pages 237–276 in this manual).

Oral Medication. Administer oral solid and liquid medication and record the procedure in the chart provided.

Reconstituting Powdered Drugs. Reconstitute a powdered drug for parenteral administration.

Preparing the Injection. Prepare an injection from an ampule and a vial.

Subcutaneous Injection. Administer a subcutaneous injection and record the procedure in the chart provided.

Intramuscular Injection. Administer an intramuscular injection using both the standard procedure and the Z-track method. Record each procedure in the chart provided.

Intradermal Injection. Administer an intradermal injection and record the procedure in the chart provided.

CHART	
Date	

Practice for Competency

TUBERCULIN SKIN TESTING

Assignment

Tine Test. Administer a tine test and record the procedure in the chart provided. Read and interpret the test results and record them in the chart.

The following values can be used for the test results:

a. 1 mm induration

b. vesiculation

c. 4 mm of induration

d. absence of induration

e. 2 mm of induration

CHART	
Date	

Evaluation of Competency

PROCEDURE 7-1: ADMINISTERING ORAL MEDICATION

Name _____   Date _____

Evaluated By _____   Score_____

Performance Objective

Outcome:	Administer oral solid and liquid medication.
Conditions:	Given the following: appropriate medication, medicine cup, and a medication tray.
Standards:	Time: 10 minutes
	Accuracy: Satisfactory score on the Performance Evaluation Checklist.

Performance Evaluation Checklist

Trial 1	Trial 2	Point Value	Performance Standards
		●	Washed hands.
		●	Assembled equipment.
		●	Worked in a quiet, well-lit atmosphere.
		★	Selected the correct medication from the shelf.
		●	Checked the drug label.
		●	Checked the expiration date.
		●	Compared the medication with the physician's instructions.
		★	Calculated the correct dose to be given, if needed.
		●	Removed the bottle cap.
		●	Checked the drug label and poured the medication.
			Solid Medication
		★	Poured the correct number of capsules or tablets into the bottle cap.
		▷	Is able to state why the medication is poured into the bottle cap.
		●	Transferred the medication to medicine cup.
			Liquid Medication
		●	Placed lid of bottle upside down on a flat surface with the open end facing up.
		●	Palmed the surface of the drug label.
		▷	Is able to state why the surface of the drug label should be palmed.

Trial 1	Trial 2	Point Value	Performance Standards
		●	Placed thumbnail at the proper calibration on medicine cup.
		●	Held medicine cup at eye level.
		★	Poured the correct amount of medication and read the dose at the lowest level of the meniscus.
		●	Checked the drug label and returned the medication to shelf.
		●	Greeted and identified the patient.
		●	Introduced yourself and explained the procedure.
		●	Handed the medicine cup to the patient.
		●	Offered water to patient.
		▷	Is able to state one instance when water should not be offered.
		●	Remained with patient until the medication was swallowed.
		●	Washed hands.
		●	Charted the procedure correctly.
		★	Completed the procedure within 10 minutes.

CHART	
Date	

Evaluation of Student Performance

EVALUATION CRITERIA			COMMENTS
Symbol	Category	Point Value	
★	Critical Step	16 points	
●	Essential Step	6 points	
▷	Theory Question	2 points	

Score calculation: 100   points

−   _____   points missed

_____ Score

Satisfactory score: 85 or above

AAMA/CAAHEP Competency Achieved:
☐ Apply pharmacology principles to prepare and administer oral and parenteral medication.

Evaluation of Competency

PROCEDURE 7-2: RECONSTITUTING POWDERED DRUGS

Name _____   Date _____

Evaluated By _____   Score_____

Performance Objective

Outcome:	Reconstitute a powdered drug for parenteral administration.
Conditions:	Given the following: vial containing the powdered drug, re-constituting liquid, and a needle and syringe.
Standards:	Time: 5 minutes
	Accuracy: Satisfactory score on the Performance Evaluation Checklist.

Performance Evaluation Checklist

Trial 1	Trial 2	Point Value	Performance Standards
		●	Withdrew an amount of air equal to the amount of liquid to be injected into the vial from the vial containing the powdered drug.
		★	Added the appropriate amount of reconstituting liquid to the powdered drug.
		●	Rolled the vial between the hands.
		●	Labeled multiple-dose vials with the name of the medication, the date of preparation, and your initials.
		●	Stored multiple-dose vials as indicated in the manufacturer's instructions.
		▷	Is able to state the importance of checking the expiration date of a re-constituted multiple dose vial before administering it.
		★	Completed the procedure within 5 minutes.

Evaluation of Student Performance

EVALUATION CRITERIA			COMMENTS
Symbol	**Category**	**Point Value**	
★	Critical Step	16 points	
●	Essential Step	6 points	
▷	Theory Question	2 points	
Score calculation: 100 points			
‾‾‾‾‾‾ points missed			
‾‾‾‾‾‾ Score			
Satisfactory score: 85 or above			

AAMA/CAAHEP Competency Achieved:

☐ Apply pharmacology principles to prepare and administer oral and parenteral medications.

Evaluation of Competency

PROCEDURE 7-3: PREPARING THE INJECTION

Name _____ Date _____

Evaluated By _____ Score_____

Performance Objective

Outcome:	Prepare an injection from an ampule and vial.
Conditions:	Given the following: medication ordered by the physician, needle and syringe, antiseptic wipe, and medication tray.
Standards:	Time: 10 minutes
	Accuracy: Satisfactory score on the Performance Evaluation Checklist.

Performance Evaluation Checklist

Trial 1	Trial 2	Point Value	Performance Standards
		●	Washed hands.
		●	Assembled equipment.
		●	Worked in a quiet, well-lit atmosphere.
		★	Selected the correct medication from the shelf.
		●	Checked the drug label.
		●	Checked the expiration date.
		●	Compared the medication with the physician's instructions.
		★	Calculated the correct dose to be given, if needed.
		●	Opened the antiseptic wipe and cleansed the vial or ampule.
		●	Opened syringe and needle package(s).
		●	Assembled needle and syringe if necessary.
		●	Removed the needle guard and checked to make sure that needle is attached firmly to syringe.
		●	Checked the drug label and withdrew the proper amount of medication.
			Withdrew Medication From a Vial
		●	Pulled back on plunger to draw an amount of air into syringe equal to the amount of medication to be withdrawn.
		●	Inserted needle through rubber stopper until it reached the empty space between stopper and the fluid level.

Trial 1	Trial 2	Point Value	Performance Standards
		●	Pushed down on plunger to inject air into the vial.
		●	Kept needle above the fluid level.
		▷	Is able to state why an equal amount of air must be injected into the vial.
		●	Inverted the vial while holding onto syringe and plunger.
		★	Held syringe at eye level and withdrew the proper amount of medication.
		●	Kept the tip of needle below the fluid level.
		▷	Is able to state why the tip of needle must be kept below the fluid level.
		●	Removed any air bubbles in syringe.
		▷	Is able to state why air bubbles should be removed from the syringe.
		●	Removed any air remaining at the top of syringe.
		●	Removed the needle from rubber stopper.
			Withdrew Medication From an Ampule
		●	Tapped the stem of ampule lightly to remove any medication in the neck of ampule.
		●	Placed piece of gauze around the neck of ampule.
		●	Held ampule firmly between the fingers.
		●	Broke off the stem by snapping it quickly and firmly away from the body.
		●	Inserted needle below the fluid level.
		★	Withdrew the proper amount of medication.
		●	Kept needle below the fluid level.
		▷	Is able to state why needle must be kept below the fluid level.
		●	Removed needle from ampule without allowing needle to touch the edge of ampule.
		●	Removed any air bubbles in syringe.
		●	Removed any air remaining at the top of syringe.
		▷	Is able to state what should be done if a filter needle was used to withdraw the medication.
		●	Replaced the needle guard on syringe.
		●	Placed syringe on a medication tray with an antiseptic wipe.
		●	Checked the drug label and returned the medication to its proper place.
		★	Completed the procedure within 10 minutes.

Evaluation of Student Performance

EVALUATION CRITERIA			COMMENTS
Symbol	**Category**	**Point Value**	
★	Critical Step	16 points	
●	Essential Step	6 points	
▷	Theory Question	2 points	

Score calculation: 100 points

_____ − points missed

_____ Score

Satisfactory score: 85 or above

AAMA/CAAHEP Competency Achieved:

☐ Apply pharmacology principles to prepare and administer medication.

Notes

Evaluation of Competency

PROCEDURE 7-4: ADMINISTERING A SUBCUTANEOUS INJECTION

Name _____   Date _____

Evaluated By _____   Score_____

Performance Objective

Outcome:	Administer a subcutaneous injection.
Conditions:	Given the following: appropriate medication, appropriate needle and syringe, antiseptic wipe, disposable gloves, and a biohazard sharps container.
Standards:	Time: 5 minutes
	Accuracy: Satisfactory score on the Performance Evaluation Checklist.

Performance Evaluation Checklist

Trial 1	Trial 2	Point Value	Performance Standards
		●	Greeted and identified the patient.
		●	Introduced yourself and explained the procedure.
		●	Selected an appropriate subcutaneous injection site.
		▷	Is able to state what tissue layer of the body the medication will be injected into.
		●	Cleansed area with an antiseptic wipe and allowed it to dry completely.
		▷	Is able to state why the site should be allowed to dry.
		●	Applied gloves.
		●	Removed needle guard.
		●	Properly positioned the hand on area surrounding the injection site.
		▷	Is able to state when it is advisable to grasp area surrounding the injection site.
		●	Inserted needle at a 45-degree or 90-degree angle (depending on the length of the needle) with a quick, smooth motion.
		●	Removed the hand from the skin.
		▷	Is able to state why the hand should be removed from the skin.
		★	Aspirated to make sure that the needle was not in a blood vessel.
		▷	Is able to state what should be done if needle is in a blood vessel.

Trial 1	Trial 2	Point Value	Performance Standards
		●	Injected the medication slowly and steadily.
		▷	Is able to state what would happen if the medication were injected too rapidly.
		●	Placed an antiseptic wipe gently over the injection site and removed needle quickly at the same angle as insertion.
		●	Gently massaged the injection site with an antiseptic wipe.
		●	Properly disposed of needle and syringe.
		▷	Is able to state why the needle and syringe should be disposed of properly.
		●	Removed gloves and washed hands.
		●	Charted the procedure correctly.
		●	Remained with patient to make sure there were no unusual reactions.
		★	Completed the procedure within 5 minutes.

CHART	
Date	

Evaluation of Student Performance

EVALUATION CRITERIA			COMMENTS
Symbol	Category	Point Value	
★	Critical Step	16 points	
●	Essential Step	6 points	
▷	Theory Question	2 points	

Score calculation: 100 points

‾‾‾‾‾‾ points missed

‾‾‾‾‾‾ Score

Satisfactory score: 85 or above

AAMA/CAAHEP Competencies Achieved:

☐ Apply pharmacology principles to prepare and administer medication.
☐ Document appropriately.

Evaluation of Competency

PROCEDURE 7-5: ADMINISTERING AN INTRAMUSCULAR INJECTION

Name _____ Date _____

Evaluated By _____ Score_____

Performance Objective

Outcome:	Administer an intramuscular injection.
Conditions:	Given the following: appropriate medication, appropriate needle and syringe, antiseptic wipe, disposable gloves, and a biohazard sharps container.
Standards:	Time: 5 minutes
	Accuracy: Satisfactory score on the Performance Evaluation Checklist.

Performance Evaluation Checklist

Trial 1	Trial 2	Point Value	*Performance Standards*
		●	Greeted and identified the patient.
		●	Introduced yourself and explained the procedure.
			Selected and properly located the intramuscular injection site.
		●	Dorsogluteal
		●	Deltoid
		●	Vastus lateralis
		●	Ventrogluteal
		▷	Is able to state what tissue layer of the body the medication will be injected into.
		●	Cleansed the area with an antiseptic wipe and allowed it to dry completely.
		●	Applied gloves.
		●	Removed needle guard.
		●	Stretched the skin taut over the injection site using the thumb and first two fingers.
		▷	Is able to explain why the skin should be stretched taut.
		●	Held the barrel of syringe like a dart and inserted needle quickly at a 90-degree angle to the patient's skin with a firm motion.

Trial 1	Trial 2	Point Value	Performance Standards
		▷	Is able to state why the needle should be inserted quickly and smoothly.
		★	Aspirated to make sure the needle was not in a blood vessel.
		▷	Is able to state what would happen if the medication was injected into a blood vessel.
		●	Injected the medication slowly and steadily.
		●	Placed an antiseptic wipe gently over the injection site and removed needle quickly at the same angle as that of insertion.
		●	Gently massaged the injection site with an antiseptic wipe.
		▷	Is able to state the reason for massaging the injection site.
		●	Properly disposed of needle and syringe.
		●	Removed gloves and washed hands.
		●	Charted the procedure correctly.
		●	Remained with the patient to make sure that there were no unusual reactions.
		★	Completed the procedure within 5 minutes.

CHART	
Date	

Evaluation of Student Performance

EVALUATION CRITERIA			COMMENTS
Symbol	Category	Point Value	
★	Critical Step	16 points	
●	Essential Step	6 points	
▷	Theory Question	2 points	

Score calculation: 100 points

_____ points missed

_____ Score

Satisfactory score: 85 or above

AAMA/CAAHEP Competencies Achieved:

☐ Identify and respond to issues of confidentiality.

☐ Perform within legal and ethical boundaries.

☐ Apply pharmacology principles to prepare and administer oral and parenteral medications.

☐ Document appropriately.

Evaluation of Competency

PROCEDURE 7-6: ADMINISTERING A Z-TRACK INTRAMUSCULAR INJECTION

Name _____   Date _____

Evaluated By _____   Score_____

Performance Objective

Outcome: Administer an intramuscular injection using the Z-track method.

Conditions: Given the following: appropriate medication, appropriate needle and syringe, antiseptic wipe, disposable gloves, and a biohazard sharps container.

Standards: Time: 5 minutes

Accuracy: Satisfactory score on the Performance Evaluation Checklist.

Performance Evaluation Checklist

Trial 1	Trial 2	Point Value	Performance Standards
		●	Greeted and identified the patient.
		●	Introduced yourself and explained the procedure.
		●	Selected and properly located the intramuscular injection site.
		●	Cleansed area with an antiseptic wipe and allowed the site to dry completely.
		●	Applied gloves.
		●	Removed needle guard.
		●	Pulled the skin away laterally from the injection site with the nondominant hand.
		●	Inserted needle quickly and smoothly at a 90-degree angle.
		★	Aspirated to make sure that the needle was not in a blood vessel.
		●	Injected the medication slowly and steadily.
		●	Waited 10 seconds before withdrawing the needle.
		▷	Is able to state why there should be a 10-second waiting period.
		●	Withdrew needle quickly at the same angle as that of insertion.
		●	Released the traction on the skin.

Trial 1	Trial 2	Point Value	Performance Standards
		▷	Is able to state what occurs when the skin traction is released.
		●	Properly disposed of needle and syringe.
		●	Did not massage the injection site.
		▷	Is able to state why the injection site should not be massaged.
		●	Applied gentle pressure if bleeding occurred.
		●	Removed gloves and washed hands.
		●	Charted the procedure correctly.
		●	Remained with patient to make sure that there were no adverse reactions.
		★	Completed the procedure within 5 minutes.

CHART	
Date	

Evaluation of Student Performance

EVALUATION CRITERIA			COMMENTS
Symbol	Category	Point Value	
★	Critical Step	16 points	
●	Essential Step	6 points	
▷	Theory Question	2 points	

Score calculation: 100   points

−

_____ points missed

_____ Score

Satisfactory score: 85 or above

AAMA/CAAHEP Competencies Achieved:

☐ Apply pharmacology principles to prepare and administer oral and parenteral medications.

☐ Document appropriately.

Evaluation of Competency

PROCEDURE 7-7: ADMINISTERING AN INTRADERMAL INJECTION

Name _____   Date _____

Evaluated By _____   Score_____

Performance Objective

Outcome: Administer an intradermal injection.

Conditions: Given the following: appropriate medication, appropriate needle and syringe, antiseptic wipe, disposable gloves, and a biohazard sharps container.

Standards: Time: 5 minutes

Accuracy: Satisfactory score on the Performance Evaluation Checklist.

Performance Evaluation Checklist

Trial 1	Trial 2	Point Value	Performance Standards
		●	Greeted and identified the patient.
		●	Introduced yourself and explained the procedure.
		●	Selected an appropriate intradermal injection site.
		▷	Is able to state what tissue layer of the body the medication will be injected into.
		●	Cleansed area with antiseptic wipe and allowed it to dry completely.
		●	Applied gloves.
		●	Removed needle guard.
		●	Stretched the skin taut at the site of administration.
		●	Inserted needle at an angle of 10 to 15 degrees, with the bevel upward.
		●	The bevel of the needle just penetrated the skin.
		●	Injected the medication slowly and steadily until a wheal formed.
		●	Placed an antiseptic wipe gently over the injection site and removed the needle quickly at the same angle as that of insertion.
		●	Did not massage the injection site.
		▷	Is able to state why the injection site should not be massaged.
		●	Properly disposed of needle and syringe.
		●	Removed gloves and washed hands.

Trial 1	Trial 2	Point Value	Performance Standards
		●	Remained with patient to make sure that there were no adverse reactions.
		●	Read the test results; or informed the patient when to return to have the test results read; or instructed patient in the proper procedure for reading test results at home and reporting them to the medical office.
		●	Charted the procedure correctly.
		★	Completed the procedure within 5 minutes.

CHART	
Date	

Evaluation of Student Performance

EVALUATION CRITERIA			COMMENTS
Symbol	Category	Point Value	
★	Critical Step	16 points	
●	Essential Step	6 points	
▷	Theory Question	2 points	

Score calculation: 100 points

  −   points missed

           Score

Satisfactory score: 85 or above

AAMA/CAAHEP Competencies Achieved:

☐ Apply pharmacology principles to prepare and administer oral and parenteral medications.

☐ Document appropriately.

Evaluation of Competency

PROCEDURE 7-8: ADMINISTERING A TINE TEST

Name _____ Date _____

Evaluated By _____ Score_____

Performance Objective

Outcome: Administer a tine test and read the test results.

Conditions: Given the following: tine test device, antiseptic wipe, disposable gloves, millimeter ruler, and a biohazard sharps container.

Standards: Time: 10 minutes

Accuracy: Satisfactory score on the Performance Evaluation Checklist.

Performance Evaluation Checklist

Trial 1	Trial 2	Point Value	Performance Standards
			TINE TEST ADMINISTRATION
		●	Washed hands.
		●	Greeted and identified the patient.
		●	Introduced yourself and explained the procedure.
		●	Selected an appropriate site to administer the tine test.
		▷	Is able to explain what type of skin areas should be avoided and why they should be avoided.
		●	Cleansed the area with an antiseptic wipe and allowed the site to dry.
		●	Applied gloves.
		●	Exposed the tuberculin tines using a twisting, pulling motion on the cap.
		●	Grasped patient's forearm with the nondominant hand and stretched the skin tightly.
		▷	Is able to explain why patient's arm should be held and the skin stretched tightly.
		●	Held the test in the dominant hand and placed the plastic disc on patient's skin for 1 to 2 seconds.
		●	Released the tension from the grasp on the patient's arm and withdrew the tine test unit.

Trial 1	Trial 2	Point Value	Performance Standards
		●	Did not massage the test site after application of the tines.
		▷	Is able to explain why the test site should not be massaged.
		●	Discarded the plastic disc.
		●	Instructed patient to return for reading of the test in 48 to 72 hours; or instructed patient in reading the test at home and reporting results to the medical office.
		●	Removed gloves and washed hands.
		●	Charted the procedure correctly.
			INTERPRETATION OF TEST RESULTS
		●	Greeted and identified the patient.
		●	Introduced yourself and explained the procedure.
		●	Worked in a quiet, well-lit atmosphere.
		●	Washed hands and applied gloves.
		●	Asked patient to flex arm at the elbow.
		●	Located the application site.
		●	Gently palpated the test site with fingertips.
		●	If induration is present, rubbed the area lightly, going from the area of normal skin to the indurated area.
		●	Measured diameter of the largest single reaction around one of the puncture sites with a millimeter ruler.
		★	The measurement was identical to the evaluator's measurement.
		●	Interpreted the test results.
		▷	Is able to state how tine test results are interpreted.
		●	Washed hands.
		●	Charted the results correctly.
		★	Completed the procedure within 10 minutes.

CHART	
Date	

Evaluation of Student Performance

EVALUATION CRITERIA			COMMENTS
Symbol	Category	Point Value	
★	Critical Step	16 points	
●	Essential Step	6 points	
▷	Theory Question	2 points	

Score calculation: 100 points

‾‾‾‾‾‾‾‾‾ points missed

‾‾‾‾‾‾‾‾‾ Score

Satisfactory score: 85 or above

AAMA/CAAHEP Competencies Achieved:

☐ Apply pharmacology principles to prepare and administer oral and parenteral medications.

☐ Document appropriately.

Notes

Drug Dosage Calculation: Supplemental Education for Chapter 7

This section is designed as supplemental education for Chapter 7 (Administration of Medication) in your textbook. Completion of the exercises in this section will enable you to calculate drug dosage effectively and accurately, which is essential for administering the proper amount of medication to patients and preventing medication errors. This section is organized so that each unit builds on the next one; therefore, it is important that you are completely familiar with each step before proceeding to the next.

Learning Objectives

After completing this chapter, you should be able to:

1. Identify metric abbreviations.
2. Indicate dose quantity using metric notation guidelines.
3. Identify apothecary abbreviations.
4. Indicate dose quantity using apothecary notations.
5. Identify common medical abbreviations used in writing medication orders.
6. Interpret medication orders.
7. Convert units of measurement within the following systems: metric, apothecary, and household.
8. Convert units of measurement using ratio and proportion.
9. Convert units of measurement between the metric, apothecary, and household systems.
10. Determine oral drug dosage.
11. Determine parenteral drug dosaging.

Unit 1: The Metric System

UNITS OF MEASUREMENT

The basic units of measurement in the metric system are the gram, liter, and meter. The gram is a unit of weight used to measure solids; the liter is a unit of measure used to measure liquids; and the meter is a unit of linear measure used to measure length or distance.

Practice Problems

In the space provided below, indicate whether each of the following metric units of measurement is a unit of weight (W), volume (V), or length (L).

_____ 1. milligram
_____ 2. cubic centimeter
_____ 3. meter
_____ 4. kilogram
_____ 5. liter
_____ 6. milliliter
_____ 7. kiloliter
_____ 8. millimeter
_____ 9. microgram
_____ 10. gram

WRITING METRIC NOTATIONS

In order to read prescriptions and medication orders, to record medication administration, and to avoid medication errors, the medical assistant must be familiar with and be able to use metric notation guidelines. Review the Metric Notation Guidelines on page 258 of your textbook before completing the following practice problems.

Metric Abbreviations-Practice Problems

In the space provided, indicate the correct abbreviation for each of the metric units of measurement listed below.

_____ 1. milligram
_____ 2. gram
_____ 3. kilogram
_____ 4. liter
_____ 5. cubic centimeter
_____ 6. microgram
_____ 7. milliliter

Metric Dose Quantity-Practice Problems

In the space provided, use metric notation guidelines to indicate the following dose quantities.

_____ 1. 25 milligrams

_____ 2. 5 grams

_____ 3. 1½ liters

_____ 4. 1 cubic centimeter

_____ 5. 10 milliliters

_____ 6. ½ gram

_____ 7. 50 milligrams

_____ 8. ½ cubic centimeter

_____ 9. 4 milliliters

_____10. 2 kilograms

_____11. 120 milliliters

_____12. 3 cubic centimeters

_____13. ¼ gram

_____14. 250 milligrams

_____15. ½ liter

_____16. 500 milliliters

_____17. 1 cubic centimeter

_____18. 5 kilograms

_____19. 2½ grams

_____20. 10 milligrams

Unit 2: The Apothecary System

UNITS OF MEASUREMENT

The basic units of measurement in the apothecary system are the grain, minim, and inch. The grain is a unit of weight used to measure solids; the minim is a unit of measure used to measure liquids; and the inch is a unit of linear measure used to measure length or distance.

Practice Problems

In the space provided, indicate whether each of the following units of measurement is a unit of weight (W), volume (V), or length (L).

_____ 1. grain

_____ 2. inch

_____ 3. minim

_____ 4. fluidram

_____ 5. foot

_____ 6. quart
_____ 7. ounce
_____ 8. gallon
_____ 9. yard
_____10. fluidounce
_____11. pound
_____12. pint
_____13. dram
_____14. mile

WRITING APOTHECARY NOTATIONS

Although the apothecary system is used less frequently than the metric system, the medical assistant must still be familiar with and be able to use apothecary notation guidelines. Review the Apothecary Notation Guidelines on pages 258 and 259 of your textbook before completing the following practice problems.

Apothecary Abbreviations-Practice Problems

In the space provided, indicate the correct abbreviation or symbol for each of the apothecary units of measurement listed below.

_____ 1. grain
_____ 2. dram
_____ 3. ounce
_____ 4. minim
_____ 5. fluidram
_____ 6. fluidounce
_____ 7. pint
_____ 8. quart
_____ 9. gallon
_____10. inch

Apothecary Dose Quantity-Practice Problems

In the space provided, use apothecary notations to indicate the following dose quantities.

_____ 1. 4 ounces
_____ 2. 10 grains
_____ 3. 5 drams
_____ 4. $\frac{1}{2}$ ounce
_____ 5. 6 fluidrams
_____ 6. $7\frac{1}{2}$ grains
_____ 7. $3\frac{1}{2}$ ounces
_____ 8. 10 minims
_____ 9. 3 fluidounces

_____10. 2 drams

_____11. ¼ grain

_____12. 16 ounces

_____13. 12 minims

_____14. 1 dram

_____15. 9 fluidrams

_____16. 4 grains

_____17. 8 drams

_____18. 32 fluidounces

_____19. 30 minims

_____20. 8 ounces

Unit 3: The Household System

The household system is more complicated and less accurate for administering medication than the metric and apothecary systems. However, most individuals are familiar with this system because of its frequent utilization in the United States. Thus, this unit of measurement may be the only one the patient can fully relate to and therefore may safely use to administer liquid medication at home.

UNITS OF MEASUREMENT

Volume is the only household unit of measurement used to administer medication. The basic unit of liquid volume is the drop. The remaining units, in order of increasing volume, are the teaspoon, tablespoon, ounce, cup, and glass.

Practice Problems

In the space provided, indicate the correct abbreviation for each of the household units of measurement listed below.

_____ 1. drop

_____ 2. teaspoon

_____ 3. tablespoon

_____ 4. ounce

Unit 4: Medication Orders

To safely administer medication, the medical assistant should be completely familiar with common medical abbreviations. Review Table 7-7 in your textbook (Abbreviations and Symbols Commonly Used in the Medical Office on Prescription Forms) before completing the following practice problems on the following page.

Medical Abbreviations-Practice Problems

In the space provided, write the meaning of the following medical abbreviations.

1. NPO _____

2. EENT _____

3. prn _____

4. ung _____

5. AS _____

6. hs _____

7. tab _____

8. OD _____

9. ac _____

10. pc _____

11. qid _____

12. $\bar{c}$ _____

13. OU _____

14. $\bar{s}$ _____

15. bid _____

16. tid _____

17. qh _____

18. gtts _____

19. qd _____

20. q4h _____

21. non rep _____

22. AU _____

23. qs _____

24. IM _____

25. caps _____

26. qod _____

27. po _____

28. OS _____

29. ad lib _____

30. $\overline{aa}$ _____

Interpreting Medication Orders-Practice Problems

Interpret the following medication orders. Using a drug reference, indicate the drug category based on action and a brand name for each medication.

1. tetracycline hydrochloride, 250 mg po, qid

   _____

   Drug category: _____

   Brand name: _____

2. cimetidine, 400 mg po, hs

   _____

   Drug category: _____

   Brand name: _____

3. alprazolam, 0.25 mg po, tid

   _____

   Drug category: _____

   Brand name: _____

4. verapamil, 240 mg po, qd, ac

   _____

   Drug category: _____

   Brand name: _____

5. erythromycin, 333 mg po, q8h

   _____

   Drug category: _____

   Brand name: _____

6. cephalexin, 250 mg po, q6h

   _____

   Drug category: _____

   Brand name: _____

7. furosemide, 40 mg po, bid

   _____

   Drug category: _____

   Brand name: _____

8. phenelzine sulfate, 15 mg po, qod

_____

Drug category: _____

Brand name: _____

9. acetaminophen, 120 mg po, q4-6h, prn

_____

Drug category: _____

Brand name: _____

10. cyclobenzaprine, 10 mg po, tid

_____

Drug category: _____

Brand name: _____

Unit 5: Converting Units of Measurement

Changing from one unit of measurement to another is known as conversion. Conversion is required when medication is ordered in one unit of measurement and the medication label expresses the drug strength in a different unit. The dose quantity must be mathematically translated or converted to the unit of measurement of the medication on hand. For example, if the physician orders 5 grams of an oral solid medication and the medication label expresses the drug strength in milligrams, the medical assistant will need to convert the grams into milligrams to know how much medication to administer.

Converting units of measurement can be classified into the following categories:

1. Conversion of units within a measurement system.
2. Conversion of units from one measurement system to another.

Converting units within a measurement system allows a quantity to be expressed in a different but equal unit of measurement within the same system. An example of converting between units of weight within the metric system is as follows: 1 gram is equal to 1000 milligrams.

Converting from one measurement system to another allows a quantity to be expressed in a unit of measurement of another system. An example of a conversion between the apothecary and metric systems is as follows: 1 grain (apothecary system) is equivalent to 60 milligrams (metric system). Methods used to convert units of measurement are presented in this unit and in Unit 6.

Conversion requires the use of a conversion table to indicate the equivalent values between units of measurement. The practice problems that follow will assist you in attaining competency in conversion table utilization.

Using Conversion Tables-Practice Problems

Refer to the conversion tables at the end of this chapter. Locate and record the equivalent value for each of the units of measurement listed on the following page. In the space provided, indicate the conversion table you used to locate the equivalent value (e.g., metric, apothecary, metric to apothecary, etc.).

	ANSWER	CONVERSION TABLE
1. 1 g	= _____ mg	_____
2. 1 ounce	= _____ drams	_____
3. 1 tablespoon	= _____ teaspoons	_____
4. 1 grain	= _____ mg	_____
5. 1 liter	= _____ ml	_____
6. 1 dram	= _____ grains	_____
7. 1 pint	= _____ fluidounces	_____
8. 1 teaspoon	= _____ drops	_____
9. 1 ml	= _____ cc	_____
10. 1 ml	= _____ minims	_____
11. 1 fluidounce	= _____ ml	_____
12. 1 kg	= _____ g	_____
13. 1 fluidram	= _____ minims	_____
14. 1 gallon	= _____ quarts	_____
15. 1 ounce	= _____ tablespoons	_____
16. 1 quart	= _____ pints	_____
17. 1 fluidram	= _____ ml	_____
18. 1 g	= _____ grains	_____
19. 1 quart	= _____ ml	_____
20. 1 drop	= _____ minims	_____
21. 1 fluidounce	= _____ tablespoons	_____
22. 1 fluidram	= _____ teaspoons	_____
23. 1 tablespoon	= _____ fluidrams	_____
24. 1 kg	= _____ pounds	_____
25. 1 glass	= _____ ml	_____

CONVERTING UNITS WITHIN THE METRIC SYSTEM

Drug administration often requires conversion within the metric system to prepare the correct dosage. Metric conversion involves either converting a larger unit to a smaller unit (e.g., grams to milligrams) or converting a smaller unit to a larger unit (e.g., milliliters to liters).

Methods used to convert one metric unit to another are described below.

Converting a Larger Unit to a Smaller Unit

Converting a larger unit to a smaller unit within the metric system can be accomplished using one of three methods of conversion, outlined below. The method you use is based on your personal preference as well as the level of difficulty of the conversion problem; for example, more difficult problems will require the use of ratio and proportion as the method of conversion.

Examples of converting a larger unit to a smaller unit are as follows:

1. grams to milligrams
2. liters to milliliters
3. kilograms to grams

METHOD OF CONVERSION. To convert a larger unit to a smaller unit within the metric system:

Method 1: Multiply the unit to be changed by 1000.
Method 2: Move the decimal point of the unit to be changed three places to the right.
Method 3: Ratio and proportion (see Unit 6).

GUIDELINE: If you are converting a larger unit to a smaller unit, you should expect the quantity to become larger. Use this guideline as a reference to assist in making accurate conversions. Refer to the example problems below as an illustration of this guideline.

Examples

PROBLEM   2 L = _____ ml
  Method 1:   Multiply the unit to be changed by 1000.
                2 × 1000 = 2000 ml
  Method 2:   Move the decimal point of the unit to be changed three places to the right.
                2.000 = 2000 ml

> *Answer*   2 L = 2000 ml

PROBLEM   4g = _____ mg
  Method 1:   Multiply the unit to be changed by 1000.
                4 × 1000 = 4000 mg
  Method 2:   Move the decimal point of the unit to be changed three places to the right.
                4.000 = 4000 mg

> *Answer*   4 g = 4000 mg

Converting a Smaller Unit to a Larger Unit

Converting a smaller unit to a larger unit within the metric system can be accomplished using one of three methods of conversion as outlined below.
    Examples of converting a smaller unit to a larger unit are as follows:

1. milligrams to grams
2. milliliters to liters
3. grams to kilograms

METHOD OF CONVERSION: To convert a smaller unit to a larger unit within the metric system:

Method 1: Divide the unit to be changed by 1000.
Method 2: Move the decimal point of the unit to be changed three places to the left.
Method 3: Ratio and proportion (see Unit 6).

GUIDELINE: If you are converting a smaller unit to a larger unit, you should expect the quantity to become smaller. Refer to the problems below as an illustration of this guideline.

Examples

PROBLEM   250 mg = _____ g
  Method 1:   Divide the unit to be changed by 1000.
        250 ÷ 1000 = 0.25 g
  Method 2:   Move the decimal point of the unit to be changed three places to the left.
        2 5 0. = 0.25 g

> *Answer*   250 mg = 0.25 g

PROBLEM   1500 ml = _____ L
  Method 1:   Divide the unit to be changed by 1000.
        1500 ÷ 1000 = 1.5 L
  Method 2:   Move the decimal point of the unit to be changed three places to the left.
        1 5 0 0. = 1.5 L

> *Answer*   1500 ml = 1.5 L

Practice Problems

Convert the following metric units of measurement using either Method 1 or Method 2. In the space provided, indicate if the conversion is going from a larger to smaller unit (L→S) or smaller to larger unit (S→L).

	ANSWER	DIRECTION OF CONVERSION
1. 1 g	= _____ mg	_____
2. 750 mg	= _____ g	_____
3. 2 kg	= _____ g	_____
4. 1000 g	= _____ kg	_____
5. 1.5 L	= _____ ml	_____
6. 250 ml	= _____ L	_____
7. 5 g	= _____ mg	_____
8. 0.25 kg	= _____ g	_____
9. 1000 mg	= _____ g	_____

	ANSWER		DIRECTION OF CONVERSION
10. 2.5 g	=	_____ mg	_____
11. 475 ml	=	_____ L	_____
12. 0.05 g	=	_____ mg	_____
13. 0.5 L	=	_____ ml	_____
14. 1000 ml	=	_____ L	_____
15. 500 g	=	_____ kg	_____
16. 50 mg	=	_____ g	_____
17. 1 L	=	_____ ml	_____
18. 40 g	=	_____ mg	_____
19. 50 ml	=	_____ L	_____
20. 1 kg	=	_____ g	_____

CONVERTING UNITS WITHIN THE APOTHECARY SYSTEM

Drug administration may sometimes require conversion within the apothecary system to prepare the correct dosage. Apothecary conversion involves converting a larger unit to a smaller unit (e.g., drams to grains) or converting a smaller unit to a larger unit (e.g., ounces to pounds). Methods used to convert one apothecary unit to another are described below.

Converting a Larger Unit to a Smaller Unit

Converting a larger unit to a smaller unit within the apothecary system is accomplished through either the equivalent value method or the ratio and proportion method. Examples of converting a larger unit to a smaller unit are as follows:

Weight:
drams to grains
ounces to drams
pounds to ounces

Volume:
fluidrams to minims
fluidounces to fluidrams
pints to fluidounces
quarts to pints
gallons to quarts

METHOD OF CONVERSION: To convert a larger unit to a smaller unit within the apothecary system:
Method 1: a. Look at the Apothecary Conversion Table at the end of this chapter to determine the equivalent value between the two units of measurement.
b. Multiply the equivalent value by the number next to the larger unit of measurement.
Method 2: Ratio and proportion (see Unit 6).

Examples

PROBLEM   4 drams = _____ grains
   Method 1:
   a. Look at the conversion table to determine the equivalent value:
      1 dram = 60 grains
      60 = the equivalent value
   b. Multiply the equivalent value by the number next to the larger unit of measurement:
      $4 \times 60 = 240$ grains

   Answer   4 drams = 240 grains

PROBLEM $1\frac{1}{2}$ pints = _____ fluidounces
   Method 1:
   a. Look at the conversion table to determine the equivalent value:
      1 pint = 16 fluidounces
      16 = the equivalent value
   b. Multiply the equivalent value by the number next to the larger unit of measurement:
      $1.5 \times 16 = 24$ fluidounces

   Answer $1\frac{1}{2}$ pints = 24 fluidounces

Converting a Smaller Unit to a Larger Unit

Converting a smaller unit to a larger unit within the apothecary system can also be accomplished using either the equivalent value method or the ratio and proportion method. Examples of converting from a smaller unit to a larger unit are as follows:

Weight:	*Volume:*
grains to drams	minims to fluidrams
drams to ounces	fluidrams to fluidounces
ounces to pounds	fluidounces to pints
	pints to quarts
	quarts to gallons

METHOD OF CONVERSION: To convert a smaller unit to a larger unit within the apothecary system:
Method 1:
   a. Look at the Apothecary Conversion Table at the end of this chapter to determine the equivalent value between the two units of measurement.
   b. Divide the equivalent value into the number next to the smaller unit of measurement.
Method 2: Ratio and proportion (see Unit 6).

Examples

PROBLEM   30 grains = _____ drams

Method 1:

a. Look at the conversion table to determine the equivalent value:

60 grains = 1 dram

60 = the equivalent value

b. Divide the equivalent value into the number next to the smaller unit of measurement:

$30 \div 60 = \frac{1}{2}$ dram

> ***Answer***   30 grains = $\frac{1}{2}$ dram

PROBLEM   16 fluidrams = _____ fluidounces

Method 1:

a. Look at the conversion table to determine the equivalent value:

8 fluidrams = 1 fluidounce

8 = the equivalent value

b. Divide the equivalent value into the number next to the smaller unit of measurement:

$16 \div 8 = 2$ fluidounces

> ***Answer***   16 fluidrams = 2 fluidounces

Practice Problems

Convert the following apothecary units of measurement using the equivalent value method of conversion. In the space provided, indicate the equivalent value for each problem.

		ANSWER	EQUIVALENT VALUE
1. 2 quarts	=	_____ pints	_____
2. 4 drams	=	_____ grains	_____
3. $\frac{1}{2}$ ounce	=	_____ drams	_____
4. 300 grains	=	_____ drams	_____
5. 2 fluidrams	=	_____ minims	_____
6. 8 pints	=	_____ quarts	_____
7. 16 drams	=	_____ ounces	_____
8. 24 fluidrams	=	_____ fluidounces	_____
9. 18 ounces	=	_____ pounds	_____
10. 32 fluidounces	=	_____ pints	_____
11. $\frac{1}{2}$ quart	=	_____ pints	_____
12. $\frac{1}{2}$ dram	=	_____ grains	_____
13. 3 ounces	=	_____ drams	_____
14. 210 grains	=	_____ drams	_____
15. $4\frac{1}{2}$ fluidrams	=	_____ minims	_____

		ANSWER	EQUIVALENT VALUE
16. 3 pints	=	_____ quarts	_____
17. 4 drams	=	_____ ounces	_____
18. 24 ounces	=	_____ pounds	_____
19. 8 fluidounces	=	_____ pints	_____
20. 2 quarts	=	_____ gallons	_____
21. 120 minims	=	_____ fluidrams	_____
22. 2 fluidounces	=	_____ fluidrams	_____
23. $\frac{1}{2}$ pound	=	_____ ounces	_____
24. 4 pints	=	_____ fluidounces	_____
25. 2 gallons	=	_____ quarts	_____

CONVERTING UNITS WITHIN THE HOUSEHOLD SYSTEM

Household system conversion involves converting a larger unit to a smaller unit (e.g., tablespoons to teaspoons) or converting a smaller unit to a larger unit (e.g., tablespoons to ounces). Methods used to convert one unit to another are described below.

Converting a Larger Unit to a Smaller Unit

Converting a larger unit to a smaller unit within the household system is accomplished using either the equivalent value method or the ratio and proportion method. The method you use is based upon your personal preference as well as the level of difficulty of the conversion problem.

Examples of converting a larger unit to a smaller unit are as follows:

Volume:
teaspoons to drops
tablespoons to teaspoons
ounces to teaspoons
ounces to tablespoons
teacup to ounces
glass to ounces

METHOD OF CONVERSION: To convert a larger unit to a smaller unit within the household system:
Method 1:
   a. Look at the Household Conversion Table at the end of this chapter
      to determine the equivalent value between the two units of measurement.
   b. Multiply the equivalent value by the number next to the larger unit
      of measurement.
Method 2: Ratio and proportion (see Unit 6).

Examples

PROBLEM   2 tablespoons = _____ teaspoons
Method 1:
a. Look at the conversion table to determine the equivalent value:
   1 tablespoon = 3 teaspoons
   3 = the equivalent value
b. Multiply the equivalent value by the number next to the larger unit of measurement:
   2 × 3 = 6 teaspoons

> ***Answer***   2 tablespoons = 6 teaspoons

PROBLEM $\frac{1}{2}$ teaspoon = _____ drops
Method 1:
a. Look at the conversion table to determine the equivalent value:
   1 teaspoon = 60 drops
   60 = the equivalent value
b. Multiply the equivalent value by the number next to the larger unit of measurement:
   $\frac{1}{2}$ × 60 = 30 drops

> ***Answer*** $\frac{1}{2}$ teaspoon = 30 drops

Converting a Smaller Unit to a Larger Unit

Converting a smaller unit to a larger unit within the household system is accomplished using either the equivalent value method or the ratio and proportion method.
   Examples of converting from a smaller unit to a larger unit are as follows:

Volume:
drops to teaspoons
teaspoons to tablespoons
teaspoons to ounces
tablespoons to ounces
ounces to teacups
ounces to glasses

> Method of Conversion: To convert a smaller unit to a larger unit within the household system:
> *Method 1:*
>   a. Look at the Household Conversion Table at the end of this chapter to determine the equivalent value between the two units of measurement.
>   b. Divide the equivalent value into the number next to the smaller unit of measurement.
> *Method 2:* Ratio and proportion (see Unit 6).

Examples

PROBLEM   4 tablespoons = _____ ounces
Method 1:
a. Look at the conversion table to determine the equivalent value:
    1 ounce = 2 tablespoons
    2 = the equivalent value
b. Divide the equivalent value into the number next to the smaller unit of measurement:
    4 ÷ 2 = 2 ounces

        Answer   4 tablespoons = 2 ounces

PROBLEM   24 ounces = _____ glasses
Method 1:
a. Look at the conversion table to determine the equivalent value:
    1 glass = 8 ounces
    8 = the equivalent value
b. Divide the equivalent value into the number next to the smaller unit of measurement:
    24 ÷ 8 = 3 glasses

        Answer   24 ounces = 3 glasses

Practice Problems

Convert the following household units of measurement using the equivalent value method of conversion. In the space provided, indicate the equivalent value for each problem.

	ANSWER	EQUIVALENT VALUE
1. 12 teaspoons	= _____ ounces	_____
2. 4 ounces	= _____ glasses	_____
3. 90 drops	= _____ teaspoons	_____
4. ½ ounce	= _____ tablespoons	_____
5. 6 teaspoons	= _____ tablespoons	_____
6. 3 tablespoons	= _____ ounces	_____
7. 18 ounces	= _____ teacups	_____
8. ½ ounce	= _____ teaspoons	_____
9. 3 tablespoons	= _____ teaspoons	_____
10. ½ teaspoon	= _____ drops	_____

Unit 6: Ratio and Proportion

Ratio and proportion are also used to convert units of measurement. This method of conversion has the advantage of clarifying the mathematical rationale for the methods of conversion previously presented. It is also useful in converting units of measurement that are more difficult to calculate, such as converting between systems, for example when converting an apothecary unit of measurement to a metric unit of measurement.

Guidelines

Some basic guidelines must be followed when using ratio and proportion. These guidelines are described below.

1. A **ratio** is composed of two related numbers separated by a colon. It indicates the relationship between two quantities or numbers. The ratio example below shows a relationship between milligrams and grams—i.e., 1000 mg = 1 g.

    EXAMPLE   1000 mg: 1 g

2. A **proportion** shows the relationship between two equal ratios. The proportion consists of two ratios separated by an equal sign (=) which indicates that the two ratios are equal. This proportion example shows the relationship between two equal ratios of milligrams and grams.

    EXAMPLE   1000 mg: 1 g = 2000 mg: 2 g

3. The units of measurement in the two ratios of a proportion must be expressed in the same sequence. The correct sequencing in the proportion example below is mg: g = mg: g, *not* mg: g = g: mg.

    EXAMPLE   *Correct*   1000 mg: 1 g = 2000 mg: 2 g
              Incorrect: 1000 mg: 1 g = 2 g: 2000 mg

4. The numbers on the ends of a proportion are called the **extremes** while the numbers in the middle of the proportion are known as the **means**. In this example, the means consist of 1 g and 2000 mg and the extremes are 1000 mg and 2 g.

    EXAMPLE   1000 mg: 1 g = 2000 mg: 2g
                     └── means ──┘
              └──────── extremes ────────┘

5. The product of the means equals the product of the extremes. The calculation of the product of the means in the example is as follows: $1 \times 2000 = 2000$. The calculation of the product of the extremes is as follows: $1000 \times 2 = 2000$. Hence, the product of the means equals the product of the extremes or $2000 = 2000$.

    EXAMPLE   1000 mg: 1 g = 2000 mg: 2 g
                     $1 \times 2000 = 1000 \times 2$
                           $2000 = 2000$

6. In setting up a proportion, one side of the equation consists of the known quantities and the other side of the equation consists of the unknown quantity. The letter **x** is commonly used to express the unknown quantity. To be consistent, the known quantities are indicated on the left side of the equation and the unknown quantity is indicated on the right side of the equation. Using the above proportion, but inserting an unknown quantity, or **x**, the equation is set up as follows:

EXAMPLE   1000 mg: 1 g   =   x mg: 2 g
                    (known quantities)   (unknown quantity)

Practice Problems

Answer the following questions:

1. What is a ratio? _____

_____

2. In the space provided, place a check mark next to each correct example of a ratio.
   _____ a. 15 drops : 15 minims: 1 ml
   _____ b. 1000 ml = 1 L
   _____ c. 1 ounce: 8 drams
   _____ d. 60 minims/1 fluidram
   _____ e. 1 dram : 60 grains
   _____ f. 1 ml : 1 cc

3. What is a proportion? _____

_____

_____

4. In the space provided, place a check mark next to each correct example of a proportion.
   _____ a. 1 ml : 1 cc
   _____ b. 1 grain : 60 mg = 4 grains: 240 mg
   _____ c. 2x = 60 mg
   _____ d. 1000 ml : 1 L = 500 ml : 0.5 L
   _____ e. 1000 mg : 1 grain = 1000 ml : 1 L

5. In the space provided, place a check mark next to each proportion that has correct sequencing for the units of measurement.
   _____ a. 1000 g : 1 kg = 1500 g : 1.5 kg
   _____ b. 60 grains : 1 dram = 2 drams : 120 grains
   _____ c. 1000 mg : 1 g = 2000 mg : x g

6. Circle the means and underline the extremes in each of the following proportions:
   a. 1000 mg: 1 g = 500 mg: 0.5 g
   b. 2 pints: 1 quart = 4 pints: 2 quarts
   c. 1 ml: 1 cc = 2 ml: 2cc

7. In each of the following proportions, what is the product of the means and the product of the extremes?

    a. 1000 g: 1 kg = 1500 g: 1.5 kg

          _____ product of the means

          _____ product of the extremes

    b. 60 minims: 1 fluidram = 120 minims: 2 fluidrams

          _____ product of the means

          _____ product of the extremes

    c. 60 mg: 1 grain = 300 mg: 5 grains

          _____ product of the means

          _____ product of the extremes

8. In each of the following proportions, circle the known quantities and underline the unknown quantity.

    a. 1000 mg:1 g = 500 mg:x g

    b. 1 g: 15 grains = 2 g: x grains

    c. 8 drams: 1 ounce = x drams: 4 ounces

CONVERTING UNITS USING RATIO AND PROPORTION

The method to follow to convert units using ratio and proportion is outlined below.

METHOD OF CONVERSION: To convert a unit of measurement using ratio and proportion:

    a. Look at the appropriate conversion table at the end of this chapter to determine what is known about the two units of measurement (equivalent value).

    b. State the known quantities as a ratio.

    c. Determine the unknown quantity.

    d. State the unknown quantity as a ratio.

    e. Set up the proportion with the known quantities on the left side and the unknown quantity on the right side of the equation.

    f. Solve the equation as follows: Multiply the product of the means and the product of the extremes. Divide the equation by the number(s) before the x.

    g. Include the unit of measure corresponding to x in the original equation with the answer.

Examples

PROBLEM   2 g = _____ mg

a. Look at the metric conversion table to determine what is known about the two units of measurement:

1000 mg = 1 g

b. State the known quantities as a ratio:

1000 mg = 1 g

c. Determine the unknown quantity:

2 g = x mg

d. State the unknown quantity as a ratio using the correct unit of measurement sequencing:

x mg : 2 g

e. Set up the proportion with the known quantities on the left side and the unknown quantity on the right side of the equation:

1000 mg : 1 g = x mg : 2 g

f. Solve the equation by multiplying the product of the means and the product of the extremes and dividing the equation by the number before the x:

1000 mg : 1 g = x mg : 2 g
1 × x = 1000 × 2
1x = 2000
x = 2000

g. Include the unit of measure corresponding to x in the original equation with answer:

x = 2000 mg

Answer   2 g = 2000 mg

PROBLEM   300 mg = _____ grains

The steps outlined above are followed here also. However, they are combined as they would be in working an actual conversion problem.

60 mg : 1 grain = 300 mg : x grains
1 × 300 = 60 × x
300 = 60x
300 ÷ 60 = 60x ÷ 60
x = 5 grains

Answer   300 mg = 5 grains

Practice Problems

A. Return to the metric conversion practice problems and the apothecary conversion practice problems and rework the first five problems in each using the ratio and proportion method of conversion. Use your previous answers to check the accuracy of your work.

B. Use ratio and proportion to convert between the apothecary, metric, and household systems by completing the problems below. In the space at the right, indicate what is known regarding the two units of measurement.

		ANSWER		KNOWN QUANTITIES
1. 30 minims	=	_____ ml		_____
2. 4 kg	=	_____ pounds		_____
3. 90 ml	=	_____ fluidounces		_____
4. 30 mg	=	_____ grains		_____
5. 60 mg	=	_____ ounces		_____
6. 250 ml	=	_____ pints		_____
7. 6 g	=	_____ drams		_____
8. 1½ quarts	=	_____ ml		_____
9. 3 g	=	_____ grains		_____
10. 5 fluidrams	=	_____ ml		_____
11. 80 pounds	=	_____ kg		_____
12. 500 ml	=	_____ quarts		_____
13. 8 ml	=	_____ teaspoons		_____
14. 4 grains	=	_____ mg		_____
15. 32 ml	=	_____ fluidrams		_____
16. 120 mg	=	_____ grains		_____
17. 30 ml	=	_____ tablespoons		_____
18. 60 drops	=	_____ ml		_____
19. 1½ fluidounces	=	_____ tablespoons		_____
20. ½ fluidounce	=	_____ ml		_____

Unit 7: Determining Drug Dosage

ORAL ADMINISTRATION

Dosage refers to the amount of medication to be administered to the patient. Each medication has a certain dosage range or range of quantities that produce therapeutic effects. It is important to administer the exact drug dosage. If the dose is too small, it will not produce a therapeutic effect, whereas too large a dose could be harmful or even fatal to the patient.

The steps to follow in determining drug dosage depend on the unit of measurement in which the drug is ordered and the unit of measurement of the drug you have available, or the dose on-hand. A general discussion of the method for determining drug dosage is as follows:

1. If the dose on-hand is the same as that which has been ordered, no calculation is required. In this example, both the dose ordered and the dose on-hand are in the same unit of measurement, and one tablet is administered to the patient.

   EXAMPLE   The physician orders 50 mg of a medication po.
   The drug label reads 50 mg/tablet.

2. If the dosage ordered is in the same unit of measurement as that indicated on the medication label, only one calculation step is required. In this example, both the dose ordered and the dose on-hand are in the same unit of measurement, or grains. The calculation step performed will be to determine the number of tablets to administer to the patient.

   EXAMPLE   The physician orders gr $\bar{\text{v}}$ of a medication po.
   The drug label reads gr $\bar{\text{x}}$/tablet.

3. If the dosage ordered is in a different unit of measurement than indicated on the drug label, two calculation steps are required to determine the amount of medication to administer to the patient. In this example, the dose ordered and the dose on-hand are stated in different units of measurement, or in grams and milligrams. The first step requires conversion of the dose ordered to the unit of measurement of the dose on-hand; in this example, grams must be converted to milligrams. The second step is to determine the number of tablets to administer to the patient.

   EXAMPLE   The physician orders 1 g of a medication po.
   The drug label reads 500 mg/tablet.

A detailed discussion of determining drug dosage for administration of oral medication follows. The method used to calculate drug dosage when the units of measurement are the same is presented first, followed by the method used when the units of measurement are different.

Determining Drug Dosage With the Same Units of Measurement

Determining the correct drug dosage to be administered when the units of measurement are the same requires the use of a formula that is explained below.

DRUG DOSAGE FORMULA

$$\frac{\text{D (dose ordered)}}{\text{H (on-hand)}} \times \text{V (vehicle)} = \text{x (Amount of medication to be administered)}$$

D (dose ordered): This is the amount of medication ordered by the physician.

H (drug strength on-hand): This is the dosage strength available as indicated on the medication label or the dose on-hand.

V (vehicle): The vehicle refers to the type of preparation containing the dose on-hand (e.g., tablet, capsule, liquid).

x: The letter x is used to express the unknown quantity or the amount of medication to be administered.

GUIDELINES

1. The units of measurement must be included when setting up the problem.
2. The values for D and H must be in the same unit of measurement.
3. The value of x is expressed in the same unit as V.
4. When determining the drug dosage for oral liquid medication, the vehicle must also include the amount of liquid in which the available drug is contained. For example, if the medication label reads 250 mg/5 ml, the value of V is 5 ml.

The method to follow to determine drug dosage using this formula is outlined below. The first example illustrates determining dosage for oral solid medication.

Examples

PROBLEM   *Oral Solid Medication:*
The physician orders 50 mg of a medication po.
The medication label reads 25 mg/tablet.
How much medication should be administered to the patient?

Drug Dosage Formula:

$$\frac{D}{H} \times V = x$$

a. Identify the dose ordered.

D= 50 mg

b. Identify the strength of the drug on-hand.

H = 25 mg

c. Determine the vehicle containing the dose on-hand.

V = 1 tablet

d. Calculate the amount of medication to administer to the patient. The units of measurement must be included when setting up the problem and the values for D and H must be in the same unit of measurement. The value of x is expressed in the same unit as V; in this problem V = 1 tablet.

$$\frac{50 \text{ mg}}{25 \text{ mg}} \times 1 \text{ tablet} = x$$

$(50 \div 25 = 2) \times 1 \text{ tablet} = x$

$2 \times 1 \text{ tablet} = x$

$x = 2 \text{ tablets}$

> ***Answer.***   2 tablets are administered to the patient.

The next problem illustrates the determination of drug dosage for oral liquid medication. The steps outlined above are followed; however, they are combined as should be done when working out drug dosage problems. Remember, with oral liquid medication, the vehicle must also include the amount of liquid in which the available drug is contained; in the problem below, V = 5 ml.

PROBLEM   *Oral liquid medication:*
The physician orders 500 mg of a medication.
The medication label reads 250 mg/5 ml.
How much medication should be administered to the patient?

$$\frac{D}{H} \times V = x$$

$$\frac{500 \text{ mg}}{250 \text{ mg}} \times 5 \text{ ml} = x$$

$$(500 \div 250 = 2) \times 5 \text{ ml} = x$$

$$2 \times 5 \text{ ml} = x$$

$$x = 10 \text{ ml}$$

> ***Answer***   10 ml of medication are administered to the patient.

Determining Drug Dosage With Different Units of Measurement

At times the medication ordered is in a different unit of measurement than indicated on the drug label. In this case, the desired dose quantity must be converted to the unit of measurement of the dose on-hand before the drug dosage is determined. The method you use to convert a unit of measurement is based on your personal preference. Refer to Units 5 and 6 to review methods of conversion before completing this section.

> The following steps are required to determine drug dosage when the units of measurement are different:
> *Step 1:* Convert the dose quantities to the same unit of measurement. For consistency, it is best to convert to the unit of measurement of the drug on-hand.
> *Step 2:* Determine the amount of medication to administer to the patient, using the drug dosage formula.

Examples

PROBLEM   *Oral solid medication:*
The physician orders gr $\bar{x}$ of medication po.
The medication label reads 300 mg/ tablet.
How much medication should be administered to the patient?

Step 1. The dosage ordered must be converted to the unit of measurement of the medication on-hand. In this problem, 10 grains must be converted to milligrams. The ratio and proportion method of conversion is used to make the conversion.

gr $\bar{x}$ = _____ mg

1 grain: 60 mg = 10 grains: x mg

600 = 1x

x = 600 mg

> ***Answer***   gr $\bar{x}$ = 600 mg

The medication ordered is now in the same unit of measurement as the medication on-hand.

Step 2: Determine the amount of medication to administer to the patient using the drug dosage formula.

$$\frac{D}{H} \times V = x$$

$$\frac{600 \text{ mg}}{300 \text{ mg}} \times 1 \text{ tablet} = x$$

$(600 \div 300 = 2) \times 1 \text{ tablet} = x$

$2 \times 1 \text{ tablet} = x$

$x = 2 \text{ tablets}$

Answer   2 tablets are administered to the patient.

PROBLEM   *Oral liquid medication:*
The physician orders gr $\overline{xv}$ of a medication po.
The medication label reads 300 mg/fluidram.
How much medication should be administered to the patient?

Step 1. Convert 15 grains to milligrams using ratio and proportion:

gr $\overline{xv}$ = _____ mg

$60 \text{ mg} : 1 \text{ grain} = x \text{ mg} : 15 \text{ grains}$

$1x = 900 \text{ mg}$

$x = 900 \text{ mg}$

Answer   gr $\overline{xv}$ = 900 mg

Step 2: Determine the amount of medication to administer to the patient using the drug dosage formula.

$$\frac{D}{H} \times V = x$$

$$\frac{900 \text{ mg}}{300 \text{ mg}} \times 1 \text{ fluidram} = x$$

$(900 \div 300 = 3) \times 1 \text{ fluidram} = x$

$3 \times 1 \text{ fluidram} = x$

$x = 3 \text{ fluidrams}$

Answer   3 fluidrams of medication are administered to the patient.

Practice Problems

Determine the drug dosage to be administered for each of the following oral medication orders and record your answer below. In the space provided, indicate the drug category based on action for each medication using a drug reference.

PROBLEM   *Oral solid medications:*

1. The physician orders Inderal, 160 mg po.
   Medication label:

   Inderal
   propranolol

   80 mg/capsule

How much medication should be administered? _____

Drug category:_____

2. The physician orders Tagamet, gr v̄ po.
   Medication label:

   Tagamet
   cimetidine

   300 mg/tablet

How much medication should be administered? _____

Drug category:_____

3. The physician orders Amcill, 0.5 g po.
   Medication label:

   Amcill
   ampicillin

   250 mg/capsule

How much medication should be administered? _____

Drug category:_____

4. The physician orders Lasix, 80 mg po.
   Medication label:

> Lasix
> furosemide
>
> 40 mg/tablet

How much medication should be administered? _____

Drug category:_____

5. The physician orders Nardil, gr $\frac{1}{4}$ po.
   Medication label:

> Nardil
> phenelzine sulfate
>
> 15 mg/tablet

How much medication should be administered? _____

Drug category:_____

6. The physician orders Gantrisin, 500 mg po.
   Medication label:

> Gantrisin
> sulfisoxazole
>
> 0.5 g/tablet

How much medication should be administered? _____

Drug category:_____

7. The physician orders Calan, gr $\overset{..}{\text{ii}}$ po.
   Medication label:

> Calan
> verapamil
>
> 240 mg/scored caplet

How much medication should be administered? _____

Drug category:_____

8. The physician orders Xanax, 0.5 mg po.
   Medication label:

> Xanax
> alprazolam
>
> 0.25 mg/tablet

How much medication should be administered? _____

Drug category: _____

9. The physician orders Antivert, 25 mg po.
   Medication label:

> Antivert
> meclizine
>
> 12.5 mg/tablet

$$\frac{25}{1} \times \frac{1}{12.5} = 2 \text{ tab}$$

$$25 \div 12.5 \text{ mg} = 2 \text{ tab}$$

How much medication should be administered? __2 tablet.__

Drug category: _____

10. The physician orders Procardia, gr $\overline{ss}$ po.
    Medication label:

> Procardia
> nifedipine
>
> 10 mg/tablet

$$gr \,\overline{ss} = gr \, 1/2 = gr . S.$$
$$.S \times 60$$
$$= 30 mg$$
$$\overline{10 mg}$$

How much medication should be administered? __3 tablets__ $= 3$

Drug category: _____

Oral liquid medications:

1. The physician orders Sumycin Syrup, 250 mg po.
   Medication label:

> Sumycin Syrup
> tetracycline oral suspension
>
> 125 mg/5 ml

$$= 2 \times 5ml$$
$$= 10ml$$
$$\frac{250mg}{125mg} \quad \frac{}{5ml}$$

$$10 ml.$$

How much medication should be administered? _____

Drug category: _____

2. The physician orders Tagamet liquid, 300 mg po.
Medication label:

Tagamet
cimetidine liquid

300 mg/5 ml

How much medication should be administered? _____

Drug category: _____

3. The physician orders Tylenol Elixir gr $\dot{\mathrm{i}}$ po.
Medication label:

Tylenol Elixir
acetaminophen

120 mg/5 ml

How much medication should be administered? _____

Drug category: _____

(handwritten) gr 1 x 60 = 6mg
$\frac{60}{120} = \frac{1}{2} \times \frac{5}{1} = \frac{5}{2} =$
2.5mg m̄ tab 2½ Ta

4. The physician orders Keflex suspension, 0.5 g po.
Medication label:

Keflex
cephalexin

100 mg/ml

How much medication should be administered? _____

Drug category: _____

(handwritten) .5g = 500mg / 100mg = 5m Tab
5. tab̄ ml

5. The physician orders Gantanol suspension, 1 g po.
Medication label:

Gantanol Suspension
sulfamethoxazole

0.5 g/5 ml

How much medication should be administered? _____

Drug category: _____

(handwritten) 1g / .5g = 2x5ml 2.5ml 10ml

PARENTERAL ADMINISTRATION

Medications for parenteral administration must be suspended in solution. The medication label indicates the amount of the drug contained in each milliliter of solution. For example, if a medication label reads 10 mg/ml, this means that there are 10 mg of medication for each ml of liquid volume. Some medications, such as penicillin, insulin, and heparin are ordered and measured in terms of units (e.g., 300,000 units/ml). This refers to their biological activity in animal tests or the amount of the drug which is required to produce a particular response.

  Parenteral medication is available in a number of dispensing forms which include ampules, single dose vials, and multiple dose vials. Once the proper drug dosage has been determined, the medication is drawn into a syringe from the dispensing unit. Since most syringes are calibrated in cubic centimeters (cc), it is important to remember the equivalent value between ml and cc, or 1 ml is equal to 1 cc.

  Determining drug dosage for parenteral administration is calculated in a similar manner as that for oral liquid medication as explained below. The first problem illustrates the determination of drug dosage when the medication is ordered in a different unit of measurement from the dose on-hand requiring two calculation steps.

Examples

PROBLEM   The physician orders 0.5 g of a medication IM.
            The medication label reads 250 mg/2 ml.
            How much medication should be administered?

Step 1: Convert 0.5 grams to milligrams.

0.5 g = _____ mg

1000 mg : 1 g = x mg : 0.5 g

1x = 500

x = 500 mg

> *Answer:*   0.5 g = 500 mg

Step 2: Determine the amount of medication to administer to the patient:

$$\frac{D}{H} \times V = x$$

$$\frac{500 \text{ mg}}{250 \text{ mg}} \times 2 \text{ ml} = x$$

$(500 \div 250 = 2) \times 2 \text{ ml} = x$

$2 \times 2 \text{ ml} = x$

$x = 4 \text{ ml (cc)}$

> *Answer:*   4 cc of medication are administered to the patient.

The next problem illustrates the determination of drug dosage with a medication ordered in units. Note that both the dose ordered and the dose on-hand are in the same unit of measurement; therefore, conversion of units of measurement is not necessary.

PROBLEM   The physician orders 600,000 units of a medication IM.
            The medication label reads 300,000 units/ml.
            How much medication should be administered?

$$\frac{D}{H} \times V = x$$

$$\frac{600,000 \text{ units}}{300,000 \text{ units}} \times 1 \text{ ml} = x$$

$$(600,000 \div 300,000 = 2) \times 1 \text{ ml} = x$$

$$x = 2 \text{ ml (cc)}$$

> ***Answer.***   2 cc of medication are administered to the patient.

Practice Problems

Determine the drug dosage to be administered for each of the following parenteral medication orders and record your answer below. In the space provided, indicate the drug category based on action using a drug reference.

1. The physician orders Vistaril, 75 mg IM.
   Medication label:

   > Vistaril
   > hydroxyzine injection
   >
   > 50 mg/ml

   How much medication should be administered? _____

   Drug category:_____

2. The physician orders Sytobex (Vitamin B_{12}), 2 mcg IM.
   Medication label:

   > Ener-B
   > cyanocobalamin injection
   >
   > 1 mcg/ml

   How much medication should be administered? _____

   Drug category:_____

3. The physician orders Decadron, 12 mg IM.
   Medication label:

Decadron
dexamethasone injection
8 mg/ml

$\frac{12\ mg}{8\ mg}$ $\frac{12}{1} \times \frac{1}{8} = 1.5$

How much medication should be administered? _____ 1 1/2 ml

Drug category:_____

4. The physician orders Duracillin, 600,000 units IM.
   Medication label:

Wycillin
procaine penicillin G injection
300,000 units/ml

$\frac{600,000}{300,000} = 2\ ml$

How much medication should be administered? _____ 2 ml

Drug category:_____

5. The physician orders Garamycin, 40 mg IM.
   Medication label:

Garamycin
gentamicin sulfate injection
80 mg/2 ml

W. 40 mg
H. 80 mg

How much medication should be administered? _____ 1 ml

Drug category:_____

6. The physician orders Imferon, 100 mg IM.
   Medication label:

Infed
iron dextran injection
50 mg/ml

$\frac{100\ mg}{50\ mg}$

2 ml.

How much medication should be administered? _____

Drug category:_____

7. The physician orders Bicillin, 1.2 million units IM.
   Medication label:

600,000 ×2 = 1.2 million

1.2 million units

$\dfrac{1.2 \text{ million units}}{600,000} = 2ml$

Bicillin
benzathine penicillin G injection
600,000 units/ml

How much medication should be administered? _____ 2ml _____

Drug category: _____

8. The physician orders Dramamine, 25 mg IM.
   Medication label:

$\dfrac{25}{50 mg} = \dfrac{1}{2}$

Dramamine
dimenhydrinate
50 mg/ml

How much medication should be administered? _____ ½ ml _____

Drug category: _____

9. The physician orders Pronestyl, 0.75 g IM.
   Medication label:

.75 g = $\dfrac{750 mg}{500 mg}$

Pronestyl
procainamide injection
500 mg/ml

How much medication should be administered? _____ 1 ½ ml _____

Drug category: _____

10. The physician orders Compazine, 7 mg IM.
   Medication label:

$\dfrac{W}{H} \dfrac{7 mg}{5 mg}$ $5\overline{)7}^{1.4}$ $\dfrac{5}{20}$

Compazine
prochlorperazine injection
5 mg/ml

How much medication should be administered? _____ 1.4 ml _____

Drug category: _____

Answers to Practice Problems

UNIT 1. THE METRIC SYSTEM

Units of Measurement

1. W
2. V
3. L
4. W
5. V
6. V
7. V
8. L
9. W
10. W

Metric Abbreviations

1. mg
2. g
3. kg
4. L
5. cc
6. mcg
7. ml

Metric Dose Quantity

1. 25 mg
2. 5 g
3. 1.5 L
4. 1 cc
5. 10 ml
6. 0.5 g
7. 50 mg
8. 0.5 cc
9. 4 ml
10. 2 kg
11. 120 ml
12. 3 cc
13. 0.25 g
14. 250 mg
15. 0.5 L
16. 500 ml
17. 1 cc
18. 5 kg
19. 2.5 g
20. 10 mg

UNIT 2. THE APOTHECARY SYSTEM

Units of Measurement

1. W
2. L
3. V
4. V
5. L
6. V
7. W
8. V
9. L
10. V
11. W
12. V
13. W
14. L

Apothecary Abbreviations

1. gr
2. ℨ
3. ℥
4. ♏
5. fℨ
6. f℥
7. pt
8. qt
9. gal
10. in

Apothecary Dose Quantity

1. $\mathfrak{Z}$ $\overline{\text{iv}}$
2. gr $\overline{\text{x}}$
3. $\mathfrak{Z}$ $\overline{\text{v}}$
4. $\mathfrak{Z}$ $\overline{\text{ss}}$
5. f$\mathfrak{Z}$ $\overline{\text{vi}}$
6. gr $\overline{\text{viiss}}$
7. $\mathfrak{Z}$ $\overline{\text{iiiss}}$
8. m $\overline{\text{x}}$
9. f$\mathfrak{Z}$ $\overline{\text{iii}}$
10. $\mathfrak{Z}$ $\overline{\text{ii}}$
11. gr $\frac{1}{4}$
12. $\mathfrak{Z}$ $\overline{\text{xvi}}$
13. m $\overline{\text{xii}}$
14. $\mathfrak{Z}$ $\overline{\text{i}}$
15. f$\mathfrak{Z}$ $\overline{\text{ix}}$
16. gr $\overline{\text{iv}}$
17. $\mathfrak{Z}$ $\overline{\text{viii}}$
18. f$\mathfrak{Z}$ $\overline{\text{xxxii}}$
19. m $\overline{\text{xxx}}$
20. $\mathfrak{Z}$ $\overline{\text{viii}}$

UNIT 3. THE HOUSEHOLD SYSTEM

Units of Measurement

1. gtt
2. t or tsp
3. T or tbs
4. oz

UNIT 4. MEDICATION ORDERS

Medical Abbreviations

1. nothing by mouth
2. ear, eyes, nose, and throat
3. as needed
4. ointment
5. left ear
6. at bedtime
7. tablet
8. right eye
9. before meals
10. after meals
11. four times a day
12. with
13. in each eye
14. without
15. twice a day
16. three times a day
17. every hour
18. drops
19. every day
20. every 4 hours
21. do not repeat
22. in each ear
23. of sufficient quantity
24. intramuscular
25. capsules
26. every other day
27. by mouth
28. left eye
29. as desired
30. of each

Interpreting Medication Orders

1. tetracycline hydrochloride, 250 mg by mouth, four times a day; antibiotic; Achromycin, Sumycin
2. cimetidine, 400 mg by mouth, at bedtime; antiulcer; Tagamet
3. alprazolam, 0.25 mg by mouth, three times a day; antianxiety; Xanax
4. verapamil, 240 mg by mouth, every day, before meals; antihypertensive; Calan, Isoptin
5. erythromycin, 333 mg by mouth, every 8 hours; antibiotic; E-Mycin, AK-Mycin, Ilotycin, Robimycin
6. cephalexin, 250 mg by mouth, every 6 hours; antibiotic, Keflex
7. furosemide, 40 mg by mouth, twice a day, diuretic; Lasix
8. phenelzine sulfate; 15 mg by mouth, every other day; antidepressant; Nardil
9. acetaminophen, 120 mg, every 4 to 6 hours as needed; analgesic; Tylenol, Genebs, Panadol, Tempra
10. cyclobenzaprine, 10 mg by mouth, three times a day; muscle relaxant; Flexeril

UNIT 5. CONVERTING UNITS OF MEASUREMENT

Using Conversion Tables

	Answer	Conversion Table
1.	1000	metric
2.	8	apothecary
3.	3	household
4.	60	metric to apothecary
5.	1000	metric
6.	60	apothecary
7.	16	apothecary
8.	60	household
9.	1	metric
10.	15	metric to apothecary
11.	30	apothecary to metric
12.	1000	metric
13.	60	apothecary
14.	4	apothecary
15.	2	household
16.	2	apothecary
17.	5(4)	apothecary to metric
18.	15	metric to apothecary
19.	1000	apothecary to metric
20.	1	household to apothecary
21.	2	apothecary to household
22.	1	apothecary to household
23.	4	household to apothecary
24.	2.2	metric to apothecary
25.	240	household to metric

Converting Units within the Metric System

	Answer	Direction of Conversion		
1.	1000	L	$\rightarrow$	S
2.	0.75	S	$\rightarrow$	L
3.	2000	L	$\rightarrow$	S
4.	1	S	$\rightarrow$	L
5.	1500	L	$\rightarrow$	S
6.	0.25	S	$\rightarrow$	L
7.	5000	L	$\rightarrow$	S
8.	250	L	$\rightarrow$	S
9.	1	S	$\rightarrow$	L
10.	2500	L	$\rightarrow$	S
11.	0.475	S	$\rightarrow$	L
12.	50	L	$\rightarrow$	S
13.	500	L	$\rightarrow$	S
14.	1	S	$\rightarrow$	L
15.	0.5	S	$\rightarrow$	L
16.	0.05	S	$\rightarrow$	L
17.	1000	L	$\rightarrow$	S
18.	40,000	L	$\rightarrow$	S
19.	0.05	S	$\rightarrow$	L
20.	1000	L	$\rightarrow$	S

Converting within the Apothecary System

	Answer	Equivalent Value
1.	4	2
2.	240	60
3.	4	8
4.	5	60
5.	120	60
6.	4	2
7.	2	8
8.	3	8
9.	$1\frac{1}{2}$	12
10.	2	16
11.	1	2
12.	30	60
13.	24	8
14.	$3\frac{1}{2}$	60
15.	270	60
16.	$1\frac{1}{2}$	2
17.	$\frac{1}{2}$	8
18.	2	12
19.	$\frac{1}{2}$	16
20.	$\frac{1}{2}$	4
21.	2	60
22.	16	8
23.	6	12
24.	64	16
25.	8	4

Converting within the Household System

	Answer	Equivalent Value
1.	2	6
2.	$\frac{1}{2}$	8
3.	$1\frac{1}{2}$	60
4.	1	2
5.	2	3
6.	$1\frac{1}{2}$	2
7.	3	6
8.	3	6
9.	9	3
10.	30	60

UNIT 6. RATIO AND PROPORTION

Ratio and Proportion Guidelines

1. Two related numbers separated by a colon that indicate the relationship between two quantities or numbers.
2. The following are examples of ratios: c, e, and f.
3. A proportion shows the relationship between two equal ratios. It consists of two ratios separated by an equals sign.
4. The following are examples of proportions: b and d.
5. The following have correct sequencing: a and c.
6. a. Means: 1 g, 500 mg; Extremes: 1000 mg, .5 g
   b. Means: 1 quart, 4 pints; Extremes: 2 pints, 2 quarts
   c. Means: 1 cc, 2 ml; Extremes: 1 ml, 2 cc
7. a. Means: 1500; Extremes: 1500
   b. Means: 120; Extremes: 120
   c. Means: 300; Extremes: 300
8. a. Known quantities: 1000 mg: 1 g; Unknown quantities: x g
   b. Known quantities: 1 g: 15 grains; Unknown quantities: x grains
   c. Known quantities: 8 drams: 1 ounce; Unknown quantities: x drams

Converting Units of Measurement Using Ratio and Proportion

	Answer	Known Quantities
1.	2	1 ml = 15 minims
2.	8.8	1 kg = 2.2 pounds
3.	3	1 fluidounce = 30 ml
4.	$\frac{1}{2}$	1 gr = 60 mg
5.	2	1 ounce = 30 mg
6.	$\frac{1}{2}$	1 pint = 500 ml
7.	$1\frac{1}{2}$	1 dram = 4 g
8.	1500	1 qt = 1000 ml
9.	45	1 g = 15 grains
10.	20	1 fluidram = 4 ml
11.	36.4	1 kg = 2.2 pounds
12.	$\frac{1}{2}$	1 qt = 1000 ml
13.	2	1 teaspoon = 4 ml
14.	240	1 gr = 60 mg
15.	8	1 fluidram = 4 ml
16.	2	1 gr = 60 mg
17.	2	1 tablespoon = 15 ml
18.	4	1 ml = 15 drops
19.	3	1 fluidounce = 2 tablespoons
20.	15	1 fluidounce = 30 ml

UNIT 7. DETERMINING DRUG DOSAGE

Oral Solid Medication

1. 2 capsules; antiarrhythmic
2. 1 tablet; antiulcer
3. 2 capsules; antibiotic
4. 2 tablets; diuretic
5. 1 tablet; antidepressant
6. 1 tablet; sulfonamide
7. $\frac{1}{2}$ caplet; antihypertensive
8. 2 tablets; antianxiety
9. 2 tablets; antiemetic
10. 3 tablets; antihypertensive

Oral Liquid Medication

1. 10 ml; antibiotic
2. 5 ml; antiulcer
3. $2\frac{1}{2}$ ml; analgesic
4. 5 ml; antibiotic
5. 10 ml; sulfonamide

Parenteral Administration

1. 1.5 cc; antiemetic, antihistamine, antianxiety
2. 2 cc; vitamin
3. $1\frac{1}{2}$ cc; glucocorticoid
4. 2 cc; antibiotic
5. 1 cc; antibiotic
6. 2 cc; iron preparation
7. 2 cc; antibiotic
8. $\frac{1}{2}$ cc; antiemetic
9. $1\frac{1}{2}$ cc; antiarrhythmic
10. 1.4 cc; antiemetic

Table 7-1. Metric System Conversion of Equivalent Values

WEIGHT
1000 micrograms = 1 milligram
1000 milligrams = 1 gram
1000 grams = 1 kilogram

VOLUME
1000 milliliters = 1 liter
1000 liters = 1 kiloliter
1 milliter = 1 cubic centimeter

Table 7-2. Apothecary System: Conversion of Equivalent Values

WEIGHT
60 grains = 1 dram
8 drams = 1 once
12 ounces = 1 pound

VOLUME
60 minims = 1 fluidram
8 fluidrams = 1 fluidounce
16 fluidounces = 1 pint
2 pints = 1 quart
4 quarts = 1 gallon

Table 7-3. Household System: Conversion of Equivalent Values

ABBREVIATIONS
drop: gtt
teaspoon: t or tsp
tablespoon: T or tbs
ounce: oz
cup: c

VOLUME
60 drops = 1 fluidram
3 teaspoons = 1 tablespoon
6 teaspoons = 1 ounce
2 tablespoons = 1 ounce
6 ounces = 1 teacup
8 ounces = 1 glass

Table 7-4. Conversion Chart for Metric and Apothecary Systems (Commonly Used Approximate Equivalents)

METRIC SYSTEM TO APOTHECARY SYSTEM	APOTHECARY SYSTEM TO METRIC SYSTEM
Weight	**Weight**
60 mg = 1 grain	15 grains = 1000 mg (1g)
1 g = 15 grains	10 grains = 600 mg
4 g = 1 dram	7.5 grains = 500 mg
30 mg = 1 ounce	5 grains = 300 mg
1 kg = 2.2 pounds	3 grains = 200 mg
Volume	1.5 grains = 100 mg
	1 grain = 60 mg
0.06 ml = 1 minim	3/4 grain = 50 mg
1 ml(cc) = 15 minims	1/2 grain = 30 mg
4 ml = 1 fluidram	1/4 grain = 15 mg
30 ml = 1 fluidounce	1/6 grain = 10 mg
500 ml = 1 pint	1/8 grain = 8.0 mg
1000 ml (1L) = 1 quart	1/12 grain = 5.0 mg
	1/15 grain = 4.0 mg
	1/20 grain = 3.0 mg
	1/30 grain = 2.0 mg
	1/40 grain = 1.5 mg
	1/50 grain = 1.2 mg
	1/60 grain = 1.0 mg
	1/100 grain = 0.6 mg
	1/120 grain = 0.5 mg
	1/150 grain = 0.4 mg
	1/200 grain = 0.3 mg
	1/300 grain = 0.2 mg
	1/600 grain = 0.1 mg

Table 7-5. Conversion Chart for Apothecary and Metric Equivalents of Household Measures (Volume)

Household	Apothecary	Metric
1 drop	= 1 minim	= .06 ml
15 drops	= 15 minims	= 1 ml (cc)
1 teaspoon	= 1 fluidram	= 5 (4) ml
1 tablespoon	= 4 fluidrams	= 15 ml
2 tablespoons	= 1 fluidounce	= 30 ml
1 ounce	= 1 fluidounce	= 30 ml
1 teacup	= 6 fluidounces	= 180 ml
2 glass	= fluidounces	= 240 ml

Eye and Ear Assessment and Procedures

## CHAPTER 8

Eye Procedures

NAME _____

Key Terminology Assessment

Directions: Match each medical term with its definition.

_____1. canthus
_____2. hyperopia
_____3. instillation
_____4. irrigation
_____5. myopia
_____6. ophthalmologist
_____7. optician
_____8. optometrist
_____9. presbyopia
_____10. refraction

A. A professional who interprets and fills ophthalmic prescriptions.
B. The washing of a body canal with a flowing solution.
C. A decrease in the elasticity of the lens due to aging, resulting in a decreased ability to focus on close objects.
D. Farsightedness.
E. The deflection or bending of light rays by a lens.
F. The junction of the eyelids at either corner of the eye.
G. A medical doctor who specializes in diagnosing and treating disorders of the eye.
H. Nearsightedness.
I. A licensed practitioner who is skilled in measuring visual acuity and is qualified to prescribe corrective lenses.
J. The dropping of a liquid into a body cavity.

Self-Evaluation

Directions: Fill in each blank with the correct answer.

1. What is the name of the tough white outer covering of the eye?

_____

2. What is the function of the lens?

_____

3. What is the function of the retina?

_____

4. What parts of the eye are covered with conjunctiva?

_____

_____

5. What is visual acuity?

_____

_____

6. What condition can be detected by measuring distance visual acuity?

_____

7. What type of patient would warrant use of the Snellen Big E eye chart? (Give two examples.)

_____

_____

8. Explain the significance of the top number and bottom number next to each line of letters of the Snellen eye chart.

_____

_____

9. List two conditions that can be detected by measuring near visual acuity.

_____

_____

10. Explain the difference between congenital and acquired color vision defects.

_____

_____

_____

11. What is a polychromatic plate?

_____

_____

_____

12. List three reasons for performing an eye irrigation.

_____

_____

_____

13. List three reasons for performing an eye instillation.

_____

_____

_____

Critical Thinking Skills

1. For each of the following situations, write **C** if the technique is correct and **I** if the technique is incorrect.

   Measuring Distance Visual Acuity

   _____ a. The patient is not given an opportunity to study the Snellen chart before beginning the test.

   _____ b. The Snellen chart is positioned at the medical assistant's eye level.

   _____ c. The patient is instructed to use his hand to cover the eye that is not being tested.

   _____ d. The medical assistant instructs the patient to close the eye that is not being tested.

   _____ e. The first line that the medical assistant asks the patient to identify is the 20/20 line.

   _____ f. The medical assistant observes the patient for signs of squinting or leaning forward during the test.

2. A patient has a distance visual acuity reading of 20/30 in the right eye. Using this information, answer the following questions:

   a. How far was the patient from the eye chart?

   _____

   b. At what distance would a person with normal acuity be able to read this line?

   _____

3. A patient has a distance visual acuity reading of 20/10 in the left eye. Using this information, answer the following questions:

   a. How far was the patient from the eye chart?

   _____

b. At what distance would a person with normal acuity be able to read this line?

_____

4. Properly chart the distance visual acuity results in the spaces provided. In all cases, the line indicated is the smallest line the patient could read at a distance of 20 feet.

a. The patient read the line marked 20/30 with the right eye with two errors, and with the left eye read the line marked 20/30 with one error. The patient was wearing corrective lenses.

_____

_____

b. The patient read the line marked 20/20 with the right eye with one error, and with the left eye read the line marked 20/20 with no errors. The patient was wearing corrective lenses.

_____

_____

c. The patient read the line marked 20/40 with the right eye with two errors, and with the left eye read the line marked 20/30 with one error. The patient exhibited squinting and frowning during the test. The patient was not wearing corrective lenses.

_____

_____

d. The patient read the line marked 20/15 with the right eye with no errors, and with the left eye read the line marked 20/20 with one error. The patient was not wearing corrective lenses.

_____

_____

5. Your patient is a 10-year-old boy named John Patterson who has conjunctivitis in the right eye caused by a bacterium. The physician prescribes Tobramycin (eye drops). Mrs. Patterson will be responsible for instilling the drops. Complete the following:

a. Give a brief description of conjunctivitis.

_____

_____

_____

b. Using a drug reference, look up the drug Tobramycin and complete the following:

Use:

_____

_____

Adverse reactions:

_____

_____

Dosage and administration:

_____

_____

c. In a role-playing situation, one person takes the role of the medical assistant, and another the role of Mrs. Patterson. The medical assistant's responsibility is to instruct Mrs. Patterson verbally about the instillation of the eye drops into her son's eyes. List below the important points that should be included.

_____

_____

_____

6. Using a reference source, look up the following eye conditions and give a brief description of each:

    a. stye

    _____

    _____

    _____

    b. blepharitis

    _____

    _____

    _____

    c. chalazion

    _____

    _____

    _____

    d. strabismus

    _____

    _____

    _____

    e. cataract

    _____

    _____

    _____

    f. glaucoma

    _____

    _____

    _____

Ear Procedures

NAME _____

Key Terminology Assessment

Directions: Match each medical term with its definition.

_____ 1. audiometer
_____ 2. cerumen
_____ 3. impacted
_____ 4. otoscope
_____ 5. tympanic membrane

A. An instrument for examining the external ear canal and tympanic membrane.
B. Ear wax.
C. An instrument used to quantitatively measure hearing acuity for the various frequencies of sound waves.
D. A thin, semitransparent membrane located between the external ear canal and the middle ear that receives and transmits sound waves.
E. Being wedged firmly together so as to be immovable.

Self-Evaluation

Directions: Fill in each blank with the correct answer.

1. What is the function of the ear auricle?

   _____

   _____

2. What is the function of cerumen?

   _____

   _____

3. Explain why the external auditory canal must be straightened when viewing it with an otoscope.

   _____

   _____

4. What is the normal appearance of the tympanic membrane?

_____

_____

5. What is the purpose of the eustachian tube?

_____

_____

6. What is the function of the semicircular canals?

_____

_____

7. What is the range of frequencies for normal speech?

_____

_____

8. List five conditions that may cause a conductive hearing loss.

_____

_____

_____

9. List four conditions that may result in a sensorineural hearing loss.

_____

_____

10. How is hearing acuity tested with the gross screening test?

_____

_____

_____

11. What are the names of the hearing acuity tests that require the use of a tuning fork?

_____

_____

12. What information is obtained through audiometry?

_____

_____

_____

13. What information is obtained through tympanometry?

_____

_____

_____

14. List three reasons for performing an ear irrigation.

_____

_____

15. List three reasons for performing an ear instillation.

_____

_____

16. Explain how impacted cerumen is removed from the ear.

_____

_____

_____

17. Explain how to straighten the external auditory canal in an adult and in children 3 years of age and younger.

_____

_____

_____

Critical Thinking Skills

1. Explain the principle for each of the following:

Ear Irrigation

    a. Positioning the patient's head so that it is tilted toward the affected ear

_____

_____

    b. Cleansing the outer ear before irrigating

_____

_____

    c. Straightening the external auditory canal

_____

_____

   d. Injecting the irrigating solution toward the roof of the ear canal

   _____

   _____

   e. Making sure not to obstruct the canal opening

   _____

   _____

Ear Instillation

   f. Positioning the patient's head so that it is tilted toward the unaffected ear

   _____

   _____

   g. Instructing the patient to lie on the unaffected side after the instillation

   _____

   _____

   h. Placing a cotton wick in the patient's ear

   _____

   _____

2. Using a reference source, look up the following common ear conditions and give a brief description of each.

   a. External otitis

   _____

   _____

   _____

   b. Serous otitis media

   _____

   _____

   _____

Practice for Competency

EYE ASSESSMENT AND PROCEDURES

Assignment

Distance Visual Acuity. Assess distance visual acuity using a Snellen eye chart and record results in the chart provided. Circle any readings that indicate distance visual acuity above or below average.

Color Vision. Assess color vision and record results in the chart provided. Circle any abnormal results.

Eye Irrigation. Perform an eye irrigation and record the procedure in the chart provided.

Eye Instillation. Perform an eye instillation and record the procedure in the chart provided.

CHART	
Date	

CHART	
Date	

Notes

Evaluation of Competency

PROCEDURE 8-1: ASSESSING DISTANCE VISUAL ACUITY-SNELLEN CHART

Name _____   Date _____

Evaluated By _____   Score_____

Performance Objective

Outcome:	Assess distance visual acuity.
Conditions:	Given the following: Snellen eye chart and an eye occluder.
Standards:	Time: 5 minutes
	Accuracy: Satisfactory score on the Performance Evaluation Checklist.

Performance Evaluation Checklist

Trial 1	Trial 2	Point Value	Performance Standards
		●	Washed hands.
		●	Assembled equipment.
		●	Greeted and identified the patient.
		●	Introduced yourself and explained the procedure.
		●	Instructed patient not to squint during the test.
		▷	Is able to state why patient should not squint during the test.
		●	Determined if patient wears corrective lenses and instructed patient to leave them on during the test.
		●	Positioned patient 20 feet from the eye chart.
		●	Positioned the center of eye chart at patient's eye level.
		●	Instructed patient to cover the left eye with the occluder and to keep left eye open.
		▷	Is able to state why patient's left eye should remain open.
		●	Asked patient to identify the 20/70 line, using the right eye.
		▷	Is able to state why the test should begin with a line that is above the 20/20 line.
		●	Proceeded down the chart if patient identified the 20/70 line or proceeded up the chart if the patient was unable to identify the 20/70 line.
		●	Continued until the smallest line of letters that patient could read was reached.

Trial 1	Trial 2	Point Value	Performance Standards
		●	Observed patient for any unusual symptoms.
		●	Asked patient to cover the right eye and to keep right eye open.
		●	Correctly measured visual acuity in the left eye.
		★	The visual acuity measurements were identical to the evaluator's measurements
		●	Charted the results correctly.
		★	Completed the procedure within 5 minutes.

CHART	
Date	

Evaluation of Student Performance

EVALUATION CRITERIA			COMMENTS
Symbol	**Category**	**Point Value**	
★	Critical Step	16 points	
●	Essential Step	6 points	
▷	Theory Question	2 points	
Score calculation: 100 points			
− _____ points missed			
_____ Score			
Satisfactory score: 85 or above			

AAMA/CAAHEP Competency Achieved:
☐ Prepare patient for and assist with routine and specialty examinations.

Evaluation of Competency

PROCEDURE 8-2: ASSESSING COLOR VISION—ISHIHARA TEST

Name _____   Date _____

Evaluated By _____   Score_____

Performance Objective

Outcome:	Assess color vision.
Conditions:	Given an Ishihara book of color plates.
Standards:	Time: 10 minutes
	Accuracy: Satisfactory score on the Performance Evaluation Checklist.

Performance Evaluation Checklist

Trial 1	Trial 2	Point Value	*Performance Standards*
		●	Washed hands.
		●	Assembled equipment.
		●	Conducted the test in a quiet room illuminated by natural daylight.
		▷	Is able to state why natural daylight should be used.
		●	Greeted and identified the patient.
		●	Introduced yourself and explained the procedure.
		●	Instructed patient to identify the number on the practice plate.
		●	Held the first plate 30 inches from patient at a right angle to patient's line of vision.
		●	Asked patient to identify the number on the plate.
		●	Continued until patient viewed all plates.
		●	Recorded the results after identification of each plate.
		★	The results were identical to the evaluator's results.
		●	Charted the procedure correctly.
		●	Returned the Ishihara book to its proper place, storing it in a closed position.
		▷	Is able to state why the book should be stored in a closed position.
		★	Completed the procedure within 10 minutes.

CHART	
Date	

Evaluation of Student Performance

EVALUATION CRITERIA			COMMENTS
Symbol	**Category**	**Point Value**	
★	Critical Step	16 points	
●	Essential Step	6 points	
▷	Theory Question	2 points	
Score calculation: 100 points			
− _____ points missed			
_____ Score			
Satisfactory score: 85 or above			

AAMA/CAAHEP Competency Achieved:
☐ Prepare patient for and assist with routine and specialty examinations.

Evaluation of Competency

PROCEDURE 8-3: EYE IRRIGATION

Name _____   Date _____

Evaluated By _____   Score_____

Performance Objective

Outcome:	Perform an eye irrigation.
Conditions:	Given the following: disposable gloves, sterile rubber bulb syringe, sterile irrigating solution, sterile container to hold the solution, basin, moisture-resistant towel, and sterile gauze pads.
Standards:	Time: 5 minutes
	Accuracy: Satisfactory score on the Performance Evaluation Checklist.

Performance Evaluation Checklist

Trial 1	Trial 2	Point Value	*Performance Standards*
		●	Washed hands.
		●	Assembled equipment.
		●	Checked to make sure that the correct solution is obtained.
		●	Checked expiration date of the solution.
		●	Warmed the irragating solution.
		●	Greeted and identified the patient.
		●	Introduced yourself and explained the procedure.
		●	Applied gloves.
		●	Positioned patient so that his/her head is turned in the direction of the affected eye.
		▷	Is able to state why patient's head is turned in the direction of the affected eye.
		●	Positioned a basin tightly against the patient's cheek.
		●	Placed a moisture resistant towel on the patient's shoulder.
		●	Cleansed the eyelids from inner to outer canthus.
		▷	Is able to state why eyelids are cleansed.
		●	Filled irrigating syringe.
		●	Separated eyelids.

Trial 1	Trial 2	Point Value	Performance Standards
		●	Held tip of syringe 1 inch above the eye at the inner canthus.
		●	Allowed solution to flow over the eye at a moderate rate from the inner canthus to the outer canthus and directed solution to the lower conjunctiva.
		▷	Is able to state why the syringe should be directed toward the lower conjunctiva.
		●	Did not allow syringe to touch the eye.
		●	Refilled the syringe and continued irrigating until the desired results were obtained or all the solution was used.
		●	Dried eyelids with grauze pad from inner to outer canthus.
		●	Removed gloves and washed hands.
		●	Charted the procedure correctly.
		▷	Is able to state the abbreviation for both eyes, the right eye, and the left eye.
		●	Returned equipment.
		★	Completed the procedure within 5 minutes.

CHART	
Date	

Evaluation of Student Performance

EVALUATION CRITERIA			COMMENTS
Symbol	Category	Point Value	
★	Critical Step	16 points	
●	Essential Step	6 points	
▷	Theory Question	2 points	

Score calculation: 100 points

—   points missed

_____ Score

Satisfactory score: 85 or above

AAMA/CAAHEP Competency Achieved:
☐ Prepare patient for and assist with routine and specialty examinations.

Evaluation of Competency

PROCEDURE 8-4: EYE INSTILLATION

Name _____   Date _____

Evaluated By _____   Score_____

Performance Objective

Outcome:	Perform an eye instillation.
Conditions:	Given the following: disposable gloves, ophthalmic medication, sterile gauze pads, and sterile tissues.
Standards:	Time: 5 minutes
	Accuracy: Satisfactory score on the Performance Evaluation Checklist.

Performance Evaluation Checklist

Trial 1	Trial 2	Point Value	Performance Standards
		●	Washed hands.
		●	Assembled equipment.
		●	Checked to make sure that the correct medication is obtained.
		●	Checked expiration date of the medication.
		●	Greeted and identified patient.
		●	Introduced yourself and explained the procedure.
		●	Positioned patient.
		●	Applied gloves.
		●	Prepared the medication.
		●	Asked patient to look up and exposed the lower conjunctival sac.
		▷	Is able to state the reason for asking patient to look up.
		●	Inserted the medication correctly.
		●	Discarded any unused solution from eye dropper.
		●	Instructed patient to close eyes and move eyeballs.
		▷	Is able to state the reason for closing the eyes and moving the eyeballs.
		●	Told patient that the instillation may temporarily blur vision.
		●	Dried eyelids with a gauze pad from inner to outer canthus.
		●	Removed gloves and washed hands.

Trial 1	Trial 2	Point Value	Performance Standards
		●	Charted the procedure correctly.
		●	Returned equipment.
		★	Completed the procedure within 5 minutes.

CHART	
Date	

Evaluation of Student Performance

EVALUATION CRITERIA			COMMENTS
Symbol	Category	Point Value	
★	Critical Step	16 points	
●	Essential Step	6 points	
▷	Theory Question	2 points	

Score calculation: 100 points

−_____ points missed

_____ Score

Satisfactory score: 85 or above

AAMA/CAAHEP Competency Achieved:

☐ Prepare patient for and assist with routine and specialty examinations.

Practice for Competency

EAR PROCEDURES

Assignment

Ear Irrigation. Perform an ear irrigation and record the procedure in the chart provided.

Ear Instillation. Perform an ear instillation and record the procedure in the chart provided.

CHART	
Date	

CHART	
Date	

Evaluation of Competency

PROCEDURE 8-5: EAR IRRIGATION

Name _____   Date _____

Evaluated By _____   Score_____

Performance Objective

Outcome: Perform an ear irrigation.

Conditions: Given the following: disposable gloves, irrigating solution, solution container, irrigating syringe, ear basin, moisture-resistant towel, and cotton balls.

Standards: Time: 10 minutes

Accuracy: Satisfactory score on the Performance Evaluation Checklist.

Performance Evaluation Checklist

Trial 1	Trial 2	Point Value	Performance Standards
		●	Washed hands.
		●	Assembled equipment.
		●	Checked to make sure that the correct solution is obtained.
		●	Checked expiration date of the solution.
		●	Warmed the irrigating solution.
		▷	Is able to state the reason for warming the irrigating solution.
		●	Greeted and identified patient.
		●	Introduced yourself and explained the procedure.
		●	Positioned patient, with the head tilted toward the affected ear.
		▷	Is able to state why the head should be tilted toward the affected ear.
		●	Placed a towel on patient's shoulder and instructed patient to hold the ear basin under the affected ear.
		●	Applied gloves.
		●	Cleansed the outer ear.
		▷	Is able to state why the outer ear should be cleansed.
		●	Filled the irrigating syringe.
		●	Expelled air from syringe.
		▷	Is able to state why air should be expelled from syringe.

Trial 1	Trial 2	Point Value	Performance Standards
		●	Properly straightened the external ear canal.
		▷	Is able to state why the canal must be straightened.
		●	Inserted syringe tip into the ear and injected irrigating solution onto roof of the ear canal.
		▷	Is able to state why solution should be injected onto roof of the canal.
		●	Did not insert the syringe too deeply.
		●	Refilled the syringe and continued irrigating until the desired results were obtained or all the solution was used.
		●	Made sure that tip of syringe did not obstruct the canal opening.
		▷	Is able to state why the canal should not be obstructed.
		●	Observed the returning solution to note the material present and the amount.
		●	Dried outside of the ear with cotton ball.
		●	Instructed patient to lie on the affected side on treatment table.
		▷	Is able to state why patient should lie on the affected side.
		●	Inserted a cotton wick loosely in the ear canal for 15 minutes.
		▷	Is able to state the purpose of the cotton wick.
		●	Removed gloves and washed hands.
		●	Charted the procedure correctly.
		▷	Is able to state the abbreviation for both ears, right ear, and left ear.
		●	Returned equipment.
		★	Completed the procedure within 10 minutes.
			**CHART**
	Date		

Evaluation of Student Performance

EVALUATION CRITERIA			COMMENTS
Symbol	Category	Point Value	
★	Critical Step	16 points	
●	Essential Step	6 points	
▷	Theory Question	2 points	
Score calculation: 100 points			
− _____ points missed			
_____ Score			
Satisfactory score: 85 or above			

AAMA/CAAHEP Competency Achieved:

☐ Prepare patient for and assist with routine and specialty examinations.

Notes

Evaluation of Competency

PROCEDURE 8-6: EAR INSTILLATION

Name _____   Date _____

Evaluated By _____   Score_____

Performance Objective

Outcome:	Perform an ear instillation.
Conditions:	Given the following: disposable gloves, otic medication, and cotton balls.
Standards:	Time: 5 minutes
	Accuracy: Satisfactory score on the Performance Evaluation Checklist.

Performance Evaluation Checklist

Trial 1	Trial 2	Point Value	*Performance Standards*
		●	Washed hands.
		●	Assembled equipment.
		●	Checked to make sure that the correct medication was obtained.
		●	Checked expiration date of the medication.
		▷	Is able to state what might occur if the medication is outdated.
		●	Greeted and identified patient.
		●	Introduced yourself and explained the procedure.
		●	Positioned patient with the head tilted in the direction of the unaffected ear.
		●	Applied gloves.
		●	Withdrew the medication into the dropper.
		●	Properly straightened the external ear canal.
		●	Placed tip of dropper in the ear canal and inserted the proper amount of medication.
		●	Instructed patient to lie on the unaffected side for 2 to 3 minutes.
		▷	Is able to state why patient should lie on the unaffected side.
		●	Placed a moistened cotton wick loosely in the ear canal for 15 minutes.
		▷	Is able to state the reason for moistening the wick.
		●	Removed gloves and washed hands.

Trial 1	Trial 2	Point Value	Performance Standards
		●	Charted the procedure correctly.
		●	Returned equipment.
		★	Completed the procedure within 5 minutes.

CHART	
Date	

Evaluation of Student Performance

EVALUATION CRITERIA			COMMENTS
Symbol	**Category**	**Point Value**	
★	Critical Step	16 points	
●	Essential Step	6 points	
▷	Theory Question	2 points	

Score calculation: 100 points
− _____ points missed
_____ Score
Satisfactory score: 85 or above

AAMA/CAAHEP Competency Achieved:
☐ Prepare patient for and assist with routine and specialty examinations.

Physical Agents to Promote Tissue Healing

NAME _____

Key Terminology Assessment

Directions: Match each medical term with its definition.

_____ 1. ambulation
_____ 2. compress
_____ 3. edema
_____ 4. erythema
_____ 5. exudate
_____ 6. inflammation
_____ 7. orthopedist
_____ 8. soak
_____ 9. sprain
_____10. strain
_____11. suppuration
_____12. toxin

A. A discharge produced by the body's tissues.
B. An overstretching of a muscle due to trauma.
C. A soft, moist, absorbent cloth that is folded in several layers and applied to a part of the body in the local application of heat or cold.
D. The ability to walk, as opposed to being confined to bed.
E. The direct immersion of a body part in water or in a medicated solution.
F. The retention of fluid in the tissues resulting in swelling.
G. A poisonous or noxious substance.
H. The protective response of the tissues to injury or destruction.
I. Redness of the skin caused by congestion of capillaries in the lower layers of skin.
J. Trauma to a joint that causes injury to the ligaments.
K. The process of pus formation.
L. A physician who deals with the prevention and correction of the locomotor structures of the body.

Self- Evaluation

Directions: Fill in each blank with the correct answer.

1. State whether the following is an example of dry heat, moist heat, dry cold, or moist cold.

    a. hot compress

_____

    b. ice bag

_____

    c. heating pad

_____

    d. hot water bag

_____

    e. cold compress

_____

2. How does the local application of heat to an affected area for a short period of time influence the following?

    a. the diameter of the blood vessels in the affected area

_____

_____

    b. the blood supply to the affected area

_____

_____

    c. tissue metabolism in the affected area

_____

_____

3. What happens to the diameter of the blood vessels if heat is applied for a prolonged period of time (more than 1 hour)?

_____

_____

4. List three reasons for applying heat locally.

_____

_____

_____

5. How does the local application of cold for a short period of time to an affected area influence the following?

    a.   the diameter of the blood vessels in the affected area

         _____

         _____

    b.   the blood supply to the affected area

         _____

         _____

    c.   tissue metabolism in the affected area

         _____

         _____

6. List two reasons for applying cold locally.

    _____

    _____

7. List three factors that must be taken into consideration when applying heat or cold.

    _____

    _____

    _____

8. Describe the general use of therapeutic ultrasound.

    _____

    _____

9. What is the purpose of the ultrasound coupling agent?

    _____

10. List two instances when the underwater ultrasound method is advocated.

    _____

    _____

11. What is the purpose of continuously moving the applicator head during the ultrasound treatment?

    _____

    _____

12. Why shouldn't the applicator head be removed from the patient's skin and held up in the air?

    _____

    _____

13. List two instances in which the medical assistant should immediately stop the ultra-sound treatment.

_____

_____

_____

14. What are three reasons for applying a cast?

_____

_____

_____

15. What are the advantages and disadvantages of a synthetic cast as compared with a plaster cast?

_____

_____

_____

_____

_____

16. What is the purpose of covering the body part with stockinette before applying a cast?

_____

_____

17. What is the purpose of applying cast padding during cast application?

_____

_____

18. What may occur if a pressure area develops after a cast has been applied?

_____

_____

19. What factors does the physician take into consideration when prescribing an ambulatory assistive device?

_____

_____

_____

20. Describe one advantage of the Lofstrand crutch.

_____

21. What may occur if axillary crutches are not fitted properly?

_____

_____

22. List eight guidelines that must be followed during crutch use to ensure safety.

_____

_____

_____

_____

_____

23. List one use of each of the following crutch gaits.

    a. four-point gait: _____

    b. three-point gait: _____

    c. swing-to gait: _____

24. List and describe the three types of canes.

_____

_____

25. List two reasons for prescribing a cane.

_____

_____

26. List one reason for prescribing a walker.

_____

_____

Critical Thinking Skills

1. Mrs. Bryan calls your office and asks what to do for her daughter Beth, age 10, who has a bleeding nose. The physician instructs you tell Mrs. Bryan to apply pressure and cold compresses to Beth's nose. Complete the following:

    a. In a role-playing situation, explain to Mrs. Bryan the procedure for applying a cold compress. In the space provided, list the important points that should be covered.

_____

_____

_____

_____

_____

b. How does the local application of cold aid in the relief of a nosebleed?

_____

_____

_____

c. Why are large ice cubes recommended for use in preparing the water for the cold compresses?

_____

_____

2. You have instructed Linda Taylor in the proper use of a heating pad for relief of her strained back. She asks you the following questions. Answer them in the spaces provided.

a. Why should I be careful not to bend or crush the heating pad?

_____

_____

b. Why shouldn't I lie on the heating pad?

_____

_____

_____

c. Why must a protective cover be used on the pad?

_____

_____

d. Why shouldn't I increase the temperature control when the pad no longer feels warm to me?

_____

_____

_____

e. How will the local application of heat aid in the relief of the injury?

_____

_____

_____

3. Mr. James Mullins calls your office and says that the hot water bag he has been using for the relief of pain on his forearm is extremely heavy and bulky and will not mold comfortably to his extremity. What questions should you ask him to determine what he may be doing wrong? Explain the principle underlying each possible cause.

_____

_____

_____

_____

_____

4. Margaret Hubble has had a short arm fiberglass cast applied to her right arm. She asks the following questions. Answer them in the spaces provided.

    a. How can I reduce the swelling in my arm?

_____

_____

_____

    b. Why can't I use a coat hanger to scratch under the cast?

_____

_____

_____

    c. What will happen if I get dirt under the cast?

_____

_____

_____

    d. How would I know if the cast is too tight or if an infection is developing?

_____

_____

_____

Practice for Competency

LOCAL APPLICATION OF HEAT AND COLD

Assignment

Hot Water Bag. Apply a hot water bag and record the procedure in the chart provided.
Heating Pad. Apply a heating pad and record the procedure in the chart provided.
Hot Soak. Apply a hot soak and record the procedure in the chart provided.
Hot Compress. Apply a hot compress and record the procedure in the chart provided.
Ice Bag. Apply an ice bag and record the procedure in the chart provided.
Cold Compress. Apply a cold compress and record the procedure in the chart provided.
Chemical Cold and Hot Pack. Apply a chemical cold and hot pack and record the procedure in the chart.

CHART	
Date	

Practice for Competency

THERAPEUTIC ULTRASOUND

Assignment

Administer an ultrasound treatment and record the procedure in the chart provided.

CHART	
Date	

Practice for Competency

AMBULATORY AIDS

Assignment

Axillary Crutch Measurement. Measure an individual for axillary crutches and record the procedure in the chart provided.

Crutch Gaits. Instruct an individual in mastering the following crutch gaits; four-point, two-point, three-point, swing-to, and swing-through. Record the procedure in the chart provided.

Cane. Instruct an individual in the use of a cane and record the procedure in the chart provided.

Walker. Instruct an individual in the use of a walker and record the procedure in the chart provided.

CHART	
Date	

Evaluation of Competency

PROCEDURE 9-1: APPLYING A HOT WATER BAG

Name _____ Date _____

Evaluated By _____ Score_____

Performance Objective

Outcome: Apply a hot water bag.

Conditions: Given the following: hot water bag and protective covering, pitcher, and a bath thermometer.

Standards: Time: 10 minutes

Accuracy: Satisfactory score on the Performance Evaluation Checklist.

Performance Evaluation Checklist

Trial 1	Trial 2	Point Value	*Performance Standards*
		●	Washed hands.
		●	Assembled equipment.
		●	Greeted and identified the patient.
		●	Introduced yourself and explained the procedure.
		●	Filled the pitcher with hot water and checked the temperature.
		▷	Is able to state the safe temperature range that should be used for adult patient.
		●	Filled the hot water bag $\frac{1}{3}$ to $\frac{1}{2}$ full of water.
		●	Expelled excess air from bag.
		▷	Is able to state the reason for expelling air from bag.
		●	Dried outside of bag and tested it for leakage.
		●	Placed bag in protective covering.
		▷	Is able to state the reason for placing bag in protective covering.
		●	Placed bag on patient's affected body area and asked patient how the temperature felt.
		●	Administered treatment for the proper length of time designated by physician.
		●	Checked patient's skin periodically.
		●	Refilled bag with hot water as needed.

Trial 1	Trial 2	Point Value	Performance Standards
		●	Washed hands.
		●	Charted the procedure correctly.
		●	Properly cared for hot water bag.
		★	Completed the procedure within 10 minutes.

CHART	
Date	

Evaluation of Student Performance

EVALUATION CRITERIA			COMMENTS
Symbol	Category	Point Value	
★	Critical Step	16 points	
●	Essential Step	6 points	
▷	Theory Question	2 points	
Score calculation: 100 points			
− _____ points missed			
_____ Score			
Satisfactory score: 85 or above			

AAMA/CAAHEP Competency Achieved:

☐ Prepare patient for and assist with procedures, treatments and minor office surgery.

Evaluation of Competency

PROCEDURE 9-2: APPLYING A HEATING PAD

Name _____   Date _____

Evaluated By _____   Score_____

Performance Objective

Outcome:	Apply a heating pad.
Conditions:	Given a heating pad with a protective covering.
Standards:	Time: 5 minutes
	Accuracy: Satisfactory score on the Performance Evaluation Checklist.

Performance Evaluation Checklist

Trial 1	Trial 2	Point Value	*Performance Standards*
		●	Washed hands.
		●	Assembled equipment.
		●	Greeted and identified patient.
		●	Introduced yourself and explained the procedure.
		▷	Is able to state why patient should be instructed not to lie on heating pad.
		●	Placed the heating pad in protective covering.
		●	Connected the plug to electrical outlet and set selector switch to the proper setting.
		●	Placed heating pad on patient's affected body area and asked how the temperature felt.
		●	Instructed patient not to turn the temperature setting higher.
		▷	Is able to state why patient may want to increase the temperature.
		●	Administered treatment for the proper length of time as designated by physician.
		●	Checked patient's skin periodically.
		●	Washed hands.
		●	Charted the procedure correctly.
		●	Returned and properly cared for equipment.
		★	Completed the procedure within 5 minutes.

CHART	
Date	

Evaluation of Student Performance

EVALUATION CRITERIA			COMMENTS
Symbol	**Category**	**Point Value**	
★	Critical Step	16 points	
●	Essential Step	6 points	
▷	Theory Question	2 points	
Score calculation: 100 points			
− _____ points missed			
_____ Score			
Satisfactory score: 85 or above			

AAMA/CAAHEP Competency Achieved:

☐ Prepare patient for and assist with procedures, treatments, and minor office surgery.

Evaluation of Competency

PROCEDURE 9-3: APPLYING A HOT SOAK

Name _____   Date _____

Evaluated By _____   Score_____

Performance Objective

Outcome:	Apply a hot soak.
Conditions:	Given the following: soaking solution, bath thermometer, basin, and bath towels.
Standards:	Time: 10 minutes
	Accuracy: Satisfactory score on the Performance Evaluation Checklist.

Performance Evaluation Checklist

Trial 1	Trial 2	Point Value	*Performance Standards*
		●	Washed hands.
		●	Assembled equipment.
		●	Greeted and identified patient.
		●	Introduced yourself and explained procedure.
		●	Filled basin half full with the warmed soaking solution.
		●	Checked temperature of the solution with a bath thermometer.
		▷	Is able to state the safe temperature range that should be used for adult patient.
		●	Placed patient in a comfortable position and padded side of the basin with towel.
		●	Slowly and gradually immersed affected body part into the solution and asked patient how the temperature felt.
		●	Kept the solution at a constant temperature.
		●	Placed a hand between patient and water when adding more water.
		●	Applied hot soak for the proper length of time as designated by physician.
		●	Checked patient's skin periodically.
		●	Completely dried affected part.
		●	Washed hands.

Trial 1	Trial 2	Point Value	Performance Standards
		●	Charted procedure correctly.
		●	Returned and properly cared for equipment.
		★	Completed the procedure within 10 minutes.

CHART	
Date	

Evaluation of Student Performance

EVALUATION CRITERIA			COMMENTS
Symbol	Category	Point Value	
★	Critical Step	16 points	
●	Essential Step	6 points	
▷	Theory Question	2 points	
Score calculation: 100 points			
− points missed			
Score			
Satisfactory score: 85 or above			

AAMA/CAAHEP Competency Achieved:
☐ Prepare patient for and assist with procedures, treatments, and minor office surgery.

Evaluation of Competency

PROCEDURE 9-4: APPLYING A HOT COMPRESS

Name _____   Date _____

Evaluated By _____   Score_____

Performance Objective

Outcome:	Apply a hot compress.
Conditions:	Given the following: solution for the compresses, bath thermometer, basin, and washcloths.
Standards:	Time: 10 minutes
	Accuracy: Satisfactory score on the Performance Evaluation Checklist.

Performance Evaluation Checklist

Trial 1	Trial 2	Point Value	Performance Standards
		●	Washed hands.
		●	Assembled equipment.
		●	Greeted and identified patient.
		●	Introduced yourself and explained procedure.
		●	Filled the basin half full with the warmed solution.
		●	Checked temperature of the solution with a bath thermometer.
		▷	Is able to state the safe temperature range that should be used for adult patient.
		●	Completely immersed the compress in the solution.
		●	Wrung out compress.
		●	Applied compress to affected body part and asked patient how the temperature felt.
		●	Placed additional compresses in the solution.
		●	Repeated the application every 2 to 3 minutes for the duration of time specified by physician.
		●	Checked patient's skin periodically.
		●	Checked temperature of the water periodically and added more hot water if needed.
		●	Thoroughly dried affected part.

Trial 1	Trial 2	Point Value	Performance Standards
		●	Washed hands.
		●	Charted the procedure correctly.
		●	Returned and properly cared for equipment.
		★	Completed the procedure within 10 minutes.

CHART	
Date	

Evaluation of Student Performance

EVALUATION CRITERIA			COMMENTS
Symbol	Category	Point Value	
★	Critical Step	16 points	
●	Essential Step	6 points	
▷	Theory Question	2 points	

Score calculation: 100 points

—_____ points missed

_____ Score

Satisfactory score: 85 or above

AAMA/CAAHEP Competency Achieved:

☐ Prepare patient for and assist with procedures, treatments, and minor office surgery.

Evaluation of Competency

PROCEDURE 9-5: APPLYING AN ICE BAG

Name _____   Date _____

Evaluated By _____   Score_____

Performance Objective

Outcome:	Apply an ice bag.
Conditions:	Given the following: ice bag and protective covering, and small pieces of ice.
Standards:	Time: 10 minutes
	Accuracy: Satisfactory score on the Performance Evaluation Checklist.

Performance Evaluation Checklist

Trial 1	Trial 2	Point Value	*Performance Standards*
		●	Washed hands.
		●	Assembled equipment.
		●	Greeted and identified patient.
		●	Introduced yourself and explained procedure.
		●	Checked ice bag for leakage.
		●	Filled bag $\frac{1}{2}$ to $\frac{2}{3}$ full with small pieces of ice.
		▷	Is able to state why small pieces of ice are used.
		●	Expelled air from bag.
		▷	Is able to state the reason for expelling air from bag.
		●	Thoroughly dried bag and placed it in protective covering.
		▷	Is able to state the purpose of placing bag in protective covering.
		●	Placed bag on affected body area and asked patient how the temperature felt.
		●	Administered treatment for the proper length of time as designated by physician.
		●	Refilled bag with ice and changed protective covering when needed.
		●	Checked patient's skin periodically.
		▷	Is able to list skin changes that would warrant removal of bag.
		●	Washed hands.

Trial 1	Trial 2	Point Value	Performance Standards
		●	Charted the procedure correctly.
		●	Properly cared for ice bag.
		★	Completed the procedure within 10 minutes.

CHART	
Date	

Evaluation of Student Performance

EVALUATION CRITERIA			COMMENTS
Symbol	Category	Point Value	
★	Critical Step	16 points	
●	Essential Step	6 points	
▷	Theory Question	2 points	
Score calculation: 100 points			
— points missed			
_____ Score			
Satisfactory score: 85 or above			

AAMA/CAAHEP Competency Achieved:

☐ Prepare patient for and assist with procedures, treatments, and minor office surgery.

Evaluation of Competency

PROCEDURE 9-6: APPLYING A COLD COMPRESS

Name _____   Date _____

Evaluated By _____   Score_____

Performance Objective

Outcome:	Apply a cold compress.
Conditions:	Given the following: ice cubes, a basin, and washcloths.
Standards:	Time: 10 minutes
	Accuracy: Satisfactory score on the Performance Evaluation Checklist.

Performance Evaluation Checklist

Trial 1	Trial 2	Point Value	*Performance Standards*
		●	Washed hands.
		●	Assembled equipment.
		●	Greeted and identified patient.
		●	Introduced yourself and explained procedure.
		●	Prepared the water by placing ice cubes in basin and adding small amount of water.
		▷	Is able to state why larger pieces of ice are used.
		●	Completely immersed the compress in the solution.
		●	Wrung out compress.
		●	Applied compress to affected body part and asked patient how the temperature felt.
		●	Placed additional compresses in the solution.
		●	Repeated the application every 2 to 3 minutes for the duration of time specified by physician.
		●	Checked patient's skin periodically.
		●	Added ice if needed to keep the water cold.
		●	Thoroughly dried affected part.
		●	Washed hands.

Trial 1	Trial 2	Point Value	Performance Standards
		●	Charted the procedure correctly.
		●	Returned and properly cared for equipment.
		★	Completed the procedure within 10 minutes.

CHART	
Date	

Evaluation of Student Performance

EVALUATION CRITERIA			COMMENTS
Symbol	Category	Point Value	
★	Critical Step	16 points	
●	Essential Step	6 points	
▷	Theory Question	2 points	
Score calculation: 100 points			
_____ points missed			
_____ Score			
Satisfactory score: 85 or above			

AAMA/CAAHEP Competency Achieved:
☐ Prepare patient for and assist with procedures, treatments, and minor office surgery.

Evaluation of Competency

PROCEDURE 9-7: APPLYING A CHEMICAL COLD AND HOT PACK

Name _____   Date _____

Evaluated By _____   Score_____

Performance Objective

Outcome:	Apply a chemical cold and hot pack.
Conditions:	Given a chemical cold and hot pack.
Standards:	Time: 5 minutes
	Accuracy: Satisfactory score on the Performance Evaluation Checklist.

Performance Evaluation Checklist

Trial 1	Trial 2	Point Value	*Performance Standards*
		●	Washed hands.
		●	Assembled equipment.
		●	Greeted and identified patient.
		●	Introduced yourself and explained the procedure.
		●	Shook the crystals to the bottom of bag.
		●	Squeezed bag firmly to break inner water bag.
		●	Shook bag vigorously to mix the contents.
		●	Applied bag to affected area.
		●	Administered treatment for the proper length of time.
		●	Discarded bag in an appropriate receptacle.
		●	Charted the procedure correctly.
		★	Completed the procedure within 5 minutes.

CHART	
Date	

Evaluation of Student Performance

EVALUATION CRITERIA			COMMENTS
Symbol	Category	Point Value	
★	Critical Step	16 points	
●	Essential Step	6 points	
▷	Theory Question	2 points	
Score calculation: 100 points			
— _____ points missed			
_____ Score			
Satisfactory score: 85 or above			

AAMA/CAAHEP Competency Achieved:
☐ Prepare patient for and assist with procedures, treatments, and minor office surgery.

Evaluation of Competency

PROCEDURE 9-8: APPLYING AN ULTRASOUND TREATMENT

Name _____   Date _____

Evaluated By _____   Score_____

Performance Objective

Outcome:	Administer an ultrasound treatment.
Conditions:	Using an ultrasound machine.
	Given the following: coupling agent and paper towels.
Standards:	Time: 15 minutes
	Accuracy: Satisfactory score on the Performance Evaluation Checklist.

Performance Evaluation Checklist

Trial 1	Trial 2	Point Value	Performance Standards
		●	Washed hands.
		●	Assembled equipment.
		●	Greeted and identified patient.
		●	Introduced yourself and explained procedure.
		●	Instructed patient to report any pain or discomfort experienced during the treatment.
		●	Asked patient to remove appropriate clothing.
		●	Positioned patient for the treatment.
		●	Applied coupling agent liberally to patient's skin.
		▷	Is able to state why coupling agent should be at room temperature.
		●	Placed the intensity control at the minimum position.
		●	Set timer to the specified amount of time.
		●	Checked to make sure that the intensity control was at zero.
		●	Advanced the intensity control to the treatment level specified by physician.
		●	Placed applicator head into coupling medium in the treatment area.
		●	Moved applicator head in a back-and-forth stroking motion or in a circular motion at rate of 1 to 2 inches per second.

Trial 1	Trial 2	Point Value	Performance Standards
		▷	Is able to explain why applicator head should be moved continuously.
		●	Continued the treatment until timer went off.
		★	Moved applicator head continuously during the treatment.
		★	Did not remove applicator head from the skin and hold it up in the air during the treatment.
		▷	Is able to state why applicator head should not be held up in the air.
		●	Stopped the treatment immediately if patient complained of any pain or discomfort.
		●	Removed applicator head from patient's skin when timer went off.
		●	Turned the intensity control to the minimum position.
		●	Wiped coupling medium from applicator head.
		●	Wiped excess coupling medium from patient's skin with paper towel and instructed patient to get dressed.
		●	Washed hands.
		●	Charted the procedure correctly.
		★	Completed the procedure within 15 minutes.

CHART	
Date	

Evaluation of Student Performance

EVALUATION CRITERIA			COMMENTS
Symbol	Category	Point Value	
★	Critical Step	16 points	
●	Essential Step	6 points	
▷	Theory Question	2 points	

Score calculation: 100 points

_____ points missed

_____ Score

Satisfactory score: 85 or above

AAMA/CAAHEP Competencies Achieved:
☐ Prepare and maintain examination and treatment areas.
☐ Prepare patient for and assist with procedures, treatments, and minor office surgery.

Evaluation of Competency

PROCEDURE 9-9: MEASURING FOR AXILLARY CRUTCHES

Name _____   Date _____

Evaluated By _____   Score_____

Performance Objective

Outcome:	Measure for axillary crutches.
Conditions:	Given the following: axillary crutches, and a tape measure.
Standards:	Time: 10 minutes
	Accuracy: Satisfactory score on the Performance Evaluation Checklist.

Performance Evaluation Checklist

Trial 1	Trial 2	Point Value	Performance Standards
		●	Instructed patient to stand erect.
		●	Positioned crutches with the tips at a distance of 2 inches in front of, and 4 to 6 inches to the side of each foot.
		●	Adjusted crutch length so that the shoulder rests were approximately $1\frac{1}{2}$ to 2 inches below the axilla.
		●	Asked the patient to support his/her weight by the handgrips.
		●	Adjusted the handgrips so that patient's elbow was flexed approximately 30 degrees.
		●	Checked the fit of crutches by placing two fingers between the top of crutch and patient's axilla.
		●	Charted the procedure correctly.
		★	Completed the procedure within 10 minutes.
CHART			
Date			

Evaluation of Student Performance

EVALUATION CRITERIA			COMMENTS
Symbol	Category	Point Value	
★	Critical Step	16 points	
●	Essential Step	6 points	
▷	Theory Question	2 points	

Score calculation: 100 points

_____ points missed

_____ Score

Satisfactory score: 85 or above

AAMA/CAAHEP Competency Achieved:

☐ Prepare patient for and assist with procedures, treatments, and minor office surgery.

Evaluation of Competency

PROCEDURE 9-10: INSTRUCTING THE PATIENT IN CRUTCH GAITS

Name _____   Date _____

Evaluated By _____   Score_____

Performance Objective

Outcome:	Instruct an individual in the following crutch gaits: four-point, two-point, three-point, swing-to, and swing-through.
Conditions:	Given axillary crutches.
Accuracy:	Time: 15 minutes
	Accuracy: Satisfactory score on the Performance Evaluation Checklist.

Performance Evaluation Checklist

Trial 1	Trial 2	Point Value	Performance Standards
			Tripod Position
		●	Instructed the patient to:
		●	Stand erect and face straight ahead.
		●	Place the tips of crutches 4 to 6 inches in front of, and 4 to 6 inches to side of each foot.
		▷	Is able to state one use of the tripod position.
			Four-point Gait
		●	Instructed the patient to:
		●	Begin in the tripod position.
		●	Move the right crutch forward.
		●	Move the left foot forward to the level of the left crutch.
		●	Move the left crutch forward.
		●	Move the right foot forward to the level of the right crutch.
		●	Repeat the above sequence.
		▷	Is able to state one use of the four-point gait.
			Two-point Gait
		●	Instructed the patient to:
		●	Begin in the tripod position.
		●	Move the left crutch and the right foot forward at the same time.

Trial 1	Trial 2	Point Value	Performance Standards
		●	Move the right crutch and left foot forward at the same time.
		●	Repeat the above sequence.
		▷	Is able to state one use of the two-point gait.
			Three-point Gait
		●	Instructed patient to:
		●	Begin in the tripod position.
		●	Move both crutches and the affected leg forward.
		●	Move the unaffected leg forward while balancing weight on both crutches.
		●	Repeat the above sequence.
		▷	Is able to state two uses of the three-point gait.
			Swing-to Gait
		●	Instructed patient to:
		●	Begin in the tripod position.
		●	Move both crutches forward together.
		●	Lift and swing body to the crutches.
		●	Repeat the above sequence.
		▷	Is able to state one use of the swing-to gait.
			Swing-through Gait
		●	Instructed patient to:
		●	Begin in the tripod position.
		●	Move both crutches forward together.
		●	Lift and swing body past the crutches.
		●	Repeat the above sequence.
		▷	Is able to state one use of the swing-through gait.
		★	Completed the procedure within 15 minutes.

Evaluation of Student Performance

EVALUATION CRITERIA			COMMENTS
Symbol	**Category**	**Point Value**	
★	Critical Step	16 points	
●	Essential Step	6 points	
▷	Theory Question	2 points	
Score calculation: 100 points			
— points missed			
Score			
Satisfactory score: 85 or above			

AAMA/CAAHEP Competency Achieved:

☐ Prepare patient for and assist with procedures, treatments, and minor office surgery.

Notes

Evaluation of Competency

PROCEDURES 9-11 AND 9-12: INSTRUCTING THE PATIENT IN USE OF A CANE AND WALKER

Name _____   Date _____

Evaluated By _____   Score_____

Performance Objective

Outcome:	Instruct an individual in the use of a cane and walker.
Conditions:	Given the following: a cane, and a walker.
Standards:	Time: 10 minutes
	Accuracy: Satisfactory score on the Performance Evaluation Checklist.

Performance Evaluation Checklist

Trial 1	Trial 2	Point Value	Performance Standards
			CANE
		●	Instructed the patient to:
		●	Hold the cane on the strong side of body.
		●	Place tip of the cane 4 to 6 inches to the side of foot.
		●	Move the cane forward approximately 12 inches.
		●	Move the affected leg forward to the level of the cane.
		●	Move strong leg forward and ahead of the cane and weak leg.
		●	Repeat the above sequence.
		▷	Is able to state one condition for which a cane is used.
			WALKER
		●	Instructed the patient to:
		●	Pick up the walker and move it forward approximately 6 inches.
		●	Move the right foot and then the left foot up to the walker.
		●	Repeat the above sequence.
		▷	Is able to state one condition for which a walker is used.
		★	Completed the procedure within 10 minutes.

Evaluation of Student Performance

EVALUATION CRITERIA			COMMENTS
Symbol	**Category**	**Point Value**	
★	Critical Step	16 points	
●	Essential Step	6 points	
▷	Theory Question	2 points	
Score calculation: 100 points			
− _____ points missed			
_____ Score			
Satisfactory score: 85 or above			

AAMA/CAAHEP Competency Achieved:

☐ Prepare patient for and assist with procedures, treatments, and minor office surgery.

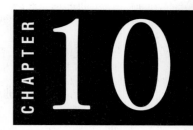

The Gynecologic Examination and Prenatal Care

The Gynecologic Examination

NAME _____

Directions: Match each medical term with its definition.

_____ 1. adnexal
_____ 2. atypical
_____ 3. cytology
_____ 4. endocervix
_____ 5. exfoliated cells
_____ 6. external os
_____ 7. gynecology
_____ 8. internal os
_____ 9. perineum
_____10. vulva

A. The opening of the cervical canal of the uterus into the vagina.
B. The mucous membrane lining the cervical canal.
C. Deviation from the normal.
D. The external region between the vaginal orifice and the anus in a female and between the scrotum and the anus in a male.
E. Adjacent
F. Cells that have been sloughed off from the surface of tissues into the secretions bathing those tissues.
G. The region of the external genital organs in the female.
H. The science that deals with the study of cells, including their origin, structure, function, and pathology.
I. The branch of medicine that deals with the diseases of the reproductive organs of women.
J. The internal opening of the cervical canal into the uterus.

Self-Evaluation

Directions: Fill in each blank with the correct answer.

1. What is the purpose of the gynecologic examination?

_____

_____

_____

2. What is the purpose of performing a breast examination?

_____

_____

_____

3. How often should a woman perform a breast self-examination at home? When should it be performed in relation to the menstrual cycle and why?

_____

_____

_____

4. What are the components of the pelvic examination?

_____

_____

5. What position is generally used for the pelvic examination?

_____

6. How can the medical assistant help the patient to relax during the pelvic examination?

_____

_____

7. What is the function of a vaginal speculum?

_____

_____

8. List two reasons for moistening a vaginal speculum with warm water before insertion.

_____

_____

9. What is the purpose of performing a visual examination of the vagina and the cervix?

_____

_____

10. What is the purpose of performing a Pap test?

_____

_____

11. Describe the schedule for having a Pap test recommended by the American Cancer Society.

_____

_____

_____

_____

12. Why should the medical assistant instruct the patient not to douche or insert vaginal medications for 48 hours before coming to the medical office to have a Pap smear taken?

_____

_____

_____

_____

13. Why shouldn't a smear for a Pap test be taken from a woman during her menstrual period?

_____

_____

14. What are the three types of specimens that may be obtained for a Pap smear?

_____

_____

_____

15. Why must the slides be fixed immediately after collection of the Pap smear?

_____

_____

_____

16. List three conditions that the maturation index can help to evaluate.

_____

_____

_____

17. Why is the Bethesda system now recommended for reporting the results of the Pap test?

_____

_____

_____

18. What is the purpose of performing the bimanual pelvic examination?

_____

_____

_____

19. Describe the laboratory procedure that can be used to identify *Trichomonas vaginalis* in the medical office.

_____

_____

_____

20. What is the name of a common drug used to treat trichomoniasis? Why must the patient's sexual partner also be treated?

_____

_____

21. Describe the laboratory procedure that can be used to identify *Candida albicans* in the medical office.

_____

_____

_____

22. What special growth conditions are required for culturing *Neisseria gonorrhoeae?*

_____

_____

_____

23. What laboratory procedure is used to detect the presence of *Neisseria gonorrhoeae* in the male? Why can't this method be used to detect its presence in the female?

_____

_____

24. What complications may result from a chlamydial infection (in both male and female patients)?

_____

_____

_____

_____

25. List the symptoms (in the female) of each of the following sexually transmitted diseases.

a. trichomoniasis: _____

_____

_____

_____

b. candidiasis: _____

_____

_____

_____

c. gonorrhea: _____

_____

_____

_____

d. chlamydia: _____

_____

_____

_____

Critical Thinking Skills

1. Susan Alland, age 19, has come to the office for a gynecologic examination. It is the first time she has had this procedure performed, and she seems apprehensive about it. Explain how you could reduce her anxiety and help her to prepare for the examination.

_____

_____

_____

_____

2. In a role-playing situation, one person takes the role of the medical assistant and another the role of Mrs. Clemmer. The medical assistant's responsibility is to verbally instruct Mrs. Clemmer in the procedure for breast self-examination. List the important points that should be included.

_____

_____

_____

_____

_____

3. The following symptomatic terms relating to gynecology may be used in the medical office. Using a reference source, define each in the space provided.

    a. amenorrhea

_____

_____

    b. dysmenorrhea

_____

_____

    c. menorrhagia

_____

_____

    d. metrorrhagia

_____

_____

4. Patients coming to the medical office for gynecologic examinations frequently ask the medical assistant questions regarding methods of contraception. The medical assistant should have a knowledge of the various types of contraceptives, how they work to prevent pregnancy, and the advantages and disadvantages of each. A list of common contraceptive methods is presented on the next page. Using a reference source, list the information requested for each in the spaces provided.

Contraceptive Method	Mode of Action	Advantages	Disadvantages
Oral Contraceptives (Birth Control Pills)			
Diaphragm			
Vaginal Spermicide			
IUD (Intrauterine Device)			
Condom			
Rhythm Method			
Sterilization (Tubal Ligation and Vasectomy)			

Prenatal Care

NAME _____

Key Terminology Assessment

Directions: Match each medical term with its definition.

_____ 1. abortion
_____ 2. Braxton Hicks contractions
_____ 3. dilation (of the cervix)
_____ 4. EDD
_____ 5. effacement
_____ 6. engagement
_____ 7. fetal heart tones
_____ 8. fetus
_____ 9. fundus
_____ 10. gestation
_____ 11. gravidity
_____ 12. high-risk
_____ 13. infant
_____ 14. lochia
_____ 15. multipara
_____ 16. multigravida
_____ 17. nullipara
_____ 18. obstetrics
_____ 19. parity
_____ 20. pelvimetry
_____ 21. postpartum
_____ 22. prenatal
_____ 23. primigravida
_____ 24. primipara
_____ 25. puerperium
_____ 26. quickening
_____ 27. trimester

A. A woman who has completed two or more pregnancies to the age of viability regardless of whether they ended in live infants or stillbirths.
B. The entrance of the fetal head or the presenting part into the pelvic inlet.
C. Before birth.
D. Three months or one-third of the gestational period of pregnancy.
E. The condition of having borne offspring who had attained the age of viability regardless of whether they were live infants or stillbirths.
F. The period of time in which the uterus and the body systems are returning to normal following delivery.
G. The loss of a pregnancy before the stage of viability.
H. The dome-shaped upper portion of the uterus between the fallopian tubes.
I. Having an increased possibility of suffering harm, damage, or death.
J. The first movements of the fetus in utero as felt by the mother.
K. The child in utero, from the third month after conception to birth.
L. A woman who has been pregnant more than once.
M. Expected date of delivery, or due date.
N. A woman who has carried a pregnancy to viability regardless of whether the infant was dead or alive at birth.
O. The stretching of the external os from an opening a few millimeters in size to an opening large enough to allow the passage of an infant.

P. The period of intrauterine development from conception to birth.

Q. A discharge from the uterus after delivery consisting of blood, tissue, white blood cells, and some bacteria.

R. The thinning and shortening of the cervical canal from its normal length to a structure in which there is no canal at all.

S. The total number of pregnancies a woman has had, regardless of duration, including a current pregnancy.

T. A woman who has not carried a pregnancy to the point of viability.

U. That branch of medicine concerned with the care of the woman during pregnancy, childbirth, and the postpartal period.

V. A woman who is pregnant for the first time.

W. Occurring after childbirth.

X. Intermittent and irregular, painless uterine contractions that occur throughout pregnancy.

Y. Measurement of the capacity and diameter of the maternal pelvis.

Z. The heart beat of the fetus as heard through the mother's abdominal wall.

AB. A child from birth to 1 year of age.

Self-Evaluation

Directions: Fill in each blank with the correct answer.

1. List the three categories of medical office visits for provision of prenatal and postnatal care to the pregnant woman.

_____
_____
_____

2. List the four components of the first prenatal visit.

_____
_____
_____
_____

3. What is the purpose of the prenatal record?

_____

_____

4. List two types of information included in the past medical history (of the prenatal record).

_____

_____

5. List three types of information included in the present pregnancy history.

_____

_____

_____

6. What is the purpose of the interval prenatal history?

_____

_____

7. Explain the importance of performing a physical examination on the prenatal patient.

_____

_____

_____

8. List the procedures generally included in the initial prenatal examination and, next to each procedure, list the purpose for performing each.

_____

_____

_____

_____

_____

_____

_____

9. What is the importance of making sure a pregnant woman does not have gonorrhea before delivery of the infant?

_____

_____

10. What is the purpose of performing a hemoglobin and hematocrit evaluation on a prenatal patient?

_____

_____

11. What is the importance of assessing the Rh factor and ABO blood type of a pregnant woman?

_____

_____

12. What is the purpose of performing a 1-hour glucose tolerance test on a pregnant woman?

_____

_____

13. What is the purpose of performing a rubella titer test on a pregnant woman?

_____

_____

14. What is the purpose of the return prenatal visit? List the usual schedule for return prenatal visits.

_____

_____

_____

15. What tests are performed on the patient's urine specimen at each return visit and why are each of these performed?

_____

_____

_____

_____

16. List two purposes of measuring the fundal height.

_____

_____

17. What is the normal range for the fetal heart rate?

_____

18. What is the purpose of performing a vaginal examination as the patient nears term?

_____

_____

19. What is the purpose for performing each of the following special tests and procedures?

Alpha-fetoprotein analysis: _____

_____

Obstetric ultrasound scanning: _____

_____

Amniocentesis: _____

_____

Fetal heart rate monitoring: _____

_____

20. What type of patient preparation is required for an obstetric ultrasound scan using an abdominal transducer?

_____

_____

21. What conditions might warrant performing an amniocentesis?

_____

_____

_____

22. What is the difference between the following fetal heart rate monitoring tests: non-stress test and contraction stress test?

_____

_____

_____

23. What occurs during the puerperium?

_____

_____

24. Explain the changes in the lochia that should normally occur during the puerperium.

_____

_____

_____

_____

25. List the procedures generally included in the 6-weeks postpartum examination.

_____

_____

_____

_____

Critical Thinking Skills

1. Listed here are common signs and symptoms of pregnancy. Using a reference source, define each and, if possible, explain what causes the sign or symptom to occur.

   a. amenorrhea

   _____

   _____

   b. fatigue

   _____

   _____

   c. urinary frequency

   _____

   _____

   d. quickening

   _____

   _____

   e. Goodell's sign

   _____

   _____

   f. Hegar's sign

   _____

   _____

   g. Braxton Hicks contractions

   _____

   _____

   h. skin changes: striae gravidarum, chloasma, linea nigra

   _____

   _____

   _____

   _____

2. Calculate the EDD of the following patients using Nägele's rule. The first day of each patient's last menstrual period (LMP) is listed here:

   a. February 10, 2002 _____

   b. April 28, 2002 _____

   c. July 20, 2002 _____

   d. October 2, 2002 _____

   e. December 22, 2002 _____

3. The following patients are in your medical office for their first prenatal visit. In the space provided, record the following information in terms of gravida, para, abortion.

   a. Mrs. Turner is pregnant for the third time. Her first pregnancy resulted in the birth of a baby boy, now alive and well. She lost her second pregnancy at 3 months' gestation.

   _____

   b. Mrs. Stewart is pregnant for the third time. Her first pregnancy resulted in the birth of twin girls, now alive and well. Her second pregnancy resulted in the birth of a baby girl, now alive and well.

   _____

   c. Mrs. Rose is pregnant for the fourth time. She lost her first pregnancy at 2 month's gestation. Her second pregnancy was carried to term, but resulted in the birth of a stillborn. Her third pregnancy resulted in the birth of a baby girl, now alive and well.

   _____

4. Mrs. Barry is in your medical office for her first prenatal visit. Her next visit has been scheduled on a Tuesday afternoon at 3:00 P.M. The medical office policy is such that a first-voided morning clean-catch midstream specimen is required for urine testing at each visit. The medical office supplies the urine specimen container for the patient. Using terms the patient would understand (and in the space provided), explain the procedure to Mrs. Barry for the proper collection and handling of this urine specimen.

   _____

   _____

   _____

   _____

   _____

5. Mrs. Daley is pregnant for the first time and is concerned about adequate nutrition during her pregnancy. Using a reference source, list the nutrients that are of particular importance during pregnancy, why each is important, and good food sources of each.

Nutrient	Importance During Pregnancy	Food Sources

6. Listed here are the minor discomforts that a prenatal patient may experience during pregnancy. Using a reference source, indicate measures the patient can take to help prevent or relieve each discomfort.

    a. morning sickness

_____

_____

    b. heartburn

_____

_____

    c. flatulence

_____

_____

    d. constipation

_____

_____

    e. backache

_____

_____

f. respiratory discomfort

_____

_____

g. varicose veins

_____

_____

h. hemorrhoids

_____

_____

i. leg cramps

_____

_____

j. edema of the lower legs

_____

_____

7. Obtain a prenatal guidebook and list the information included in it regarding guidelines the patient should follow with respect to each of the following areas:

a. nutrition

_____

_____

b. employment

_____

_____

c. exercise

_____

_____

d. travel

_____

_____

e. smoking

_____

_____

f. alcohol

_____

_____

g. medication

_____

_____

8. Mrs. Clark asks you for information regarding the advantages and disadvantages of
    both breast-feeding and bottle feeding. Using a reference source, list these in the fol-
    lowing chart.

Breast-feeding	
Advantages	*Disadvantages*

Bottle feeding	
Advantages	*Disadvantages*

Practice for Competency

BREAST SELF-EXAMINATION

Assignment

Instruct an individual in the procedure for performing a breast self-examination and record the procedure in the chart provided.

CHART	
Date	

Practice for Competency

GYNECOLOGICAL EXAMINATION

Assignment

1. Complete the cytology request form provided on the next page, using a female classmate as the patient.
2. Practice the procedure for assisting with a gynecologic examination. Record the vital signs and height and weight in the chart provided.

CHART	
Date	

Cytology Request Form

Please Print or Type
NAME OF
PATIENT _____

DO NOT WRITE HERE	Last	First	Date of Birth	Age
	Number and Street	City	State	Zip

TYPE OF SPECIMEN
☐ Vaginal   ☐ Maturation Index
☐ Cervical   ☐ Other

Last Menstrual Period

_____
Month   Day   Year

☐ Abnormal Vaginal Bleeding   ☐ Hormone Therapy
☐ Abnormal Vaginal Discharge   ☐ Pregnancy
☐ Previous Pelvic Surgery (Type) _____
☐ Radiation Therapy Date _____ ☐ Previous Cytology_____
Clinical Diagnosis and Remarks_____

Physicians Name and Address

BILLING INFORMATION:

☐ Bill Patient   ☐ Bill Physician   ☐ Bill Medicare #
☐ Bill Welfare # _____
Case Name _____ Pt. 2 Digit #_____
Other _____

CYTOPATHOLOGY CONSULTATION REQUEST   Date _____

Evaluation of Competency

INSTRUCTING A PATIENT ON BREAST SELF-EXAMINATION

Name _____   Date _____

Evaluated By _____   Score_____

Performance Objective

Outcome:	Instruct an individual in the procedure for performing a breast self-examination.
Conditions:	No equipment or supplies required.
Standards:	Time: 5 minutes
	Accuracy: Satisfactory score on the Performance Evaluation Checklist.

Performance Evaluation Checklist

Trial 1	Trial 2	Point Value	Performance Standards
		●	Greeted and identified the patient.
		●	Introduced yourself and explained that you will be instructing the patient in a BSE.
			Instructed the Patient as Follows:
			Before a Mirror
		●	Inspect the breasts with arms at sides.
		●	Raise arms high over head.
		●	Look for any change in shape or contour of each breast.
		●	Observe for swelling, dimpling of skin, or changes in the nipple.
		●	Rest palms on hips and press down firmly to flex chest muscles.
		●	Observe for swelling, dimpling of skin, or changes in the nipple.
		●	Gently squeeze the nipple and look for a discharge.
			Lying Down
		●	Put a pillow under right shoulder to examine the right breast.
		▷	Is able to state the purpose of the pillow.
		●	Place right hand behind head.
		●	Use the finger pads of the middle three fingers of the left hand to feel for lumps or changes using a rubbing motion.
		●	Press firmly enough to feel the different breast tissues.

Trial 1	Trial 2	Point Value	Performance Standards
		●	Pay special attention to the area between the breast and underarm including the underarm itself.
		●	Use one of the following patterns to move around the breast: circular, vertical, strip, or the wedge.
		●	Choose the method that is easiest for you.
		●	Completely feel all of the breast and chest area from your collarbone to the base of a properly fitted bra and from the breast bone to the underarm.
		●	Continue the examination until every part of the right breast has been examined, including the nipple.
		●	Repeat the procedure on the left breast, with a pillow under left shoulder and using right hand.
			In the Shower
		●	Examine breasts in the bath or shower.
		▷	Is able to state why the breasts should be examined in the bath or shower.
		●	Holding fingers flat, move gently over every part of each breast.
		●	Use right hand to examine the left breast and left hand to examine the right breast.
		●	Check for lumps, hard knots, or thickening.
		●	Report any abnormalities to the physician.
		●	Charted the patient instructions correctly.
		★	Completed the procedure within 5 minutes.

CHART	
Date	

Evaluation of Student Performance

EVALUATION CRITERIA			COMMENTS
Symbol	**Category**	**Point Value**	
★	Critical Step	16 points	
●	Essential Step	6 points	
▷	Theory Question	2 points	

Score calculation: 100 points

— _____ points missed

_____ Score

Satisfactory score: 85 or above

AAMA/CAAHEP Competency Achieved:

☐ Provide instructions for health maintenance and disease prevention.

Notes

Evaluation of Competency

PROCEDURE 10-1: ASSISTING WITH A GYNECOLOGIC EXAMINATION

Name _____   Date _____

Evaluated By _____   Score_____

Performance Objective

Outcome:	Assist with a gynecologic examination.
Conditions:	Using an examining table.
	Given the following: disposable gloves, examining gown and drape, vaginal speculum, cervical scraper, cotton-tipped applicator or cytology brush, glass slides with a frosted edge, cytology fixative, lubricant, tissues, and a biohazard waste container.
Standards:	Time: 15 minutes
	Accuracy: Satisfactory score on the Performance Evaluation Checklist

Performance Evaluation Checklist

Trial 1	Trial 2	Point Value	*Performance Standards*
		●	Washed hands.
		●	Assembled equipment.
		●	Identified the slides on the frosted edge.
		●	Completed the cytology request form.
		●	Greeted and identified patient.
		●	Introduced yourself and explained procedure.
		●	Asked patient if she needs to empty bladder.
		▷	Is able to state why bladder should be empty for the examination.
		●	Prepared and instructed the patient for the examination.
		●	Measured vital signs and height and weight and charted the results correctly.
		●	Assisted patient onto examining table.
		●	Positioned and draped patient in a supine position for the breast examination.

Trial 1	Trial 2	Point Value	Performance Standards
		●	Positioned and draped patient in the lithotomy position for the pelvic examination.
		●	Adjusted and focused the light for physician.
		●	Reassured patient and helped her to relax during the examination.
		▷	Is able to explain why patient should be relaxed during the examination.
			Assisted the physician during the examination as follows:
		●	Warmed vaginal speculum before insertion.
		▷	Is able to state why a cold speculum should not be inserted into the vagina.
		●	Assisted physician with application of gloves.
		●	Applied gloves and assisted with Pap smear.
		●	Immediately fixed the slides.
		▷	Is able to explain why the slides should be fixed immediately after collection.
		●	Applied lubricant to physician's glove for the bimanual and rectal examinations.
		●	Instructed patient to move back on examining table, pulled out the footrest and the table extension and removed both of the patient's legs from the stirrups simultaneously.
		●	Allowed patient to rest in the supine position.
		●	Returned stirrups to the normal position.
		●	Offered patient tissues to remove lubricant from the perineum.
		●	Assisted patient into sitting position.
		●	Pushed in table extension while supporting patient's lower legs.
		●	Assisted patient from examining table.
		●	Instructed patient to get dressed.
		●	Informed patient of the method used by the medical office to relay test results.
		●	Prepared Pap slide for transport to the laboratory, making sure to include the completed cytology request form.
		●	Correctly charted the transport of the Pap slides to an outside laboratory.
		●	Cleaned the examining room in preparation for the next patient.
		●	Sanitized and sterilized the vaginal speculum.
		★	Completed the procedure within 15 minutes.

CHART	
Date	

Evaluation of Student Performance

EVALUATION CRITERIA			COMMENTS
Symbol	Category	Point Value	
★	Critical Step	16 points	
●	Essential Step	6 points	
▷	Theory Question	2 points	

Score calculation: 100 points

− _____ points missed

_____ Score

Satisfactory score: 85 or above

AAMA/CAAHEP Competencies Achieved:
- ☐ Obtain vital signs.
- ☐ Prepare and maintain examination and treatment areas.
- ☐ Prepare patient for and assist with routine and specialty examinations.
- ☐ Instruct individuals according to their needs.

Cytology Request Form

Please Print or Type
NAME OF
PATIENT _____

DO
NOT
WRITE
HERE

Last	First	Date of Birth	Age

Number and Street	City	State	Zip

TYPE OF SPECIMEN
☐ Vaginal   ☐ Maturation Index
☐ Cervical   ☐ Other

Last Menstrual Period

Month   Day   Year

☐ Abnormal Vaginal Bleeding   ☐ Hormone Therapy
☐ Abnormal Vaginal Discharge   ☐ Pregnancy
☐ Previous Pelvic Surgery (Type) _____
☐ Radiation Therapy Date _____ ☐ Previous Cytology _____
Clinical Diagnosis and Remarks _____

Physicians Name and Address

BILLING INFORMATION:

☐ Bill Patient   ☐ Bill Physician   ☐ Bill Medicare #
☐ Bill Welfare # _____
Case Name _____ Pt. 2 Digit # _____
Other _____

CYTOPATHOLOGY CONSULTATION REQUEST   Date _____

Practice for Competency

ASSISTING WITH A RETURN PRENATAL EXAMINATION

Assignment

1. Complete the prenatal health history form on the following pages using a female classmate as the patient.

2. Prepare the patient and assist with a return prenatal examination. Record the results of procedures you performed on the form provided below.

INTERVAL PRENATAL HISTORY

Flow Chart Date	Year Weight this visit	Pre-gravid Blood pressure	Protein	Urine Sugar	Est. weeks gestation (dates/sizes)	Fundal height	Fetal heart rate	Edema	PROGRESS NOTES	See Add Prog Note

Prenatal Health History Summary

Date:

Patient's name _____

_____

_____

Age____ Race____ Religion _____ Marital status _____ Years married ____ Education _____ Occupation _____

Home address _____ Home tel. _____ Work tel. _____

Nearest relative _____ Relative's employer _____ Work tel. _____

Referring physician _____ Attending physician _____

PAST MEDICAL HISTORY

Check and detail positive findings including date and place of treatment. Precede findings by reference number.

#		Patient	Family
1.	Congenital anomalies		
2.	Genetic diseases		
3.	Multiple births		
4.	Diabetes mellitus		
5.	Malignancies		
6.	Hypertension		
7.	Heart disease		
8.	Rheumatic fever		
9.	Pulmonary disease		
10.	GI problems		
11.	Renal disease		
12.	Other urinary tract problems		
13.	Genitourinary anomalies		
14.	Abnormal uterine bleeding		
15.	Infertility		
16.	Venereal disease		
17.	Phlebitis, varicosities		
18.	Nervous/mental disorders		
19.	Convulsive disorders		
20.	Metabol./endocrine disorders		
21.	Anemia/hemoglobinopathy		
22.	Blood dyscrasias		
23.	Drug addiction		
24.	Smoking/alcohol		
25.	Infectious diseases		
26.	Operations/accidents		
27.	Blood transfusions		
28.	Other hospitalizations		
29.	**No known disease**		

Menstrual History   Onset ____ age   Cycle ____ q.   ____ days   Length ____ days   Amount

Last contraceptive ☐ None   Type _____   Last used _____

PAST OBSTETRICAL HISTORY

Grav | Para | Pret | Abort | Live

No.	Month/year	Sex	Weight at birth	Wks. gest.	Hrs. in labor	Type of delivery	Details of delivery: include anesthesia and maternal or newborn complications. Use Risk Guide numbers where applicable
1							
2							
3							
4							
5							
6							
7							
8							

Sensitivities (detail positive findings)

30. ☐ **None known**
31. ☐ Antibiotics
32. ☐ Analgesics
33. ☐ Sedatives
34. ☐ Anesthesia
35. ☐ Other

Preexisting Risk Guide

Indicates pregnancy/outcome at risk

36. ☐ Age < 15 or > 35
37. ☐ < 8th grade education
38. ☐ Cardiac disease (class I or II)
39. ☐ Tuberculosis, active
40. ☐ Chronic pulmonary disease
41. ☐ Thrombophlebitis
42. ☐ Endocrinopathy
43. ☐ Epilepsy (on medication)
44. ☐ Infertility (treated)
45. ☐ 2 abortions (spontaneous/induced)
46. ☐ ≥ 7 deliveries
47. ☐ Previous preterm or SGA infants
48. ☐ Infants ≥ 4,000 gms
49. ☐ Iosimmunization (ABO, etc.)
50. ☐ Hemorrhage during previous preg
51. ☐ Previous preeclampsia
52. ☐ Surgically scarred uterus
53. ☐ _____

Indicates pregnancy/outcome at **high risk**

54. ☐ Age ≥ 40
55. ☐ Diabetes mellitus
56. ☐ Hypertension
57. ☐ Cardiac disease (class III or IV)
58. ☐ Chronic renal disease
59. ☐ Congenital/chromosomal anomalies
60. ☐ Hemoglobinopathies
61. ☐ Isoimmunization (Rh)
62. ☐ Drug addiction/alcoholism
63. ☐ Habitual abortions
64. ☐ Incompetent cervix
65. ☐ Prior fetal or neonatal death
66. ☐ Prior neurologically damaged infant
67. ☐ _____

Initial Risk Assessment

68. ☐ No risk factors noted
69. ☐ At risk
70. ☐ At high risk

Signature

PRESENT PREGNANCY HISTORY

History Since LMP	Patient
1. Headaches	
2. Nausea/vomiting	
3. Abdominal pain	
4. Urinary complaints	
5. Vaginal discharge	
6. Vaginal bleeding	
7. Edema (specify area)	
8. Febrile episode	
9. Rubella exposure	
10. Other viral exposure	
11. Drug exposure	
12. Radiation exposure	
13. Other	

L
M
P   date   quality
E
D
C

16. Medications Since LMP

(Rx, non-Rx, vitamins) ☐ None

Describe: _____

_____

_____

_____

Comments:

Initial Physical Examination			Height	Weight	Pregravid weight	B.P.	Pulse	
SYSTEM	Normal	ABN	Check and detail all positive findings below. Use reference numbers.					
17. Skin								
18. EENT								
19. Mouth								
20. Neck								
21. Chest								
22. Breast								
23. Heart								
24. Lungs								
25. Abdomen								
26. Musculoskeletal								
27. Extremities								
28. Neurologic								
Pelvic Examination								
29. Ext. genitalia								
30. Vagina								
31. Cervix								
32. Uterus (describe)								
33. Adnexa								
34. Rectum								
35. Other								

Bony	36. Diag. conj.	37. Shape sacrum	38. S.S. notch	39. Ischial spines
Pelvis	40. Pubic arch	41. Trans. outlet	42. Post. sag. diam.	43. Coccyx

44. Classification:	☐ Gynecoid	☐ Android	☐ Anthropoid	☐ Platypelloid
45. Estimation:	☐ Adequate	☐ Borderline	☐ Contracted	

Exam by:

INTERVAL PRENATAL HISTORY

Flow Chart Date	Weight this visit	Year Pre-gravid	Blood pressure	Protein	Sugar	Urine Est. weeks gestation (dates/sizes)	Fundal height	Fetal heart rate	Edema	PROGRESS NOTES	See Add Pro Not

Risk Guide for Pregnancy and Outcome

Risk Guide for Pregnancy and Outcome

☐ (0) No risk factors noted _____

☐ (1) At risk _____

☐ (2) **High risk**

Continuing Risk Guide

Mo/day	Potential risk factors	Mo/day	High risk factors
/	3. Preg. without familial support	/	18. Diabetes mellitis
/	4. Second pregnancy in 12 months	/	19. Hypertension
/	5. Smoking (≥ 1 pack per day)	/	20. Thrombophlebitis
/	6. Rh negative (nonsensitized)	/	21. Herpes (type 2)
/	7. Uterine/cervical malformation	/	22. Rh sensitization
/	8. Inadequate pelvis	/	23. Uterine bleeding
/	9. Venereal disease	/	24. Hydramnois
/	10. Anemia (Hct < 30%:Hgb < 10%)	/	25. Severe preeclampsia
/	11. Acute pyelonephritis	/	26. Fetal growth retardation
/	12. Failure to gain weight	/	27. Premature rupt. membranes
/	13. Multiple pregnancy (term)	/	28. Multiple pregnancy (preterm)
/	14. Abnormal presentation	/	29. Low/failing estriols
/	15. Postterm pregnancy	/	30. Significant social problems
/	16.	/	31. Alcohol and drug abuse
/	17.	/	32.

Comments:

Evaluation of Competency

PROCEDURE 10-2: ASSISTING WITH A RETURN PRENATAL EXAMINATION

Name _____   Date _____

Evaluated By _____   Score_____

Performance Objective

Outcome:	Prepare the patient and assist with a return prenatal examination.
Conditions:	Using an examining table.
	Given the following: patient gown, patient drape, flexible, nonstretchable centimeter tape measure, Doppler fetal pulse detector, ultrasound coupling agent, vaginal speculum, disposable gloves, lubricant, and a biohazard waste container.
Standards:	Time: 15 minutes
	Accuracy: Satisfactory score on the Performance Evaluation Checklist.

Performance Evaluation Checklist

Trial 1	Trial 2	Point Value	Performance Standards
		●	Washed hands.
		●	Set up the tray for the prenatal examination.
		●	Greeted and identified the patient.
		●	Introduced yourself and obtained the urine specimen from her.
		●	Asked the patient if she has experienced any problems since her last prenatal visit and recorded information in the prenatal record.
		●	Measured patient's blood pressure and charted the results correctly.
		●	Weighed the patient and charted the results correctly.
		▷	Is able to state the importance of weighing the patient.
		●	Asked patient if she needs to empty her bladder.
		●	Instructed and prepared patient for the examination.
		●	Tested the urine specimen for glucose and protein and charted the results correctly.
		●	Assisted patient onto examining table.
		●	Positioned patient in a supine position and properly draped her.

Trial 1	Trial 2	Point Value	Performance Standards
		●	Placed patient's chart in a convenient location for review by physician and informed physician that patient was ready to be examined.
		●	Assisted physician as required during the examination.
		●	Handed physician the tape measure for determination of fundal height.
		●	Handed physician Doppler device.
		●	Assisted patient into the lithotomy position if a vaginal specimen is to be obtained or if vaginal examination is to be performed.
		●	Assisted physician with glove application and lubricants as required for a vaginal examination.
		●	Assisted patient into a sitting position and allowed her to rest.
		●	Assisted patient from examining table.
		●	Provided patient teaching and explanation of physician's instructions as required.
		●	Cleaned the examining room in preparation for the next patient.
		●	Prepared any specimens collected for transport to an outside laboratory, including the completed laboratory request form.
		★	Completed the procedure within 15 minutes.

INTERVAL PRENATAL HISTORY

Flow Chart	Date	Weight this visit	Year Pre-gravid	Blood pressure	Protein	Sugar	Urine	Est. weeks gestation (dates/sizes)	Fundal height	Fetal heart rate	Edema	PROGRESS NOTES

Evaluation of Student Performance

EVALUATION CRITERIA			COMMENTS
Symbol	**Category**	**Point Value**	
★	Critical Step	16 points	
●	Essential Step	6 points	
▷	Theory Question	2 points	

Score calculation: 100 points

  −_____ points missed

  _____ Score

Satisfactory score: 85 or above

AAMA/CAAHEP Competencies Achieved:

☐ Respond to and initiate written communications.
☐ Recognize and respond to verbal communications.
☐ Recognize and respond to nonverbal communications.
☐ Obtain vital signs.
☐ Obtain and record patient history.
☐ Prepare and maintain examination and treatment areas.
☐ Prepare patient for and assist with routine and specialty examinations.
☐ Provide instruction for health maintenance and disease prevention.

Notes

The Pediatric Examination

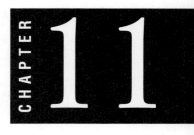

CHAPTER 11

NAME _____

Key Terminology Assessment

Directions: Match each medical term with its definition.

_____ 1. immunity
_____ 2. immunization
_____ 3. infant
_____ 4. length
_____ 5. pediatrician
_____ 6. pediatrics
_____ 7. stature
_____ 8. toxoid
_____ 9. vaccine
_____10. vertex

A. A medical doctor who specializes in the care and development of children and the diagnosis and treatment of diseases of children.
B. The height of the body in a standing position.
C. The summit, or top, especially the top of the head.
D. The resistance of the body to the effects of a harmful agent such as a pathogenic microorganism or its toxins.
E. The branch of medicine dealing with the care and development of children and the diagnosis and treatment of diseases of children.
F. A suspension of attenuated or killed microorganisms administered to an individual to prevent an infectious disease by stimulating the production of antibodies in that individual.
G. The process of becoming immune or of rendering an individual immune through the use of a vaccine or toxoid.
H. The measurement from the vertex of the head to the heel of the foot in a supine position.
I. A toxin that has been treated by heat or chemicals to destroy its harmful properties. It is administered to an individual to prevent an infectious disease by stimulating the production of antibodies in that individual.
J. A child from birth to 1 year of age.

Self-Evaluation

Directions: Fill in each blank with the correct answer.

1. What are the components of the health maintenance visit?

    _____

    _____

    _____

    _____

2. What is the usual schedule for health maintenance visits?

    _____

    _____

    _____

3. What is the purpose of the sick-child visit?

    _____

    _____

4. What procedures are often performed by the medical assistant during pediatric office visits?

    _____

    _____

    _____

5. Why is it important for the medical assistant to develop a rapport with the pediatric patient?

    _____

    _____

    _____

6. List the two positions that can be used to safely carry the infant.

    _____

    _____

7. Why is it important to measure the growth (weight and height or length) of the child during each office visit?

    _____

    _____

8. What is the difference between stature (height) and recumbent length?

_____

_____

9. What is the purpose of measuring head circumference?

_____

_____

10. According to the American Academy of Pediatrics, how often should blood pressure be measured in children?

_____

_____

11. List three purposes for collecting a urine specimen from a child.

_____

_____

_____

12. Why should the child's genitalia be cleansed before applying a pediatric urine collector?

_____

_____

13. Why is the dorsogluteal site *not* recommended for use as an intramuscular injection site in infants and young children?

_____

_____

_____

14. Why is the vastus lateralis muscle recommended as a good site for giving an intramuscular injection to an infant or young child?

_____

_____

_____

15. What is the difference between a vaccine and a toxoid?

_____

_____

_____

16. List the schedule for each of the following pediatric immunizations as recommended by the American Academy of Pediatrics.

DTaP: _____

_____

Polio: _____

_____

MMR: _____

_____

Hib: _____

_____

17. What information must be provided to parents as required by the National Childhood Vaccine Injury Act?

_____

_____

18. According to the NCVIA, what information must be recorded in the patient's medical record after a pediatric immunization has been administered?

_____

_____

_____

19. What is the purpose of the PKU screening test?

_____

_____

20. Why can the PKU screening test be performed earlier on infants on formula as compared with breast-fed babies?

_____

_____

_____

Critical Thinking Skills

1. Why would it be better for the medical assistant to take the temperature of an infant or young child before procedures are performed that are apt to make him or her cry?

_____

_____

2. Locate the following weight values on your pediatric scale. Place a check mark next to each one after it has been correctly located.

a. 7 pounds, 9 ounces _____   e. 19 pounds, 7 ounces _____
b. 8 pounds, 5 ounces _____   f. 23 pounds, 6 ounces _____
c. 12 pounds, 10 ounces _____   g. 25 pounds, 3 ounces _____
d. 15 pounds, 11 ounces _____

3. Locate the following length values on your pediatric measuring device. Place a check mark next to each after it has been correctly located.

a. $20\frac{1}{2}$ inches _____   e. $28\frac{1}{2}$ inches _____
b. $22\frac{1}{4}$ inches _____   f. 31 inches _____
c. 24 inches _____   g. $33\frac{1}{4}$ inches _____
d. $25\frac{3}{4}$ inches _____   h. $36\frac{1}{2}$ inches _____

4. Teresa Fulk, age 4, is apprehensive about standing on the scale and having her weight taken and appears reluctant to participate. What could you do to help gain her cooperation?

_____

_____

_____

5. Matthew Williams, age 2 years (24 months), has had health maintenance visits at the intervals listed below. His length and weight measurements were taken during each visit and are recorded here. Plot these on the growth chart on page 419 of your textbook. Calculate the percentile for each and record it in the space provided. *Note:* His birth weight was 7 pounds, 8 ounces, and his length was 20 inches.

Health Maintenance Visit

	WEIGHT	PERCENTILE	LENGTH	PERCENTILE
1 month	9 lb, 10 oz	_____	22 in	_____
2 months	12 lb, 4 oz	_____	$23\frac{1}{2}$ in	_____
4 months	16 lb, 5 oz	_____	$25\frac{1}{4}$ in	_____
6 months	18 lb, 8 oz	_____	27 in	_____
9 months	22 lb, 4 oz	_____	$29\frac{1}{4}$ in	_____
12 months	24 lb, 4 oz	_____	$30\frac{1}{2}$ in	_____
15 months	26 lb, 8 oz	_____	$31\frac{1}{2}$ in	_____
18 months	27 lb	_____	$32\frac{1}{2}$ in	_____
24 months	28 lb	_____	$35\frac{3}{4}$ in	_____

6. Using a reference source, describe the motor and social development of the age groups listed here. The first one is done for you.

AGE	MOTOR AND SOCIAL DEVELOPMENT
Birth to 3 months	Raises head but not stable, can turn head from side to side, activities are limited to reflexes, cries when hungry, responsive social smile, coos, eyes can focus on an object and follow a moving object 180 degrees.
4 to 6 months	
7 to 9 months	
10 to 12 months	
1 year	
2 years	
3 years	
4 years	
5 years	

AGE	MOTOR AND SOCIAL DEVELOPMENT
6 years	
7 years	
8 to 10 years	
Preadolescent	
Adolescent	

7. How would you prepare the following children for an intramuscular injection of penicillin in order to reduce apprehension and fear?

　　a.　Katie Waugh, age 3:

_____

_____

_____

　　b.　Patrick Williams, age 6:

_____

_____

_____

　　c.　Julie Andrew, age 12:

_____

_____

_____

8. Following is a list of childhood immunizations frequently administered in the medical office. Obtain a drug reference such as the *Physician's Desk Reference*, look up the information requested for each immunization, and record it in the appropriate space.

Immunizations

NAME OF IMMUNIZATION	USE	MEDICAL ASSISTING IMPLICATIONS	SIDE EFFECTS
DTaP			
Polio			
MMR			
Hib			
Hepatitis			
Varicella			

Practice for Competency

Assignment

Practice the procedure for carrying an infant, using a pediatric training mannequin in the following positions: cradle and upright. In the space provided below, indicate the name of the position and the number of times you practiced it.

CARRYING POSITION   **NUMBER OF PRACTICES**

Practice for Competency

WEIGHT AND LENGTH OF AN INFANT

Assignment

Weight. Measure the weight of an infant using a pediatric training mannequin. Record the results in the chart provided. The following values can be used for the weight measurements:

a. 9 pounds, 10 ounces

b. 12 pounds, 5 ounces

c. 16 pounds, 2 ounces

d. 20 pounds, 8 ounces

e. 24 pounds, 6 ounces

Length. Measure the length of an infant using a pediatric training mannequin. Record the results in the chart provided. The following values can be used as values for the length measurements:

a. $21^3/_4$ inches

b. $22^1/_2$ inches

c. $24^1/_4$ inches

d. 28 inches

e. $34^1/_2$ inches

CHART	
Date	

Practice for Competency

PEDIATRIC URINE COLLECTOR

Assignment

Practice the procedure for applying a pediatric urine collector, using a pediatric training mannequin. Record the procedure in the chart provided.

CHART	
Date	

Notes

Practice for Competency

PKU SCREENING TEST

Assignment

1. Complete the information section of the PKU Test Card on the following page.

2. Practice the procedure for specimen collection for the PKU screening test using a pediatric training mannequin. Record the procedure in the chart provided.

Date	CHART

ALL INFORMATION MUST BE PRINTED

DO NOT WRITE IN BLUE SHADED AREAS – DO NOT WRITE ON BARCODE

Birthdate: MM/DD/YY Time (Use 24 hour time only)

Baby's name:
(last, first)

Hospital provider number: (Mandatory)

Hospital name:

Mother's name:
(last, first, initial)

Mother's ID: Baby's ID:

Mother's address:

Mother's phone: ( ) –

Specimen date MM/DD/YY Time (Use 24 hour time only)

Physician name:

Physician address:
Physician name:

City: Ohio zip

Physician phone: ( ) –

Physician provider number (Mandatory)

ODH COPY: SPECIAL:

ODH COPY

HEA 2518

C004OH10884-2C

TEST RESULTS

Screening test normal for
PKU, HOM, GAL, Hypothyroidism

Screening test normal for
PKU and HOM only

Screening test normal:
PKU HOM GAL
Hypothyroidism

Screening test abnormal

See footnote ——— on back
Specimen rejected for reason:

Baby sex: Male Female

Birth weight: grams

Premature: Yes No
Antibiotics: Yes No
Transfusion: Yes No

Specimen: First Second

Submittor: Hospital Physician Health department Other (name below)

FILL ALL CIRCLES WITH BLOOD

BLOOD MUST SOAK COMPLETELY THROUGH

DO NOT APPPLY BLOOD TO THIS SIDE

Evaluation of Competency

CARRYING AN INFANT

Name _____   Date _____

Evaluated By _____   Score_____

Performance Objective

Outcome:	Carry an infant in the following positions: cradle and upright.
Conditions:	Given a pediatric training mannequin.
Standards:	Time: 5 minutes.
	Accuracy: Satisfactory score on the Performance Evaluation Checklist.

Performance Evaluation Checklist

Trial 1	Trial 2	Point Value	Performance Standards
			CRADLE POSITION
		●	Slid the left hand and arm under infant's back.
		●	Grasped infant's upper arm from behind.
		●	Encircled infant's upper arm with the thumb and fingers.
		●	Supported infant's head, shoulders, and back on your arm.
		●	Slipped the right arm up and under the infant's buttocks.
		●	Cradled infant in your arms with the infant's body resting against your chest.
			UPRIGHT POSITION
		●	Slipped the right hand under infant's head and shoulders.
		●	Spread the fingers apart to support infant's head and neck.
		●	Slipped the left forearm under infant's buttocks.
		●	Allowed infant to rest against your chest.
		★	Completed the procedure within 5 minutes.

CHART	
Date	

Evaluation of Student Performance

EVALUATION CRITERIA			COMMENTS
Symbol	**Category**	**Point Value**	
★	Critical Step	16 points	
●	Essential Step	6 points	
▷	Theory Question	2 points	

Score calculation: 100 points

_____ − points missed

_____ Score

Satisfactory score: 85 or above

AAMA/CAAHEP Competency Achieved:

☐ Prepare patient for and assist with routine and specialty examinations.

Evaluation of Competency

PROCEDURE 11-1: MEASURING THE WEIGHT OF AN INFANT

Name _____   Date _____

Evaluated By _____   Score_____

Performance Objective

Outcome:	Measure the weight of an infant and plot the value on a pediatric growth chart.
Conditions:	Using a pediatric training mannequin and a pediatric balance scale.
	Given a paper protector, and a pediatric growth chart.
Standards:	Time: 5 minutes.
	Accuracy: Satisfactory score on the Performance Evaluation Checklist.

Performance Evaluation Checklist

Trial 1	Trial 2	Point Value	Performance Standards
		●	Washed hands.
		●	Greeted the child's parent.
		●	Identified the child.
		●	Introduced yourself and explained the procedure.
		●	Unlocked pediatric scale and placed a clean paper protector on it.
		▷	Is able to state the purpose of the paper protector.
		●	Checked the balance scale for accuracy.
		●	Compensated for weight of paper.
		▷	Is able to state the function of paper protector.
		●	Removed infant's clothing, including diaper.
		●	Gently placed infant on his/her back on the scale.
		●	Placed one hand slightly above infant.
		●	Balanced scale.

Trial 1	Trial 2	Point Value	Performance Standards
		●	Read results while infant was lying still.
		★	The reading was identical to the evaluator's reading.
		●	Returned balance to its resting position and locked the scale.
		●	Removed the infant from the scale and charted the results correctly.
		●	Plotted the weight on growth chart and charted the results correctly.
		★	The growth plot determination was within ±2 percentile points of the evaluator's determination.
		★	Completed the procedure within 5 minutes.

CHART	
Date	

Evaluation of Student Performance

EVALUATION CRITERIA			COMMENTS
Symbol	Category	Point Value	
★	Critical Step	16 points	
●	Essential Step	6 points	
▷	Theory Question	2 points	
Score calculation: 100 points			
— _____ points missed			
_____ Score			
Satisfactory score: 85 or above			

AAMA/CAAHEP Competency Achieved:
☐ Prepare patient for and assist with routine and specialty examinations.

Evaluation of Competency

PROCEDURE 11-2: MEASURING THE LENGTH OF AN INFANT

Name _____   Date _____

Evaluated By _____   Score_____

Performance Objective

Outcome:	Measure the length of an infant and plot the value on a pediatric growth chart.
Conditions:	Using a pediatric training mannequin and a pediatric balance scale.
	Given a pediatric growth chart.
Standards:	Time: 5 minutes.
	Accuracy: Satisfactory score on the Performance Evaluation Checklist.

Performance Evaluation Checklist

Trial 1	Trial 2	Point Value	Performance Standards
		●	Washed hands.
		●	Placed infant on his/her back on a flat table.
		●	Placed the vertex of infant's head against the headboard at the zero mark.
		●	Asked parent to hold infant's head in position.
		●	Straightened infant's knees and placed soles of infant's feet firmly against an upright foot board.
		●	Read infant's length in inches from the measure.
		★	The reading was identical to the evaluator's reading.
		●	Returned foot board to its resting position.
		●	Removed infant from the table.
		●	Charted the results correctly.
		●	Plotted the length on a growth chart and charted the results correctly.

Trial 1	Trial 2	Point Value	Performance Standards
		★	The growth plot determination was within ± 2 percentile points of the evaluator's determination.
		★	Completed the procedure within 5 minutes.

CHART	
Date	

Evaluation of Student Performance

EVALUATION CRITERIA			COMMENTS
Symbol	Category	Point Value	
★	Critical Step	16 points	
●	Essential Step	6 points	
▷	Theory Question	2 points	
Score calculation: 100 points			
— points missed			
_____ Score			
Satisfactory score: 85 or above			

AAMA/CAAHEP Competency Achieved:

☐ Prepare patient for and assist with routine and specialty examinations.

Evaluation of Competency

PROCEDURE 11-3: MEASURING HEAD AND CHEST CIRCUMFERENCE OF AN INFANT

Name _____ Date _____

Evaluated By _____ Score_____

Performance Objective

Outcome:	Measure the head and chest circumference of an infant.
Conditions:	Given a flexible nonstretch tape measure.
Standards:	Time: 5 minutes
	Accuracy: Satisfactory score on the Performance Evaluation Checklist.

Performance Evaluation Checklist

Trial 1	Trial 2	Point Value	Performance Standards
			MEASUREMENT OF HEAD CIRCUMFERENCE
		●	Washed hands.
		●	Assembled equipment.
		●	Positioned the infant.
		▷	Is able to state what positions can be used to measure head circumference.
		●	Positioned the tape measure around the infant's head.
		●	The tape measure was placed slightly above the eyebrows and pinna of the ears and around the occipital prominence at the back of the skull.
		●	Read the results in centimeters (or inches).
		★	The reading was identical to the evaluator's reading.
		●	Charted the results correctly.
		●	Plotted the head circumference value on the infant's growth chart.
		★	The growth plot determination was within ± 2 percentile points of the evaluator's determination.

Trial 1	Trial 2	Point Value	Performance Standards
			MEASUREMENT OF CHEST CIRCUMFERENCE
		●	Positioned the infant on his or her back on the examining table.
		●	Encircled the tape around the infant's chest.
		●	The tape was snug but not too tight.
		●	Read the results in centimeters (or inches).
		★	The reading was identical to the evaluator's reading.
		●	Charted the results correctly.
		★	Completed the procedure within 5 minutes.

CHART	
Date	

Evaluation of Student Performance

EVALUATION CRITERIA			COMMENTS
Symbol	Category	Point Value	
★	Critical Step	16 points	
●	Essential Step	6 points	
▷	Theory Question	2 points	

Score calculation: 100 points

−   points missed

_____ Score

Satisfactory score: 85 or above

AAMA/CAAHEP Competency Achieved:
☐ Prepare patient for and assist with routine and specialty examinations.

Evaluation of Competency

PROCEDURE 11-4: APPLYING A PEDIATRIC URINE COLLECTOR

Name _____   Date _____

Evaluated By _____   Score_____

Performance Objective

Outcome:	Apply a pediatric urine collector.
Conditions:	Using a pediatric training mannequin.
	Given the following: disposable gloves, personal wipes or gauze squares and an antiseptic solution, pediatric urine collector bag, urine specimen container, and a biohazard waste container.
Standards:	Time: 10 minutes.
	Accuracy: Satisfactory score on the Performance Evaluation Checklist.

Performance Evaluation Checklist

Trial 1	Trial 2	Point Value	Performance Standards
		●	Washed hands.
		●	Assembled equipment.
		●	Greeted the child's parent and identified the child.
		●	Introduced yourself and explained the procedure.
		●	Applied gloves.
		●	Positioned child on his/her back with legs spread apart.
		●	Cleansed child's genitalia.
			Females
		●	Cleansed each side of the meatus with a separate wipe using a front-to-back motion.
		●	Cleansed directly down the middle with a third wipe.
		●	Rinsed area and thoroughly wiped it dry.
		●	Removed paper backing from urine collector bag.
		●	Positioned urine collector bag so that the round opening of bag covered upper half of the external genitalia, with the opening of bag placed directly over the urinary meatus.

Trial 1	Trial 2	Point Value	Performance Standards
			Males
		●	Retracted the foreskin of penis if the child is not circumcised.
		●	Cleansed area around the meatus and the urethral orifice.
		●	Used a separate wipe for each swipe.
		●	Cleansed the scrotum.
		●	Rinsed area and thoroughly wiped it dry.
		▷	Is able to state the reason for cleansing the urinary meatus and surrounding area.
		●	Removed the paper backing from urine collector bag.
		●	Positioned so that child's penis and scrotum are projected through the opening of the bag.
		●	Loosely diapered child.
		●	Checked bag every 15 minutes until urine specimen was obtained.
		●	Gently removed collector bag.
		●	Cleansed genital area and rediapered child.
		●	Transferred urine specimen into specimen container and tightly applied the lid.
		●	Labeled container.
		●	Disposed of collector bag in a biohazard waste container.
		●	Tested the specimen or prepared it for transfer to an outside laboratory.
		●	Removed gloves and washed hands.
		●	Charted the procedure correctly.
		★	Completed the procedure within 10 minutes.
CHART			
	Date		

Evaluation of Student Performance

EVALUATION CRITERIA			COMMENTS
Symbol	**Category**	**Point Value**	
★	Critical Step	16 points	
●	Essential Step	6 points	
▷	Theory Question	2 points	

Score calculation: 100 points
_____ − points missed
_____ Score
Satisfactory score: 85 or above

AAMA/CAAHEP Competency Achieved:

☐ Prepare patient for and assist with procedures, treatments, and minor office surgery.

Notes

Evaluation Of Competency

PROCEDURE 11-5: PKU SCREENING TEST

Name _____   Date _____

Evaluated By _____   Score_____

Performance Objective

Outcome: Collect a capillary blood specimen for a PKU screening test.

Conditions: Using a pediatric training mannequin.

Given the following: disposable gloves, sterile lancet, heel warmer or warm compress, antiseptic wipe, PKU testing card, mailing envelope, sterile gauze and a biohazard sharps container.

Standards: Time: 10 minutes.

Accuracy: Satisfactory score on the Performance Evaluation Checklist.

Performance Evaluation Checklist

Trial 1	Trial 2	Point Value	*Performance Standards*
		●	Washed hands.
		●	Assembled equipment.
		●	Greeted the infant's parent and identified the infant.
		●	Introduced yourself and explained the procedure.
		●	Completed the information section of the PKU card.
		●	Applied gloves.
		●	Selected an appropriate puncture site.
		▷	Is able to name the sites that can be used for the puncture.
		●	Warmed the puncture site.
		▷	Is able to state the purpose for warming the site.
		●	Cleaned the puncture site with an anitseptic wipe allowed it to dry.
		●	Grasped infant's foot around the puncture site.
		●	Punctured the heel or toe using a sterile lancet.

Trial 1	Trial 2	Point Value	Performance Standards
		●	Wiped away the first drop of blood with a gauze pad.
		▷	Is able to state why the first drop of blood should be wiped away.
		●	Completely filled each circle on the PKU test card with a large drop of blood.
		●	Allowed the blood to completely soak through the filter paper.
		●	Held a gauze pad over the puncture site and applied pressure.
		●	Remained with infant until bleeding stopped.
		●	Removed gloves and washed hands.
		●	Allowed test card to air dry for 2 hours at room temperature.
		●	Did not stack cards together while drying.
		●	Placed test card in envelope for transport to an outside laboratory.
		●	Charted the procedure correctly.
		★	Completed the procedure within 10 minutes.

CHART	
Date	

Evaluation of Student Performance

EVALUATION CRITERIA			COMMENTS
Symbol	Category	Point Value	
★	Critical Step	16 points	
●	Essential Step	6 points	
▷	Theory Question	2 points	

Score calculation: 100 points

− _____ points missed

_____ Score

Satisfactory score: 85 or above

AAMA/CAAHEP Competency Achieved:
☐ Prepare patient for and assist with procedures, treatments, and minor office surgery.

ALL INFORMATION MUST BE PRINTED

DO NOT WRITE IN BLUE SHADED AREAS – DO NOT WRITE ON BARCODE

Birthdate:

Baby's name:
(last, first)

Hospital provider number:

Hospital name:

Mother's name:
(last, first, initial)

Mother's ID:

Mother's address:

Mother's phone:

Specimen date

Physician name:

Physician address:
Physician name:

City:

Physician phone:

Physician provider number

ODH COPY:

SPECIAL:

MM/DD/YY   Time   (Use 24 hour time only)

(Mandatory)

Baby's ID:

MM/DD/YY   Time   (Use 24 hour time only)

Ohio zip

ODH COPY

(Mandatory)

HEA 2518

CC04OH10884462C

TEST RESULTS

Screening test normal for
PKU, HOM, GAL, Hypothyroidism

Screening test normal for
PKU and HOM only

Screening test normal for
PKU only

Screening test normal:
PKU   HOM   GAL
Hypothyroidism

Screening test abnormal

See footnote _____ on back
Specimen rejected for reason:

Baby sex: Male   Female

Birth weight: _____ grams

Premature: Yes   No
Antibiotics: Yes   No
Transfusion: Yes   No

Specimen: First   Second

Submittor:
Hospital
Physician
Health department
Other (name below)

FILL ALL CIRCLES WITH BLOOD

BLOOD MUST SOAK COMPLETELY THROUGH

DO NOT APPPLY BLOOD TO THIS SIDE

Notes

Cardiopulmonary Procedures

NAME _____

Key Terminology Assessment

Directions: Match each medical term with its definition.

_____ 1. artifact
_____ 2. baseline
_____ 3. cardiac cycle
_____ 4. ECG cycle
_____ 5. electrocardiogram
_____ 6. electrocardiograph
_____ 7. electrode
_____ 8. electrolyte
_____ 9. interval
_____10. ischemia
_____11. normal sinus rhythm
_____12. segment
_____13. spirometer

A. A chemical substance that promotes conduction of an electrical current.
B. The flat horizontal line that separates the various waves of the ECG cycle.
C. The instrument used to record the electrical activity of the heart.
D. Additional electrical activity that is picked up by the electrocardiograph that interferes with the normal appearance of the ECG cycles.
E. Refers to an electrocardiogram that is within normal limits.
F. One complete heart beat.
G. The graphic representation of the electrical activity of the heart.
H. The length of a wave or the length of a wave with a segment.
I. The graphic representation of a cardiac cycle.
J. A conductor of electricity that is used to promote contact between the body and the electrocardiograph.
K. The portion of the ECG between two waves.
L. Deficiency of blood in a part.
M. An instrument for measuring air taken into and expelled from the lungs.

Self-Evaluation

Directions: Fill in each blank with the correct answer.

1. What is the purpose of electrocardiography?

_____

_____

_____

2. Trace the path the blood takes through the heart, starting with the right atrium.

_____

_____

_____

3. What is the function of the SA node?

_____

_____

4. Why is the impulse (initiated by the SA node) delayed momentarily by the AV node?

_____

_____

5. What is the cardiac cycle?

_____

_____

6. Label the following on the ECG cycle:

      P wave   P-R interval

      QRS complex   Q-T interval

      T wave   P-R segment

                    S-T segment

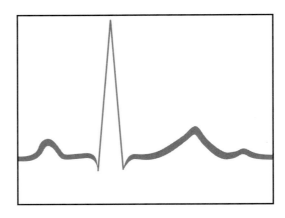

7. Explain what each component of the ECG cycle represents.

P wave _____

QRS complex _____

T wave_____

P-R interval_____

Q-T interval _____

P-R segment _____

S-T segment _____

8. What is the purpose of standardizing the electrocardiograph?

_____

_____

_____

9. How high should the standardization mark be when the ECG is standardized?

_____

10. What is the function of an electrode?

_____

_____

11. Why must an electrolyte be used when recording an ECG?

_____

_____

_____

12. Diagram the bipolar leads on the following illustration:

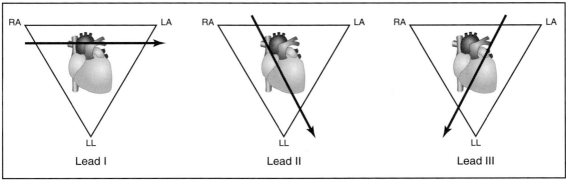

Lead I   Lead II   Lead III

13. Locate and label the chest leads on the following illustration:

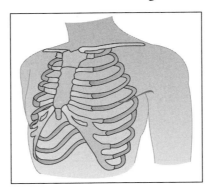

14. A normal ECG is recorded with the paper moving at a speed of

_____

15. What is the difference between a three-channel and a single-channel electrocardio-graph?

_____

_____

_____

16. What is the purpose of each of the following electrocardiographic capabilities?
    a. telephone transmission

    _____

    _____

    b. interpretive capability

    _____

    _____

17. Why should artifacts be eliminated if they occur in an ECG recording?

_____

_____

_____

18. What is the function of an artifact filter?

_____

19. List three possible causes of muscle artifacts.

_____

_____

_____

20. List three possible causes of wandering baseline.

_____
_____
_____

21. List three possible causes of AC artifacts.

_____
_____
_____

22. List three uses of Holter monitor electrocardiography.

_____
_____
_____

23. Explain the use of the patient activity diary in Holter monitor electrocardiography.

_____
_____
_____

24. List five guidelines that should be relayed to the patient undergoing Holter monitor electrocardiography.

_____
_____
_____
_____
_____

25. List the distinguishing characteristics of each of the following cardiac arrhythmias.

Paroxysmal atrial tachycardia

_____
_____

Atrial flutter

_____
_____

Premature ventricular contraction

_____
_____

Ventricular fibrillation

_____

_____

_____

Critical Thinking Skills

1. Obtain the instruction manual that comes with your electrocardiograph. Using the information in the manual, answer the following questions:

    a. List the names of the controls on the electrocardiograph and state the function of each.

        Control   **Function**

        _____

        _____

        _____

        _____

        _____

        _____

        _____

        _____

    b. Explain how to correct the standardization on the electrocardiograph if it is more or less than 10 mm.

        More than 10 mm

        _____

        _____

        Less than 10 mm

        _____

        _____

    c. Whom would you contact if the machine were in need of repair?

        _____

        _____

    d. Read how to change the paper in the machine and describe the procedure in the space provided below. If the opportunity arises, change the paper.

        _____

        _____

2. Practice locating the six chest leads on five different individuals. Try to select individuals of both sexes of various ages and body contours. Record each individual's name here after you have successfully located the chest leads. Also record any problems you encountered locating the leads.

   a. _____

   b. _____

   c. _____

   d. _____

   e. _____

3. Record a 12-lead ECG. Identify and label the various waves, intervals, and segments making up an ECG cycle on each lead.

4. While recording a 12-lead ECG, ask the patient to breathe deeply, talk, cough, and move an extremity. What type of artifact occurred with each?

   a. breathing deeply _____

   b. talking _____

   c. coughing _____

   d. moving an extremity _____

5. If possible, attach examples of the following types of artifacts here:

   a. Muscle artifact

   b. Wandering baseline

   c. Alternating current artifact

Notes

Practice for Competency

12-LEAD ELECTROCARDIOGRAM

Assignment

ECG Form. Complete the patient information section of the ECG form on the following page.

12-Lead Electrocardiogram. Practice the procedure for running a 12-lead electrocardiogram and record the procedure in the chart provided.

CHART	
Date	

PATIENT _____ AGE ___ SEX ___ DATE ___ CASE NO. ___

ADDRESS _____ HEIGHT ___ WEIGHT ___ ECG NO. ___

BUILD { LINEAR ___ / INTERMEDIATE ___ / LATERAL ___

_____

TELEPHONE NO. _____ BLOOD PRESSURE ___ ROOM NO. ___

OCCUPATION _____ MEDICATION _____

DUTIES _____ DOCTOR(S) _____

PRE TEST HISTORY
Check ☒ if yes:

PAST HISTORY:
(Have you ever had?)
Rheumatic fever ☐
Heart murmur ☐
High Blood Pressure ☐
Any Heart Trouble ☐
Disease of Arteries ☐
Varicose Veins ☐
Lung Disease ☐
Operations ☐
Injuries to back, etc. ☐
Epilepsy ☐
Arthritis or Rheumatism ☐
Other Illnesses ☐
EXPLAIN: _____

FAMILY HISTORY:
(Have you or any relative had?)
Heart Attacks ☐
High Blood Pressure ☐
Too Much Cholesterol ☐
Diabetes ☐
Congenital Heart Disease ☐
Heart Operation ☐
Early Sudden Death ☐

PRESENT SYMPTOMS REVIEW:
(Have you recently had?)
Chest Discomfort ☐
Shortness of breath ☐
Heart Palpitations ☐
Cough on Exertion ☐
Coughing up blood ☐
Back, Shoulder or arm discomfort ☐
"Indigestion" ☐
Joint Problems ☐
Urinating at Night ☐
Fainting Spells ☐
Other Illnesses ☐

RESTING ECG: COMMENTS _____

PERMISSION FOR STRESS TESTING

I _____ , do hereby request and authorize Dr.: _____
to administer a cardiac stress test on _____ . The nature of this
assurance has been made concerning the results of this test.

DATE: _____ SIGNATURE OF PATIENT OR LEGAL GUARDIAN: _____

TIME: _____ WITNESS SIGNATURE: _____

BURDICK 007883
ODN912

BURDICK **ExTOL** PROGRAM/RECORD
PRODUCT NUMBER 007883

COPYRIGHT © 1978 • THE BURDICK CORPORATION

Courtesy of Spacelabs Burdick, Inc., Deerfield, Wisconsin.

Practice for Competency

HOLTER MONITOR

Assignment

Activity Diary. Complete the patient information section on the Holter Activity Diary on the following page.

Holter Monitor. Practice the procedure for applying the Holter monitor and record the procedure in the chart provided.

	CHART
Date	

HOLTER MONITOR

PATIENT ACTIVITY DIARY

☐ 10 Hr.   ☐ 12 Hr.   ☐ 24 Hr.   ☐ 26 Hr.

Patient's Name: _____

Patient's Address: _____

_____

Age: _____ **Sex:** _____ **Phone:** _____

Date of Birth: _____ **Soc. Sec. #:** _____

Medication: _____

Doctor: _____ **Phone:** _____

Hospital: _____ **Room:** _____

Date or Recording: _____ **Started:** _____ **AM PM**

Serial Numbers
  Recorder: _____

  Battery: _____

Connected by: _____

_____

Evaluation of Competency

PROCEDURE 12-1: RECORD A 12-LEAD ELECTROCARDIOGRAM (THREE-CHANNEL)

Name _____ Date _____

Evaluated by_____ Score_____

Performance Objective

Outcome:	Record a 12-lead electrocardiogram.
Conditions:	Using a three-channel electrocardiograph.
	Given ECG paper and disposable electrodes.
Standards:	Time: 15 minutes.
	Accuracy: Satisfactory score on the Performance Evaluation Checklist.

Performance Evaluation Checklist

Trial 1	Trial 2	Point Value	Performance Standards
		●	Worked in a quiet atmosphere away from sources of electrical interference.
		●	Washed hands.
		●	Greeted and identified the patient.
		●	Introduced yourself and explained the procedure.
		●	Asked patient to remove appropriate clothing.
		●	Placed patient in a supine position on the table.
		●	Draped patient properly.
		●	Made sure that patient's arms and legs were adequately supported on the table.
		●	Explained procedure to patient.
		●	Instructed patient to lie still and not to talk.
		▷	Is able to state why the patient should lie still.
		●	Properly positioned the electrocardiograph with the power cord pointing away from patient and not passing under the table.
		●	Prepared the patient's skin for application of the disposable electrodes.
		▷	Is able to state why the patient's skin must be prepared properly.

Trial 1	Trial 2	Point Value	Performance Standards
		●	Applied the limb electrodes.
		●	Properly located each chest position and applied the chest electrodes.
		▷	Is able to state why the tabs of the electrodes should point downward.
		●	Connected the lead wires to the electrodes.
		●	Arranged lead wires to follow body contour.
		▷	Is able to state why the lead wires should follow body contour.
		●	Plugged the patient cable into machine and properly supported the cable.
		●	Turned on the electrocardiograph.
		●	Entered patient data using the soft-touch keypad.
		▷	Is able to state the purpose of entering patient data.
		●	Pressed the AUTO button and ran the recording.
		●	Watched for artifacts and corrected them if they occurred.
		●	Turned off the electrocardiograph.
		●	Disconnected the lead wires.
		●	Removed and discarded the disposable electrodes.
		●	Assisted patient from the table.
		●	Washed hands.
		●	Charted the procedure correctly.
		●	Placed the recording in the appropriate place to be reviewed by physician.
		●	Returned equipment to proper place.
		★	Completed the procedure within 15 minutes.

CHART			
Date			

Evaluation of Student Performance

EVALUATION CRITERIA			COMMENTS
Symbol	**Category**	**Point Value**	
★	Critical Step	16 points	
●	Essential Step	6 points	
▷	Theory Question	2 points	

Score calculation: 100 points

− _____ points missed

_____ Score

Satisfactory score: 85 or above

AAMA/CAAHEP Competency Achieved:

☐ Perform electrocardiograms.

Notes

Evaluation of Competency

PROCEDURE 12-2: APPLYING A HOLTER MONITOR

Name _____ Date _____

Evaluated by_____ Score_____

Performance Objective

Outcome:	Apply a Holter monitor.
Conditions:	Using a Holter monitor.
	Given the following: blank magnetic tape, battery, carrying case, belt or shoulder strap, disposable electrodes, alcohol swabs, gauze, razor, nonallergenic tape, patient diary, and a liquid skin abrasive.
Standards:	Time: 20 minutes.
	Accuracy: Satisfactory score on the Performance Evaluation Checklist.

Performance Evaluation Checklist

Trial 1	Trial 2	Point Value	Performance Standards
		●	Assembled equipment.
		●	Installed a new battery.
		●	Inserted a blank magnetic tape into recorder.
		●	Washed hands.
		●	Greeted and identified patient.
		●	Introduced yourself and explained procedure.
		●	Instructed patient in the guidelines for wearing a Holter monitor.
		●	Asked patient to remove clothing from waist up.
		●	Positioned patient in a sitting position.
		●	Located electrode placement sites.
		●	Shaved patient's chest, if needed.
		●	Swabbed skin with alcohol and allowed it to dry.
		●	Slightly abraded skin.
		▷	Is able to state why skin should be abraded.
		●	Removed electrodes from package.
		●	Peeled off the adhesive backing and checked to make sure that electrolyte was moist.

Trial 1	Trial 2	Point Value	Performance Standards
		●	Properly applied electrodes.
		▷	Is able to state why electrodes should be firmly attached.
		●	Attached the lead wires to electrodes.
		●	Formed a loop in each lead wire.
		●	Attached the loop to the patient with tape.
		●	Placed tape over each electrode.
		▷	Is able to state why tape should be applied over electrodes.
		●	Connected the lead wires to patient cable.
		●	Checked the recorder's effectiveness, using the test cable connected to an ECG machine and running a short baseline recording.
		▷	Is able to state why recorder should be checked.
		●	Instructed patient to dress and properly positioned patient cable.
		●	Inserted recorder into its carrying case and strapped it over the patient's clothing.
		●	Made sure that strap was properly adjusted.
		●	Plugged electrode cable into the recorder.
		●	Checked the time and turned on the recorder.
		●	Recorded the starting time in the diary.
		●	Completed patient information section of the diary.
		●	Provided patient with instructions on completing the diary.
		●	Instructed patient when to return for removal of monitor.
		●	Washed hands.
		●	Charted the procedure correctly.
		★	Completed the procedure within 20 minutes.

CHART

Date	

Evaluation of Student Performance

EVALUATION CRITERIA			COMMENTS
Symbol	**Category**	**Point Value**	
★	Critical Step	16 points	
●	Essential Step	6 points	
▷	Theory Question	2 points	
Score calculation: 100 points			
− _____ points missed			
_____ Score			
Satisfactory score: 85 or above			

AAMA/CAAHEP Competency Achieved:

☐ Perform electrocardiograms.

Notes

Colon Procedures

NAME _____

Key Terminology Assessment

Directions: Match each medical term with its definition.

_____ 1. biopsy
_____ 2. endoscope
_____ 3. insufflate
_____ 4. melena
_____ 5. occult blood
_____ 6. peroxidase
_____ 7. proctoscope
_____ 8. proctoscopy
_____ 9. sigmoidoscope
_____ 10. sigmoidoscopy

A. The visual examination of the rectum using a proctoscope.
B. Blood occurring in such a small amount that it is not visually detectable to the unaided eye.
C. The surgical removal and examination of tissue from the living body.
D. The visual examination of the rectum and sigmoid colon using a sigmoidoscope.
E. The darkening of the stool due to the presence of blood in an amount of 50 ml or greater.
F. An instrument consisting of a tube and an optical system, which is used for direct visual inspection of organs or cavities.
G. An endoscope that is specially designed for passage through the anus to permit visual inspection of the rectum.
H. A substance which is able to transfer oxygen from hydrogen peroxide to oxidize guaiac causing the guaiac to turn a blue color.
I. An endoscope that is specially designed for passage through the anus to permit visualization of the rectum and sigmoid colon.
J. To blow a powder, vapor, or gas into a body cavity.

Self-Evaluation

Fill in each blank with the correct answer.

1. List five causes of blood in the stool.

   _____

   _____

   _____

2. Define the term *melena* and explain what causes it.

   _____

   _____

   _____

   _____

3. What is the primary reason for screening patients for the presence of fecal occult blood?

   _____

   _____

4. Why must three consecutive stool specimens be obtained for the guaiac slide test?

   _____

   _____

   _____

5. List two reasons for placing the patient on a high-fiber diet when testing for fecal occult blood.

   _____

   _____

   _____

6. List three examples of medications that must be discontinued prior to guaiac slide testing.

   _____

   _____

7. List two factors that could cause false-positive test results on a guaiac slide test.

   _____

   _____

8. List three examples of diagnostic tests that may be performed if the guaiac slide test is positive.

_____

_____

_____

9. Why is it important to perform quality control methods when developing the guaiac slide test?

_____

_____

10. What is the purpose of the digital rectal examination?

_____

_____

_____

11. What is the purpose of performing a proctoscopy?

_____

_____

_____

12. What is the purpose of performing a sigmoidoscopy?

_____

_____

_____

13. Why is the 65-cm flexible fiberoptic sigmoidoscope preferred by physicians for performing a sigmoidoscopy?

_____

_____

_____

14. What is the purpose of insufflating air into the colon during a sigmoidoscopy?

_____

_____

15. What is the purpose of suctioning during sigmoidoscopy?

_____

_____

16. Describe the advance patient preparation that may be required for a sigmoidoscopy.

_____

_____

_____

_____

17. What is the recommended patient position for flexible fiberoptic sigmoidoscopy?

_____

18. How can the medical assistant help the patient relax during the sigmoidoscopy?

_____

_____

Critical Thinking Skills

1. Mr. Morrison has been given a Hemoccult slide kit for fecal occult blood testing. In the space provided, plan a breakfast, lunch, and dinner meal for him following the guidelines in Table 13-1 of your textbook.

_____

_____

_____

_____

_____

2. Mr. Hofmann has been scheduled to have a sigmoidoscopy. He asks for your help in planning a light evening meal containing low-residue foods. In the space provided, plan a balanced evening meal for Mr. Hofmann.

_____

_____

_____

_____

_____

Practice for Competency

Assignment

Patient Instructions. Instruct an individual in the specimen collection procedure for the Hemoccult slide test. Record patient instructions in the chart provided.

Developing the Test. Develop the Hemoccult slides and record the results in the chart provided.

CHART	
Date	

Practice for Competency

SIGMOIDOSCOPY

Assignment

Practice the procedure for assisting with a sigmoidoscopy. Record advance patient preparation instructions in the chart provided.

Date	CHART

Evaluation of Competency

PROCEDURES 13-1 AND 13-2: HEMOCCULT SLIDE TEST

Name _____   Date _____

Evaluated By _____   Score_____

Performance Objective

Outcome:	Instruct an individual in the specimen collection procedure for a Hemoccult slide test and develop the test.
Conditions:	Given the following: Hemoccult slide testing kit, developing solution, reference card, and a biohazard waste container.
Standards:	Time: 15 minutes
	Accuracy: Satisfactory score in the Performance Evaluation Checklist.

Performance Evaluation Checklist

Trial 1	Trial 2	Point Value	*Performance Standards*
			INSTRUCTIONS FOR THE HEMOCCULT SLIDE TEST
		●	Obtained the Hemoccult slide testing kit.
		●	Checked expiration date of the slides.
		●	Greeted and identified patient.
		●	Introduced yourself and explained purpose of the test.
		●	Informed patient when the test should not be performed.
		●	Instructed patient in the proper preparation required for the test.
		●	Encouraged patient to comply with the diet modifications.
		▷	Is able to state the reason that the patient should follow the diet modifications.
		●	Provided patient with envelope containing the slide test kit.
		●	Instructed patient in completion of the information on the front flap of each card.
		●	Provided instructions on the proper care and storage of the slides.
		▷	Is able to explain why the slides must be stored properly.
			Instructed the patient in the initiation of the test by:
		●	Beginning the diet modifications.
		●	Collecting a stool specimen from the first bowel movement after the 2-day preparatory period.

Trial 1	Trial 2	Point Value	Performance Standards
			Instructed the patient in the proper collection and processing of the stool specimen as follows:
		●	Obtain a sample of the stool from the commode, using wooden applicator.
		●	Open the front flap of the first cardboard slide.
		●	Spread a thin smear of the specimen over the filter paper in the square labeled "A".
		●	Obtain another specimen from a different area of the stool, using the same wooden applicator.
		●	Spread a thin smear of the specimen over the filter paper in the square labeled "B".
		●	Close the front flap of the cardboard slide and fill in the date.
		●	Discard the applicator in a waste container.
		▷	Is able to state why a sample is collected from two different parts of the stool.
		●	Instructed the patient to continue the testing period until all 3 specimens have been obtained.
		●	Instructed the patient to allow the slides to air-dry overnight.
		●	Instructed patient to place the cardboard slides in the envelope and return them to the medical office.
		●	Provided patient with an opportunity to ask questions.
		●	Made sure the patient understood the instructions.
		●	Charted patient instructions.
			DEVELOPING THE HEMOCCULT SLIDE TEST
		●	Assembled equipment.
		●	Checked expiration date on the developing solution bottle.
		●	Applied gloves.
		●	Opened the back flap of the cardboard slides.
		●	Applied 2 drops of the developing solution to the guaiac test paper.
		●	Did not allow the developing solution to come in contact with skin or eyes.
		●	Read results within 60 seconds.
		▷	Is able to state why the slides should be read within 60 seconds.
		●	Performed the quality control procedure.
		▷	Is able to state the purpose of the quality control procedure.
		▷	Is able to state what is observed during a positive and negative reaction.
		●	Properly disposed of the slides in a biohazard waste container.
		●	Removed gloves and washed hands.
		●	Charted the results correctly.
		★	Completed the procedure within 15 minutes.

CHART	
Date	

Evaluation of Student Performance

EVALUATION CRITERIA			COMMENTS
Symbol	**Category**	**Point Value**	
★	Critical Step	16 points	
●	Essential Step	6 points	
▷	Theory Question	2 points	
Score calculation: 100 points			
− _____ points missed			
_____ Score			
Satisfactory score: 85 or above			

AAMA/CAAHEP Competency Achieved:

☐ Instruct patients in the collection of fecal specimens.

Notes

Evaluation of Competency

PROCEDURE 13-3: ASSISTING WITH A SIGMOIDOSCOPY

Name _____   Date _____

Evaluated By _____   Score_____

Performance Objective

Outcome:	Assist with a sigmoidoscopy.
Conditions:	Given the following: disposable gloves, flexible sigmoido-scope, lubricant, a drape, biopsy forceps, sterile specimen container with a preservative, tissue wipes, and a biohazard waste container.
Standards:	Time: 15 minutes
	Accuracy: Satisfactory score on the Performance Evaluation Checklist.

Performance Evaluation Checklist

Trial 1	Trial 2	Point Value	Performance Standards
		●	Washed hands.
		●	Assembled equipment.
		●	Checked to make sure that light bulb of the endoscope was working.
		●	Labeled specimen container.
		●	Greeted and identified the patient.
		●	Introduced yourself and explained the procedure.
		●	Asked patient if he or she needs to empty bladder.
		▷	Is able to state the reason for the patient to have an empty bladder.
		●	Instructed and prepared patient for the examination.
		●	Assisted patient onto examining table.
		●	Assisted patient into the Sim's position.
		●	Properly draped patient.
		●	Reassured patient and helped him or her to relax during the examination.
			Assisted physician as required during the examination including:
		●	Lubricated physician's gloved finger for the digital rectal examination.
		●	Placed lubricant on the sigmoidoscope.

Trial 1	Trial 2	Point Value	Performance Standards
		●	Assisted with the suction equipment as required.
		▷	Is able to state the purpose of the suctioning equipment.
		●	Assisted with the collection of a biopsy.
		●	After the examination, applied gloves and cleaned patient's anal region of excess lubricant.
		●	Removed gloves, washed hands, and assisted patient from examining table.
		●	Instructed patient to get dressed.
		●	Transported any specimens to laboratory, along with a completed laboratory request form.
		●	Cleaned the examining room.
		●	Sanitized and disinfected the sigmoidoscope according to the manufacturer's instructions.
		★	Completed the procedure within 15 minutes.

Evaluation of Student Performance

EVALUATION CRITERIA			COMMENTS
Symbol	Category	Point Value	
★	Critical Step	16 points	
●	Essential Step	6 points	
▷	Theory Question	2 points	

Score calculation: 100 points
− _____ points missed
_____ Score
Satisfactory score: 85 or above

AAMA/CAAHEP Competencies Achieved:
☐ Prepare and maintain examination and treatment areas.
☐ Prepare patient for and assist with routine and specialty examinations.

Radiology and Diagnostic Imaging

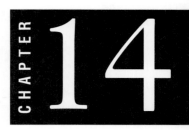

NAME _____

Key Terminology Assessment

Directions: Match each medical term with its definition.

_____ 1. contrast medium
_____ 2. echocardiogram
_____ 3. enema
_____ 4. fluoroscope
_____ 5. fluoroscopy
_____ 6. radiograph
_____ 7. radiography
_____ 8. radiologist
_____ 9. radiology
_____ 10. radiolucent
_____ 11. radiopaque
_____ 12. sonogram
_____ 13. ultrasonography

A. A permanent record of a picture of an internal body organ or structure produced on radiographic film.
B. A medical doctor who specializes in the diagnosis and treatment of disease, using radiant energy such as x-rays, radium, and radioactive material.
C. A substance that is used to make a particular structure visible on a radiograph.
D. The record obtained by the use of ultrasonography.
E. Injection of fluid into the rectum to aid in the elimination of feces from the colon.
F. The branch of medicine that deals with the use of radiant energy in the diagnosis and treatment of disease.
G. An instrument used to view internal organs and structures directly.
H. Describing a structure that obstructs the passage of x-rays.
I. The taking of permanent records of internal body organs and structures by passing x-rays through the body to act on a specially sensitized film.
J. Describing a structure that permits the passage of x-rays.
K. Examination of a patient using the fluoroscope.
L. An ultrasound examination of the heart.
M. The use of high-frequency sound waves to produce an image of an organ or tissue.

Self-Evaluation

Directions: Fill in each blank with the correct answer.

1. Who discovered x-rays?

_____

2. What is the function of x-rays?

_____

_____

3. Why is it so important for a patient to prepare properly for an x-ray examination?

_____

_____

4. What is the function of a radiopaque contrast medium?

_____

_____

5. How is a patient positioned to obtain an anteroposterior view?

_____

_____

6. What is the purpose of mammography?

_____

_____

_____

7. Why must the breasts be compressed during mammography?

_____

_____

8. What is the purpose of the upper GI x-ray examination?

_____

_____

_____

9. Why must the GI tract be free of food and fluid before an upper GI x-ray examination is performed?

_____

_____

10. What is the purpose of the lower GI x-ray examination?

_____

_____

11. What is cholecystography?

_____

_____

12. What is an intravenous pyelogram?

_____

_____

13. What type of patient preparation is required for an IVP?

_____

_____

_____

_____

14. Define the following:

    a.   angiocardiogram

_____

_____

    b.   bronchogram

_____

_____

    c.   cardiac arteriogram

_____

_____

    d.   cerebral angiogram

_____

_____

    e.   cystogram

_____

_____

15. What are the primary uses of ultrasonography?

_____

_____

16. What are the advantages of ultrasonography?

_____

_____

_____

17. What is the purpose of performing obstetric ultrasonography?

_____

_____

_____

18. What are the primary uses of computed tomography?

_____

_____

_____

19. What type of images are produced by computed tomography?

_____

20. What type of patient preparation is required for computed tomography?

_____

_____

_____

_____

21. What are the primary uses of magnetic resonance imaging?

_____

_____

_____

Critical Thinking Skills

1. Dr. Tristen instructs you to schedule Phyllis Ray for cholecystography at Grant Hospital. After you have explained the instructions for preparing for the examination to Ms. Ray, she asks you the following questions. Respond to them in the space provided.

   a. Why must a fat-free evening meal be consumed the day before the exam?

   _____

   _____

   _____

b. Why must I take special tablets after the evening meal?

_____

_____

_____

c. Why must I take a cathartic and perform a cleansing enema before the examination?

_____

_____

_____

d. Why must I consume a meal containing fat on the day of the examination?

_____

_____

_____

e. Ms. Ray asks you to help her plan a fat-free evening meal. Using a nutrition reference source, plan a balanced fat-free meal for Ms. Ray.

_____

_____

_____

_____

2. Trent Douglas has been having pain in his lower abdomen and occult blood in his stool. Dr. Hartman tells you to schedule him for a lower GI colon x-ray examination at Grant Hospital. In the space provided, explain how you would instruct Mr. Douglas to prepare for this examination. Include both the patient preparation and the reason for each of the measures.

_____

_____

_____

_____

_____

_____

3. Jason Zindra, a competitive swimmer, has been experiencing pain in his left shoulder joint. Dr. Baker schedules him for magnetic resonance imaging of the left shoulder. Mr. Zindra asks you the following questions regarding this procedure. Respond to them in the space provided.

a. Is this a safe procedure?

_____

_____

b. Will there be any pain involved with this procedure?

_____

_____

c. Will I be exposed to x-rays?

_____

_____

d. What should I wear to the test?

_____

_____

e. I'm going to wear my watch during the procedure to keep track of the time.

_____

_____

f. I have trouble with claustrophobia.

_____

_____

g. Does the MRI machine make any noise?

_____

_____

h. Will the technician be in the room with me?

_____

_____

Practice for Competency

RADIOLOGY AND DIAGNOSTIC IMAGING

Assignment

Radiology Examinations. Instruct a patient in the proper preparation required for each of the following types of x-ray examinations: mammogram, upper GI, lower GI, cholecystogram, and intravenous pyelogram. Record the procedure in the chart provided.

Diagnostic Imaging Procedures. Instruct a patient in the proper preparation required for each of the following types of diagnostic imaging procedures: ultrasonography, computed tomography, and magnetic resonance imaging. Record the procedure in the chart provided.

CHART	
Date	

CHART	
Date	

Evaluation of Competency

PREPARATION FOR RADIOLOGY EXAMINATIONS

Name _____   Date _____

Evaluated by_____   Score_____

Performance Objective

Outcome:	Instruct a patient in the proper preparation required for each of the following x-ray examinations: mammogram, upper GI, lower GI, cholecystogram, and intravenous pyelogram.
Conditions:	Given a patient instruction sheet for each x-ray examination.
Standards:	Time: 15 minutes
	Accuracy: Satisfactory score on the Performance Evaluation Checklist.

Performance Evaluation Checklist

Trial 1	Trial 2	Point Value	*Performance Standards*
		●	Greeted and identified patient.
		●	Introduced yourself.
			Instructed patient in the proper preparation for each of the following x-ray examinations:
		●	Mammogram
		●	Upper GI
		●	Lower GI
		●	Cholecystogram
		●	Intravenous pyelogram
		●	Charted the procedure correctly.
		★	Completed the procedure within 15 minutes.
CHART			
	Date		

Evaluation of Student Performance

EVALUATION CRITERIA			COMMENTS
Symbol	**Category**	**Point Value**	
★	Critical Step	16 points	
●	Essential Step	6 points	
▷	Theory Question	2 points	
Score calculation: 100 points			
− points missed			
Score			
Satisfactory score: 85 or above			

AAMA/CAAHEP Competencies Achieved:

☐ Instruct individuals according to their needs.

☐ Provide instructions for health maintenance and disease prevention.

Evaluation of Competency

PREPARATION FOR DIAGNOSTIC IMAGING PROCEDURES

Name _____   Date _____

Evaluated by_____   Score_____

Performance Objective

Outcome:	Instruct a patient in the proper preparation required for each of the following diagnostic imaging procedures: ultrasonography, computed tomography, and magnetic resonance imaging.
Conditions:	Given a patient instruction sheet for each diagnostic imaging procedure.
Standards:	Time: 15 minutes
	Accuracy: Satisfactory score on the Performance Evaluation

Performance Evaluation Checklist

Trial 1	Trial 2	Point Value	*Performance Standards*
		●	Greeted and identified patient.
		●	Introduced yourself.
			Instructed patient in the proper preparation for each of the following diagnostic imaging procedures:
		●	Ultrasonography
		●	Computed tomography
		●	Magnetic resonance imaging
		●	Charted the procedure correctly.
		★	Completed the procedure within 15 minutes.
CHART			
Date			

Evaluation of Student Performance

EVALUATION CRITERIA			COMMENTS
Symbol	**Category**	**Point Value**	
★	Critical Step	16 points	
●	Essential Step	6 points	
▷	Theory Question	2 points	
Score calculation: 100 points			
− _____ points missed			
_____ Score			
Satisfactory score: 85 or above			

AAMA/CAAHEP Competencies Achieved:

☐ Instruct individuals according to their needs.

☐ Provide instructions for health maintenance and disease prevention.

Introduction to the Clinical Laboratory

NAME _____

Key Terminology Assessment

Directions: Match each medical term with its definition.

_F_ 1. fasting
_C_ 2. homeostasis
_G_ 3. in vivo
_F_ 4. laboratory test
_A_ 5. normal range
___ 6. plasma
_B_ 7. profile
___ 8. quality control
_H_ 9. routine test
_B_ 10. serum
_I_ 11. specimen

A. A certain established and acceptable parameter within which the laboratory test results of a healthy individual are expected to fall.

B. Plasma from which the clotting factor fibrinogen has been removed.

C. The state in which body systems are functioning normally and the internal environment of the body is in equilibrium.

D. A number of laboratory tests providing related or complementary information used to determine the health status of a patient.

E. Abstaining from food or fluids (except water) for a specified amount of time prior to the collection of a specimen.

F. The clinical analysis and study of material, fluids, or tissues obtained from patients to assist in diagnosing and treating disease.

G. Occurring in the living body or organism.

H. Laboratory tests performed on a routine basis on apparently healthy patients to assist in the early detection of disease.

I. The liquid part of the blood, consisting of a clear yellowish fluid that makes up approximately 55% of the total blood volume.

J. A small sample of something taken to show the nature of the whole.

K. The application of methods to ensure that test results are reliable and valid and that errors are detected and eliminated.

Self-Evaluation

Directions: Fill in each blank with the correct answer.

1. What is the general purpose of a laboratory test?

   assist in diagnosis of a pt's condition.

2. List five specific uses of laboratory test results.

   - assist in the diagnosis of conditions - evaluate the pts progress to regulate trmx - establish each pts baseline or normal level, - prevent or reduce disease - requirement by state law

3. What is the purpose of performing a routine test?

   to assist in the diagnosis of a patient's condition / to detect an early disease

4. What information is included in a laboratory directory?

   names of the tests performed by the lab, normal range for each test, instructions on completion of forms, patient preparation required for each test, supplies required for the collection of each spec

5. What is the purpose of a laboratory request?

   is required when the specimen is collected at the medical office + transferred to an outside lab for testing or when

6. What is the reason for indicating the following information on the laboratory request form?

   a. Patient's age and gender

   the normal ranges for some tests vary, depending on the pts age + sex

b. Date and time of collection of the specimen

indicates the # of days that have passed since collected.

c. Source of the specimen

Certain tests require that the source of the speciman be recorded on lab request form.

d. Physician's clinical diagnosis

assists the lab in correlating the clinical laboratory data c̄ the needs of the physician.

e. Any medications the patient is taking

Certain medications the pt is taking may interfere c̄ the accuracy of results

7. What tests are included in the following profiles?

a. Health screen profile

Glucose, B.U.N, Creatinine, Cholest Calcium, Phos, electrolytes

b. Liver function profile

Bilirubin, Alk Phos, Alt, Ast

c. Prenatal profile

d. Lipid profile

Triglycerides, Cal, Phos,

_Pg. 509_

8. What information is included on laboratory reports?

Name, Address, Physicians Name +#
Pts name, sex, date of speciman,
Names of tests performed,

9. Why must the test results of specimens tested by an outside laboratory be compared with the normal ranges supplied by the laboratory?

Normal ranges differ from one lab to another + reagents to perform tests.

10. Why do some laboratory tests require advance patient preparation?

leads to accuracy, assists the physician in accurate diagnosis + treatment

11. Why is it important to explain the reason for the advance preparation to the patient?

do to accuracy + prevent from calling pt back + redoing test

12. What is a specimen?

a small sample or part taken from the body to represent the nature of the whole.

13. List ten examples of specimens.

blood, urine, feces, sputum + cervical + Vaginal scraping of cells secretion from parts of the body gastric juices, cerebrospinal fluid, Pleural fluid, + tissue Bx's

14. List and explain five guidelines that should be followed during specimen collection and handling.

- Review + follow OSHA Standards
- Review requirements for collection
- Assemble equipment + supplies
- Identify pt. + explain procedure.
- Collection of speciman
- + proper handling of speciman

15. Why must a specimen be properly handled and stored?

certain specimans may be more sensitive to the environment + special handling required

16. Define each of the following categories of laboratory tests based on function and list three examples of tests included in each.

    a. Hematology

    _____

    _____

    _____

    b. Clinical Chemistry

    _____

    _____

    _____

    c. Serology and Blood Banking

    _____

    _____

    _____

d. Urinalysis

_____

_____

_____

e. Microbiology

_____

_____

_____

17. What are the six basic steps involved in testing a specimen?

-the specific amount of speciman required is measured, - nessary chemical reagents required for speciman, - specimans may require further processing, - the substance is either manually or automatically measured, - results are obtained from readout, - results are recorded on lab report form

18. What is the purpose of quality control?

the application of methods, + means to ensure that test results are reliable + valid + that errors that may interfere c obtaining accurate test results

19. List four quality control methods that should be employed in testing a specimen.

-check precision +accuracy of lab equip -discarding outdated reagents - following procedure exactly, -performing test in duplicate, -maintaing equipment

20. List ten laboratory safety guidelines that should be followed in the medical office to prevent accidents from occurring.

- Follow OSHA Guidlines, -hands should be washed, - Avoid hand to mouth contact - do not pipet any speciman by mouth, - immediately cleanup, - properly dispose of all contaminated needles, - cover any break in skin. - - -

Critical Thinking Skills

1. Refer to Table 15-1 in your textbook and list the specimen requirements for each of the following tests:

a. Albumin, serum _____

   b. ALT _____

   c. Bilirubin, total _____

   d. Blood group (ABO) _____

   e. BUN, serum _____

   f. Calcium _____

   g. CBC (with differential) _____

   h. CPK _____

   i. Glucose, plasma _____

   j. LD _____

   k. Sedimentation rate (ESR) _____

   l. Thyroxine (T_4) _____

   m. Triglycerides _____

   n. Uric acid, serum_____

   o. Urinalysis _____

2. Your physician has ordered an FBS on Mrs. Wright. The blood specimen is to be collected at 9 A.M. at the medical office. In the space provided, indicate the information you would relay to Mrs. Wright regarding the advance preparation required for this test.

   do not eat any sugar before
   test, + do not eat or
   drink anything after midnight

3. Refer to the laboratory report in your textbook (Fig. 15-2). Using the normal values listed on this report, determine if the following tests fall within normal range or if they are high or low. Mark each test according to the following: **N** = normal, **H** = high, **L** = low. Your patient is an adult female.

   a. Glucose: 140 mg/dl ___H_____

   b. BUN: 15 mg/dl ___N_____

   c. Creatinine: 1.7 mg/dl___H_____

   d. Potassium: 5.5 ___H_____

   e. Triglycerides: 140 mg/dl ___N_____

   f. Total protein: 4.0 g/dl ___L_____

   g. Albumin: 3.5 g/dl ___N_____

   h. Alkaline phosphatase: 80 U/L ___N_____

   i. LD: 132 U/L___N_____

   j. ALT: 44 U/L _____

   k. Uric acid: 5.2 mg/dl___N_____

   l. Neutrophils: 84% ___H_____

   m. WBC: 15.5 ___H_____

    n. RBC: 3.7 _____

    o. Hgb: 10.8 _____

    p. Hct: 32 _____

4. Refer to the laboratory report in your textbook (Fig. 15-2) and circle any abnormal values using a red pen.

Notes

Practice for Competency

COLLECTING SPECIMEN FOR TRANSPORT TO AN OUTSIDE LABORATORY

Assignment

Laboratory Requisition. Complete the Laboratory Request Form on the following page using a classmate as a patient. The tests that have been ordered by the physician include the following: CBC (with differential), cholesterol, HDL cholesterol, and glucose.

Specimen Collection. Practice the procedure for collecting a specimen for transport to an outside laboratory and record the procedure in the chart provided.

CHART	
Date	

Biomedical Laboratories, Inc.

☐ Fax — Send additional copy of report to:

☐ Call — Client Number/Physician's Name — Phone/Fax Number — ( )

☐ Mail — Physician's Address — City, State, Zip

Patient's Name (Last)	(First)	(M)	Sex	Date of Birth MO DAY YR	Collection Time AM PM :	Fasting ☐YES ☐NO	Collection Date MO DAY YR

NPI/UPIN	Physician's ID #	Patient's SS #	Patient's ID #	Urine hrs/vol hrs___ vol___

PATIENT / RESP. PARTY

Physician's Name (Last, First) — X _____ Physician's Signature

Medicare # (Include prefix/suffix) — ☐ Primary ☐ Secondary

Medicaid # — State — Physician's Provider #

Diagnosis/Signs/Symptoms in ICD-9 Format(Highest Specificity)

REQUIRED

Patient's Address — Phone
City — State — ZIP
Name of Responsible Party (if different from patient)
Address of Responsible Party — APT #
City — State — ZIP

Patient's Relationship to Responsible Party: ■ 1 - Self ■ 2 - Spouse ■ 3 - Child ■ 4 - Other

Perform-ance Lab — Carrier — Group # — Employee # — Mem

I hereby authorize the release of medical information related to the service described herein and authorize payment directed to LabCorp.
X _____ Patient's Signature — Date

INSURANCE

Insurance Company Name — Plan — Carrier Code
Subsciber/Member # — Location — Group #
Insurance Address — Physician's Provider #
City — State — ZIP
Employer's Name or Number — Insured SS# (If Not Patient) — Worker's Comp ☐ Yes ☐ No

MEDICARE ADVANCE BENEFICIARY NOTICE (ABN)

I have read the ABN on the reverse. If Medicare denies payment, I agree to pay for the identified test(s).
X _____ Patient's Signature — Date

@ : Carrier-specific limited coverage test
# : Investigational test per Medicare

INDIVIDUAL COMPONENTS OF TEST COMBINATIONS/PROFILES LISTED IN THE SECTION ABOVE CAN BE ORDERED BELOW.

NOTE: WHEN ORDERING TESTS FOR WHICH MEDICARE OR MEDICAID REIMBURSEMENT WILL BE SOUGHT, PHYSICIANS SHOULD ONLY ORDER TESTS THAT ARE MEDICALLY NECESSARY FOR THE DIAGNOSIS OR TREATMENT OF THE PATIENT. COMPONENTS OF THE ORGAN OR DISEASE PANELS/COMBINATIONS PRINTED BELOW ARE SHOWN ON THE REVERSE SIDE AND MAY ALSO BE ORDERED INDIVIDUALLY BELOW. COMPONENTS MAY BE BILLED SEPARATELY PER CARRIER POLICY.

ORGAN OR DISEASE PANELS (See reverse for components)

Code	Test		
303758	Basic Metabolic Panel	80049	SST
302085	Comp Metabolic Panel	80054	SST
303754	Electrolyte Panel	80051	SST
303755	Hepatic Function Panel	80058	SST
303744	Hepatitis Panel	80059	SST
303756	Lipid Panel	@ 80061	SST
235010	Lipid Panel w/LDL/HDL Ratio	@ 80061	SST
000455	Thyroid Panel	@ 80091	SST
000620	Thyroid Panel w/ TSH	@ 80092	SST

HEMATOLOGY

005009	CBC w Diff w Plt	@ 85025	LAV
115907	CBC w Diff w/o Plt	@ 85022	LAV
028142	CBC w/o Diff w Plt	@ 85027	LAV
005017	CBC w/o Diff w/o Plt	@ 85021	LAV
005058	Hematocrit	@ 85014	LAV
005041	Hemoglobin	@ 85018	LAV
005249	Platelet Count	@ 85595	LAV
005033	RBC Count	85041	LAV
005025	WBC Count	85048	LAV
005090	WBC Differential	@ 85007	LAV

ALPHABETICAL/COMBINATION TESTS

006049	ABO and Rh (see reverse)	86900 86901	LAV
001081	Albumin	82040	SST
001107	Alkaline Phosphatase	84075	SST
001545	ALT (SGPT)	84460	SST
001396	Amylase	82150	SST
006254	Antinuclear Antibodies	86038	SST
001123	AST (SGOT)	84450	SST
000810	B12 and Folate (see reverse)	82607 82746	SST
001099	Bilirubin, Total	82250	SST

ALPHABETICAL TESTS CON'T

001040	BUN	84520	SST
001016	Calcium	82310	SST
007419	Carbamazepine (Tegretol®)	80156	SER
002139	CEA	@ 82378	SST
001065	Cholesterol, Total	@ 82465	SST
001370	Creatinine	82565	SST
007385	Digoxin (Lanoxin)	@ 80162	SER
004515	Estradiol	82670	SST
004598	Ferritin	@ 82728	SST
100800	Fructosamine	@ 82985	SST
004309	FSH	83001	SST
028481	FSH and LH (see reverse)	83001 83002	SST
001958	GGT	82977	SST
001818	Glucose, Plasma	@ 82947	GRY
001032	Glucose, Serum	@ 82947	SST
002022	Glucose, 2-hr. PP	82950	SST
001693	Glycohemoglobin, Total	@ 83036	LAV
004556	hCG, Beta Subunit, Qual	@ 84703	SST
004416	hCG, Beta Subunit, Quant	@ 84702	SST
001925	HDL Cholesterol	@ 83718	SST
162289	Helicobacter pylori, IgG	@ 86677	SST
006395	Hep B Surface Antibody	86706	SST
006510	Hep B Surface Antigen	87340	SST
140608	Hep C Antibody	86803	SST
001453	Hemoglobin A1C	@ 83036	LAV
083824	HIV Antibodies *	86701	SST
001339	Iron	@ 83540	SST
001321	Iron and IBC (see reverse)	@ 83540 83550	SST
001115	LDH	83615	SST

ALPHABETICAL TESTS CON'T

004283	LH	83002	SST
001404	Lipase	83690	SER
007708	Lithium (Eskalith®)	80178	SER
001537	Magnesium	@ 83735	SST
007823	Phenobarbital (Luminal®)	80184	SER
0007401	Phenytoin (Dilantin®)	80185	SER
001180	Potassium	84132	SST
004465	Prolactin, Serum	84146	SST
010322	Prostate-Specific Antigen	@ 84153	SST
004747	Prostatic Acid Phos	@ 84066	SST
001073	Protein, Total	84155	SST
005199	Prothrombin Time (PT)	85610	BLU
020321	PT and PTT Activated	85610 85730	BLU
005207	PTT Activated	85730	BLU
006502	Rheumatoid Arthritis Factor	86431	SST
006072	RPR	@ 86592	SST
006197	Rubella Antibodies, IgG	86762	SST
005215	Sed Rate, Westergren	85651	LAV
001198	Sodium	84295	SST
004226	Testosterone	84403	SST
007336	Theophylline	80198	SER
001149	Thyroxine (T4)	@ 84436	SST
001172	Triglycerides	@ 84478	SST
002188	Triiodothyronine (T3)	84480	SST
004259	TSH, High Sensitivity	@ 84443	SST
001057	Uric Acid	84550	SST
003038	Urinalysis Microscopic on Positives	81003	URN
003772	Urinalysis with Microscopic	81001	URN
007260	Valproic Acid (Depakene®)	80164	SER

MICROBIOLOGY - See Reverse Side

☐ ENDOCERVICAL ☐ THROAT ☐ URINE
☐ STOOL ☐ URETHRAL INDICATE SOURCE

OTHER

008649	Aerobic Bacterial Culture †	87070	Bact Trnspt
164160	Chlamydia/GC DNA Probe W/ Confirmation on Positives *	87490 87590	Probe Trnspt
096479	Chlamydia/GC DNA Probe Without Confirmation	87490 87590	Probe Trnspt
164202	Chlamydia DNA Probe *	87490	Probe Trnspt
180745	Genital, Beta-Hemolytic Strep Cult, Group B	87081	Bact Trnspt
008334	Genital Culture, Routine †	87070	Bact Trnspt
180810	Lower Respiratory Culture †	87070	Steril Trnspt
164210	N. gonorrhoeae DNA Probe *	87590	Probe Trnspt
008623	Ova and Parasites	87015 87211	O & P Kit
008144	Stool Culture †	87081 X2 87045	Fecal Trnspt
008169	Throat, Beta-Hemolytic Strep Cult, Group A	87081	Bact Trnspt
008342	Upper Respiratory Culture, Routine	87060	Bact Trnspt
008847	Urine Culture, Routine † @	87086	Urn Cul Trnsp

† = ID/Susceptibility at Additional Charge
* = Confirmation at Additional Charge

Clinical Information/Comments

OTHER TESTS/INDIVIDUAL PROFILE COMPONENTS
TEST# — TEST NAMES

LABCORP USE ONLY	STAT ☐ 998074	VENIPUNCTURE ☐ 998085	TRAVEL ☐ 998096	NON LABCORP ☐ 998239	VERBAL ORDER ☐ 998250	CHART ORDER ☐ 998261	HANDWRITTEN ☐ 998272	24 HR TUV ☐ 998283	PST/PSC #

CONTAINERS RECEIVED	SST SPUN	USST UNSPUN	SER SERUM TRNSPT	FRZ FRZ TRNS	RED RED	LAV LAVENDER	SLD SLIDE	BLU LT. BLUE	GRY GREY	GRN GREEN	RYB RYL BLU	YEL ACD	PLS PLASMA	URN URINE	24U 24 HR URINE	TA-U TART. ACID	FL FLUID	OT OTHER	BACT TRNSP	O & P KIT	PROBE TRNSP	URN CUL TRNSP	STERIL TRNSP	FECAL TRNSP	VIRAL TRNSP

Evaluation of Competency

PROCEDURE 15-1: COLLECTING A SPECIMEN FOR TRANSPORT TO AN OUTSIDE LABORATORY

Name _____ Date _____

Evaluated by_____ Score_____

Performance Objective

Outcome:	Collect a specimen for transport to an outside laboratory.
Conditions:	Given the appropriate supplies for the specimen collection and transport (will be based upon the type of specimen collected).
Standards:	Time: 10 minutes
	Accuracy: Satisfactory score on the Performance Evaluation Checklist.

Performance Evaluation Checklist

Trial 1	Trial 2	Point Value	Performance Standards
		●	Informed patient of any advance preparation or special instructions.
		▷	Is able to state why patient should prepare properly.
		●	Reviewed requirements in the laboratory directory for the collection and handling of specimen.
		●	Completed laboratory request form.
		●	Washed hands.
		●	Assembled equipment and supplies.
		●	Clearly labeled the tubes and containers with patient's name, date, and initials.
		●	Greeted and identified patient. Identified yourself and explained procedure.
		▷	Is able to state why it is important to correctly identify patient.
		●	Collected specimen incorporating the following guidelines:
		●	Followed the OSHA Standard.
		●	Collected specimen using proper technique.
		●	Collected the proper type and amount of specimen required for the test.
		●	Processed specimen further if required by the outside laboratory.

Trial 1	Trial 2	Point Value	Performance Standards
		●	Placed the lid tightly on specimen container.
		●	Charted the procedure correctly.
		●	Properly handled and stored specimen according to the laboratory specifications.
		●	Prepared specimen for transport to the outside laboratory, making sure to include the completed laboratory request.
		●	Reviewed laboratory report when it was returned and notified physician of any abnormal results.
		●	Filed laboratory report in patient's chart.
		★	Completed the procedure within 10 minutes.

CHART	
Date	

Evaluation of Student Performance

EVALUATION CRITERIA			COMMENTS
Symbol	Category	Point Value	
★	Critical Step	16 points	
●	Essential Step	6 points	
▷	Theory Question	2 points	

Score calculation: 100 points

−_____ points missed

_____ Score

Satisfactory score: 85 or above

AAMA/CAAHEP Competencies Achieved:
☐ Use methods of quality control.
☐ Screen and follow-up test results.

## CHAPTER 16

Urinalysis

NAME _____

Key Terminology Assessment:

Directions: Match each medical term with its definition.

_____ 1. agglutination
_____ 2. bilirubinuria
_____ 3. glycosuria
_____ 4. ketonuria
_____ 5. ketosis
_____ 6. meniscus
_____ 7. micturition
_____ 8. nephron
_____ 9. oliguria
_____10. pH
_____11. polyuria
_____12. proteinuria
_____13. refractive index
_____14. refractometer
_____15. renal threshold
_____16. specific gravity
_____17. supernatant
_____18. urinalysis
_____19. void

A. Decreased or scanty output of urine.
B. The presence of protein in the urine.
C. The clear liquid that remains at the top after a precipitate settles.
D. The presence of bilirubin in the urine.
E. Increased output of urine.
F. The curved upper surface of a liquid in a container.
G. The concentration at which a substance in the blood that is not normally excreted by the kidneys begins to appear in the urine.
H. The presence of sugar in the urine.
I. The physical, chemical, and microscopic analysis of urine.
J. The presence of ketone bodies in the urine.
K. The act of voiding urine.
L. The accumulation of large amounts of ketone bodies in the tissues and body fluids.
M. The weight of a substance as compared with the weight of an equal volume of a substance known as the standard.

N. The unit that describes the acidity or alkalinity of a solution.
O. The functional unit of the kidney.
P. An instrument used to measure the refractive index of urine, which is an indirect measurement of the specific gravity of urine.
Q. The ratio of the velocity of light in air to the velocity of light in a solution.
R. The aggregation or uniting of separate particles into clumps or masses.
S. To empty the bladder.

Self-Evaluation

Directions: Fill in each blank with the correct answer.

1. List two functions of the urinary system.

2. What is the function of the urinary bladder?

3. How does the function of the urethra differ in the male and female?

4. What is the urinary meatus?

5. Most of the urine (95%) is composed of what substance?

6. List two conditions that may cause polyuria.

7. List two conditions that may cause oliguria.

8. What is the term used to describe painful urination?

_____

9. What is the term used to describe a condition of frequent urination?

_____

10. What is the term used to describe excessive (voluntary) urination during the night?

_____

11. The inability to retain urine is known as

_____

12. What type of urine specimen is required for the detection of a urinary tract infection (UTI)?

_____

13. List three changes that may take place in a urine specimen if it is allowed to stand for more than 1 hour.

_____

_____

14. Why is a first-voided morning specimen often preferred for urine testing?

_____

_____

15. What condition is a twenty-four hour urine specimen often used to diagnose?

_____

_____

16. Why does concentrated urine tend to be dark in color?

_____

_____

17. List two factors that may cause a urine specimen to become cloudy.

_____

_____

18. What type of odor will a urine specimen have that has been allowed to stand out for a long period of time?

_____

19. What is the purpose of testing the specific gravity of urine?

_____

20. What is the normal range for specific gravity of urine?

_____

21. What is the difference between a qualitative test and a quantitative test?

_____

_____

_____

22. What may cause an increase in the pH of the urine?

_____

_____

23. Why does urine become more alkaline if it is not preserved?

_____

_____

_____

24. What may cause glycosuria?

_____

_____

25. What may cause ketosis?

_____

_____

26. What may cause blood to appear in the urine?

_____

_____

27. Why should a nitrite test *not* be performed on a urine specimen that has been left standing out?

_____

_____

28. How should urine reagent strips be stored?

_____

_____

29. What is the purpose of performing a microscopic examination of the urine?

_____

_____

_____

30. Why is a first-voided urine specimen recommended for a microscopic examination of the urine?

_____

_____

31. What effect does concentrated urine have on red blood cells present in it?

_____

_____

32. What is a urinary cast?

_____

_____

33. List one condition that may cause yeast cells to appear in the urine.

_____

34. List two reasons for performing a urine culture test.

_____

35. List three reasons for performing a pregnancy test.

_____

36. What is the name of the hormone that is present only in the urine and blood of a pregnant woman?

_____

37. List five guidelines that should be followed when performing a pregnancy test.

_____

_____

_____

_____

_____

Critical Thinking Skills

1. You have instructed Mr. Pratt to collect a first-voided morning urine specimen, which will be brought to the medical office for testing. The patient asks the following questions. Respond to them in the spaces provided.

   a. Why is a first-voided specimen desired?

   _____

   _____

   b. Why must the specimen be preserved until it is brought to the medical office?

   _____

   _____

2. You have jut instructed Mrs. Berger to obtain a clean-catch midstream specimen at the medical office. The patient asks the following questions. Respond to them in the spaces provided.

   a. What is the purpose of cleansing the urinary meatus?

   _____

   _____

   b. Why must a front-to-back motion be used to clean the urinary meatus?

   _____

   _____

c. Why must a small amount of urine first be voided into the toilet?

_____

_____

d. Why shouldn't the inside of the specimen cup be touched?

_____

_____

3. Obtain the instructions that come with any type of commercially prepared diagnostic kit for the chemical testing of urine (e.g., Multistix 10 SG). Using the instructions, answer the following questions in the spaces provided.

a. What is the brand name of the test?

_____

b. This test is used to detect the presence of what substance(s)?

_____

_____

_____

c. Explain how to perform the test.

_____

_____

_____

d. Explain the proper storage and handling of this test.

_____

_____

_____

e. List any medications or other substances that may interfere with the test results.

_____

_____

_____

f. List any technique that may interfere with obtaining an accurate reading. (Example: not reading the test at the prescribed time.)

_____

_____

_____

g. If possible, perform this test on a urine specimen and record the results below:

_____

_____

Practice for Competency

URINE SPECIMEN COLLECTION

Assignment

Clean Catch Midstream Urine Specimen. Instruct an individual in the procedure for collecting a clean-catch midstream specimen and record the procedure in the chart provided.

Twenty-Four Hour Urine Specimen. Instruct an individual in the procedure for collecting a 24-hour urine specimen and record the procedure in the chart provided.

CHART	
Date	

Practice for Competency

PHYSICAL EXAMINATION OF URINE

Assignment

Color and Clarity. Assess the color and clarity of a urine specimen and record the results in the chart provided.

Measuring the Specific Gravity of Urine. Measure the specific gravity of a urine specimen using a refractometer. Record the results in the chart provided.

CHART	
Date	

Practice for Competency

CHEMICAL EXAMINATION OF URINE

Assignment

Multistix 10 SG Reagent Strip. Perform a chemical assessment of a urine specimen using a Multistix 10 SG reagent strip. Record the results on the laboratory report form provided. Circle any abnormal results.

Multistix® 10 SG Reagent Strips for Urinalysis

PATIENT

DATE   TIME

LEUKOCYTES	NEGATIVE		TRACE	SMALL +	MODERATE ++	LARGE +++	
NITRATE	NEGATIVE		POSITIVE	POSITIVE	(Any degree of uniform pink color is positive)		
UROBILINOGEN	NORMAL 0.2	NORMAL 1	mg/dL 2	4	8	(1 mg = approx. 1 EU)	
PROTEIN	NEGATIVE	TRACE	mg/dL 30 +	100 ++	300 +++	2000 or more ++++	
pH	5.0	6.0	6.5	7.0	7.5	8.0	8.5
BLOOD	NEGATIVE	NON-HEMOLYZED TRACE	NON-HEMOLYZED MODERATE	HEMOLYZED TRACE	SMALL +	MODERATE ++	LARGE +++
SPECIFIC GRAVITY	1.000	1.005	1.010	1.015	1.020	1.025	1.030
KETONE	NEGATIVE	mg/dL	TRACE 5	SMALL 15	MODERATE 40	LARGE 80	LARGE 160
BILIRUBIN	NEGATIVE		SMALL +	MODERATE ++	LARGE +++		
GLUCOSE	NEGATIVE	g/dL (%) mg/dL	1/10 (tr.) 100	1/4 250	1/2 500	1 1000	2 or more 2000 or more

Printed by permission of Bayer Corporation, Diagnostic Division, Tarrytown, NY, 10591

Multistix® *10 SG* *Reagent Strips for Urinalysis*

PATIENT

DATE   **TIME**

LEUKOCYTES	NEGATIVE ☐		TRACE ☐	SMALL + ☐	MODERATE ++ ☐	LARGE +++ ☐	
NITRATE	NEGATIVE ☐		POSITIVE ☐	POSITIVE ☐	(Any degree of uniform pink color is positive)		
UROBILINOGEN	NORMAL 0.2 ☐	NORMAL 1 ☐	mg/dL 2 ☐	4 ☐	8 ☐	(1 mg = approx. 1 EU)	
PROTEIN	NEGATIVE ☐	TRACE ☐	mg/dL 30 + ☐	100 ++ ☐	300 +++ ☐	2000 or more ++++ ☐	
pH	5.0 ☐	6.0 ☐	6.5 ☐	7.0 ☐	7.5 ☐	8.0 ☐	8.5 ☐
BLOOD	NEGATIVE ☐	NON-HEMOLYZED TRACE ☐	NON-HEMOLYZED MODERATE ☐	HEMOLYZED TRACE ☐	SMALL + ☐	MODERATE ++ ☐	LARGE +++ ☐
SPECIFIC GRAVITY	1.000 ☐	1.005 ☐	1.010 ☐	1.015 ☐	1.020 ☐	1.025 ☐	1.030 ☐
KETONE	NEGATIVE ☐	mg/dL	TRACE 5 ☐	SMALL 15 ☐	MODERATE 40 ☐	LARGE 80 ☐	LARGE 160 ☐
BILIRUBIN	NEGATIVE ☐		SMALL + ☐	MODERATE ++ ☐	LARGE +++ ☐		
GLUCOSE	NEGATIVE ☐	g/dL (%) mg/dL	1/10 (tr.) 100 ☐	1/4 250 ☐	1/2 500 ☐	1 1000 ☐	2 or more 2000 or more ☐

Multistix® *10 SG* *Reagent Strips for Urinalysis*

PATIENT

DATE   **TIME**

LEUKOCYTES	NEGATIVE ☐		TRACE ☐	SMALL + ☐	MODERATE ++ ☐	LARGE +++ ☐	
NITRATE	NEGATIVE ☐		POSITIVE ☐	POSITIVE ☐	(Any degree of uniform pink color is positive)		
UROBILINOGEN	NORMAL 0.2 ☐	NORMAL 1 ☐	mg/dL 2 ☐	4 ☐	8 ☐	(1 mg = approx. 1 EU)	
PROTEIN	NEGATIVE ☐	TRACE ☐	mg/dL 30 + ☐	100 ++ ☐	300 +++ ☐	2000 or more ++++ ☐	
pH	5.0 ☐	6.0 ☐	6.5 ☐	7.0 ☐	7.5 ☐	8.0 ☐	8.5 ☐
BLOOD	NEGATIVE ☐	NON-HEMOLYZED TRACE ☐	NON-HEMOLYZED MODERATE ☐	HEMOLYZED TRACE ☐	SMALL + ☐	MODERATE ++ ☐	LARGE +++ ☐
SPECIFIC GRAVITY	1.000 ☐	1.005 ☐	1.010 ☐	1.015 ☐	1.020 ☐	1.025 ☐	1.030 ☐
KETONE	NEGATIVE ☐	mg/dL	TRACE 5 ☐	SMALL 15 ☐	MODERATE 40 ☐	LARGE 80 ☐	LARGE 160 ☐
BILIRUBIN	NEGATIVE ☐		SMALL + ☐	MODERATE ++ ☐	LARGE +++ ☐		
GLUCOSE	NEGATIVE ☐	g/dL (%) mg/dL	1/10 (tr.) 100 ☐	1/4 250 ☐	1/2 500 ☐	1 1000 ☐	2 or more 2000 or more ☐

Printed by permission of Bayer Corporation, Diagnostic Division, Tarrytown, NY, 10591

Practice for Competency

MICROSCOPIC ANALYSIS OF URINE

Assignment

Urine Sediment. Practice the procedure for preparing a urine specimen for a microscopic analysis of the urine sediment. Examine the specimen and record the results in the chart provided.

Urine Culture. Perform a rapid urine culture test and record the results in the chart provided.

CHART	
Date	

Practice for Competency

URINE PREGNANCY TESTING

Assignment

Pregnancy Testing. Perform a urine pregnancy test and record results in the chart provided.

CHART	
Date	

Evaluation of Competency

PROCEDURE 16-1: CLEAN CATCH MIDSTREAM SPECIMEN COLLECTION INSTRUCTIONS

Name _____   Date _____

Evaluated By _____   Score_____

Performance Objective

Outcome:	Instruct a patient in the procedure for collecting a clean-catch midstream urine specimen.
Conditions:	Given the following: sterile specimen container, antiseptic solution, and cotton balls or tissues.
Standards:	Time: 10 minutes
	Accuracy: Satisfactory score on the Performance Evaluation Checklist

Performance Evaluation Checklist

Trial 1	Trial 2	Point Value	Performance Standards
		●	Washed hands.
		●	Assembled supplies.
		●	Greeted and identified the patient.
		●	Introduced yourself and explained the procedure.
			Instructed the female patient by telling her to:
		●	Wash hands and remove undergarments.
		●	Expose the urinary meatus by spreading the labia apart with one hand.
		●	Cleanse each side of the urinary meatus with a front-to-back motion, using a fresh cotton ball or antiseptic wipe on each side of the meatus.
		▷	Is able to state why a front-to-back motion should be used.
		●	Cleanse directly across the meatus using a third cotton ball or antiseptic wipe.
		●	Rinse with water to remove all traces of soap (soap solution method only).
		●	Dry area with a cotton ball, using a single front-to-back motion (soap solution method only).
		●	Continuing to hold the labia apart, void a small amount of urine into the toilet.

Trial 1	Trial 2	Point Value	Performance Standards
		▷	Is able to state the purpose of voiding into the toilet.
		●	Collect the next amount of urine by voiding a small amount into the sterile container without touching the inside of the container.
		●	Void the last amount of urine into the toilet.
		●	Wipe area dry with a tissue and wash the hands with soap and water.
			Instructed the male patient by telling him to:
		●	Wash hands and remove undergarments.
		●	Retract the foreskin of the penis if uncircumcised.
		●	Cleanse area around the meatus and the urethral opening by washing each side of the meatus with a separate cotton ball or antiseptic wipe.
		●	Cleanse directly across the meatus, using a third cotton ball or antiseptic wipe.
		●	Rinse with water to remove all traces of soap (soap solution method only).
		●	Dry area with a cotton ball, using a single front-to-back motion (soap solution method only).
		●	Void a small amount of urine into the toilet.
		●	Collect the next amount of urine by voiding into the sterile container without touching the inside of the container.
		●	Void the last amount of urine into the toilet.
		●	Wipe area dry with a tissue and wash the hands with soap and water.
			Performed the following:
		●	Provided patient with instructions on what to do with specimen.
		●	Immediately capped and labeled specimen container.
		●	Washed hands.
		●	Completed a laboratory requisition, if required.
		●	Charted the procedure correctly.
		★	Completed the procedure within 10 minutes.

CHART	
Date	

Evaluation of Student Performance

EVALUATION CRITERIA			COMMENTS
Symbol	**Category**	**Point Value**	
★	Critical Step	16 points	
●	Essential Step	6 points	
▷	Theory Question	2 points	

Score calculation: 100 points

          − _____ points missed

          _____ Score

Satisfactory score: 85 or above

AAMA/CAAHEP Competency Achieved:

☐ Instruct patient in the collection of a clean-catch midstream urine specimen.

Notes

Evaluation of Competency

PROCEDURE 16-2: COLLECTION OF A 24-HOUR URINE SPECIMEN

Name _____   Date _____

Evaluated By _____   Score _____

Performance Objective

Outcome: Collect a 24-hour urine specimen.

Conditions: Given a large urine collection container, written instructions, and a laboratory requisition.

Standards: Time: 5 minutes

Accuracy: Satisfactory score on the Performance Evaluation Checklist.

Performance Evaluation Checklist

Trial 1	Trial 2	Point Value	Performance Standards
		●	Washed hands.
		●	Assembled equipment.
		●	Greeted and identified patient.
		●	Introduced yourself and explained the procedure.
			Instructed the patient in the collection of the specimen:
		●	Empty your bladder when you get up in the morning.
		●	Make a note of what time it is and write it down.
		●	The next time you need to urinate, void the urine into the plastic container.
		●	Tightly screw the lid onto the container.
		●	Store the container in the refrigerator or in an ice chest.
		●	Repeat these steps each time you urinate.
		●	Instructed the patient to collect all of his/her urine in a 24-hour period.
		▷	Is able to state when the patient should begin the collection again from the beginning.
		●	On the following morning, get up at the same time.
		●	Void into the container for the last time.

Trial 1	Trial 2	Point Value	Performance Standards
		●	Put the lid on the container tightly.
		●	Return the urine collection container to the office the same morning as completing the test.
		●	Provided the patient with the collection container and written instructions.
		●	Charted instructions given to the patient in his/her medical record.
			Processing the specimen:
		●	Asked the patient if there were any problems when he/she returned the collection container.
		▷	Is able to state what should be done if the specimen was undercollected or overcollected.
		●	Prepared the specimen for transport to the laboratory.
		●	Completed a laboratory request form.
		●	Charted the results correctly.
		★	Completed the procedure within 5 minutes.

CHART	
Date	

Evaluation of Student Performance

EVALUATION CRITERIA			COMMENTS
Symbol	**Category**	**Point Value**	
★	Critical Step	16 points	
●	Essential Step	6 points	
▷	Theory Question	2 points	
Score calculation: 100 points			
− _____ points missed			
_____ Score			
Satisfactory score: 85 or above			

AAMA/CAAHEP Competency Achieved:
☐ Instruct individuals according to their needs.

Evaluation of Competency

ASSESSING COLOR AND APPEARANCE OF A URINE SPECIMEN

Name _____   Date _____

Evaluated By _____   Score_____

Performance Objective

Outcome:	Assess the color and appearance of a urine specimen.
Conditions:	Given a transparent container, and a urine specimen.
Standards:	Time: 5 minutes
	Accuracy: Satisfactory score on the Performance Evaluation Checklist.

Performance Evaluation Checklist

Trial 1	Trial 2	Point Value	Performance Standards
			COLOR
		●	Transferred urine specimen to a transparent container.
		●	Assessed the color of the urine specimen.
		★	The assessment was identical to the evaluator's assessment.
		●	Charted the results correctly.
			CLARITY
		●	Assessed the appearance of the urine specimen in the transparent container.
		★	The assessment was identical to the evaluator's assessment.
		●	Charted the results correctly.
		●	Properly disposed of urine specimen.
		●	Washed hands.
		★	Completed the procedure within 5 minutes.

CHART	
Date	

Evaluation of Student Performance

EVALUATION CRITERIA			COMMENTS
Symbol	Category	Point Value	
★	Critical Step	16 points	
●	Essential Step	6 points	
▷	Theory Question	2 points	
Score calculation: 100 points			
− _____ points missed			
_____ Score			
Satisfactory score: 85 or above			

AAMA/CAAHEP Competency Achieved:

☐ Perform urinalysis.

Evaluation of Competency

PROCEDURE 16-3 AND 16-4: MEASURING THE SPECIFIC GRAVITY OF URINE – REFRACTOMETER METHOD

Name _____ Date _____

Evaluated By _____ Score_____

Performance Objective

Outcome: Calibrate the refractometer and measure the specific gravity of a urine specimen.

Conditions: Given the following: disposable gloves, refractometer, urine specimen, disposable pipet, lint-free tissues, antiseptic wipe, distilled water, and a biohazard waste container.

Standards: Time: 5 minutes

Accuracy: Satisfactory score on the Performance Evaluation Checklist.

Performance Evaluation Checklist
Measuring Specific Gravity

Trial 1	Trial 2	Point Value	Performance Standards
			MEASURING SPECIFIC GRAVITY
		●	Washed hands.
		●	Assembled equipment.
		●	Calibrated the refractometer.
		●	Applied gloves.
		●	Prepared the urine specimen.
		●	Mixed the urine specimen with the pipet.
		▷	Is able to state why the specimen must be well-mixed.
		●	Withdrew a small amount of urine into the pipet.
		●	Held the pipet in a vertical position.
		●	Placed drop of urine on the surface of prism of the refractometer.
		●	Pointed the refractometer toward a light source.
		●	Rotated eyepiece to bring the calibrated scale clearly into view.
		●	Read the value on the scale at boundary line between the light and dark areas.

Trial 1	Trial 2	Point Value	Performance Standards
		★	The reading was within ± .002 of the evaluator's reading.
		●	Cleaned the prism with a lint-free tissue.
		●	Disinfected the prism surface with an alcohol wipe.
		●	Removed gloves and washed hands.
			CALIBRATION OF THE REFRACTOMETER
		●	Placed a drop of distilled water on the surface of the prism.
		●	Pointed the refractometer toward a light source.
		●	Rotated the eye piece to bring the calibrated scale clearly into view.
		●	Read the value on the scale at boundary line between the light and dark areas.
		●	Determined if the calibration is correct.
		▷	Is able to state the value of correct calibration.
		●	Corrected calibration if necessary.
		▷	Is able to state how calibration is corrected.
		●	Cleaned prism surface with a lint-free tissue.
		★	Completed the procedure within 5 minutes.

CHART	
Date	

Evaluation of Student Performance

Symbol	Category	Point Value
★	Critical Step	16 points
●	Essential Step	6 points
▷	Theory Question	2 points

EVALUATION CRITERIA / **COMMENTS**

Score calculation: 100 points
− _____ points missed
_____ Score

Satisfactory score: 85 or above

AAMA/CAAHEP Competency Achieved:
☐ Perform urinalysis.

Evaluation of Competency

PROCEDURE 16-5: CHEMICAL TESTING OF URINE USING THE MULTISTIX 10 SG REAGENT STRIP

Name _____   Date _____

Evaluated By _____   Score_____

Performance Objective

Outcome: Perform a chemical assessment of a urine assessment.

Conditions: Given the following: disposable gloves, Multistix 10 SG reagent strips, urine container, laboratory report form, and a biohazard waste container.

Standards: Time: 5 minutes

Accuracy: Satisfactory score on the Performance Evaluation Checklist.

Performance Evaluation Checklist

Trial 1	Trial 2	Point Value	Performance Standards
		●	Obtained a freshly voided urine specimen from patient.
		▷	Is able to explain why the container used to collect specimen should be clean.
		●	Washed hands.
		●	Assembled equipment.
		●	Checked expiration date of the reagent strips.
		▷	Is able to state why expiration date should be checked.
		●	Applied gloves.
		●	Removed a reagent strip from bottle and recapped bottle immediately.
		▷	Is able to explain why bottle should be recapped immediately.
		●	Did not touch the test areas with fingers.
		▷	Is able to explain why the test areas should not be touched with fingers.
		●	Completely immersed the reagent strip in urine specimen.
		●	Removed the strip immediately and ran the edge against the rim of urine container.

Trial 1	Trial 2	Point Value	Performance Standards
		▷	Is able to state why excess urine should be removed from the strip.
		●	Held the reagent strip in a horizontal position and placed it adjacent to the corresponding color blocks on color chart.
		▷	Is able to state why the strip should be held in a horizontal position.
		●	Read the results at the exact reading times specified on color chart.
		▷	Is able to state why the results must be read at specified times.
		★	The results were identical to the evaluator's results.
		●	Disposed of the strip in a biohazard waste container.
		●	Removed gloves and washed hands.
		●	Charted the results correctly.
		★	Completed the procedure within 5 minutes.

Multistix® 10 SG *Reagent Strips for Urinalysis*

PATIENT _____

DATE _____ **TIME** _____

LEUKOCYTES	NEGATIVE ☐		TRACE ☐	SMALL + ☐	MODERATE ++ ☐	LARGE +++ ☐
NITRATE	NEGATIVE ☐		POSITIVE ☐	POSITIVE ☐	(Any degree of uniform pink color is positive)	
UROBILINOGEN	NORMAL 0.2 ☐	NORMAL 1 ☐	mg/dL 2 ☐	4 ☐	8 ☐	(1 mg = approx. 1 EU)
PROTEIN	NEGATIVE ☐	TRACE ☐	mg/dL 30 + ☐	100 ++ ☐	300 +++ ☐	2000 or more ++++ ☐
pH	5.0 ☐	6.0 ☐	6.5 ☐	7.0 ☐	7.5 ☐	8.0 ☐	8.5 ☐
BLOOD	NEGATIVE ☐	NON-HEMOLYZED TRACE ☐	NON-HEMOLYZED MODERATE ☐	HEMOLYZED TRACE ☐	SMALL + ☐	MODERATE ++ ☐	LARGE +++ ☐
SPECIFIC GRAVITY	1.000 ☐	1.005 ☐	1.010 ☐	1.015 ☐	1.020 ☐	1.025 ☐	1.030 ☐
KETONE	NEGATIVE ☐	mg/dL	TRACE 5 ☐	SMALL 15 ☐	MODERATE 40 ☐	LARGE 80 ☐	LARGE 160 ☐
BILIRUBIN	NEGATIVE ☐		SMALL + ☐	MODERATE ++ ☐	LARGE +++ ☐	
GLUCOSE	NEGATIVE ☐	g/dL (%) mg/dL	1/10 (tr.) 100 ☐	1/4 250 ☐	1/2 500 ☐	1 1000 ☐	2 or more 2000 or more ☐

Printed by permission of Bayer Corporation, Diagnostic Division, Tarrytown, NY, 10591

Evaluation of Student Performance

EVALUATION CRITERIA			COMMENTS
Symbol	**Category**	**Point Value**	
★	Critical Step	16 points	
●	Essential Step	6 points	
▷	Theory Question	2 points	

Score calculation: 100 points

− _____ points missed

_____ Score

Satisfactory score: 85 or above

AAMA/CAAHEP Competency Achieved:

☐ Perform urinalysis.

Notes

Evaluation of Competency

PROCEDURE 16-6: MICROSCOPIC EXAMINATION OF URINE – KOVA METHOD

Name _____   Date _____

Evaluated By _____   Score_____

Performance Objective

Outcome:	Prepare a urine specimen for microscopic analysis and examine the specimen under the microscope.
Conditions:	Given the following: disposable gloves, first-voided morning urine specimen, Kova urine centrifuge tube, Kova cap, Kova pipet, Kova slide, Kova stain test tube rack, urine centrifuge, mechanical stage microscope, and biohazard waste container.
Standards:	Time: 15 minutes
	Accuracy: Satisfactory score on the Performance Evaluation Checklist.

Performance Evaluation Checklist

Trial 1	Trial 2	Point Value	Performance Standards
		●	Washed hands.
		●	Assembled equipment.
		●	Applied gloves.
		●	Mixed urine specimen with pipet.
		▷	Is able to state the purpose of mixing the specimen.
		●	Poured urine specimen into urine centrifuge tube to the 12-ml mark.
		●	Capped the tube.
		●	Centrifuged specimen for 5 minutes.
		▷	Is able to state the purpose of centrifuging specimen.
		●	Removed the tube from the centrifuge without disturbing the sediment.
		●	Removed the cap.
		●	Inserted Kova pipet into the urine tube and seated it firmly.

Trial 1	Trial 2	Point Value	Performance Standards
		●	Poured off the supernatant fluid.
		●	Removed pipet from the tube.
		●	Added one drop of Kova stain to tube.
		▷	Is able to state the purpose of the stain.
		●	Placed pipet back in tube and mixed specimen thoroughly.
		●	Placed urine tube in test tube rack.
		●	Transferred a sample of the specimen to the Kova slide.
		●	Did not overfill or underfill the well of the Kova slide.
		●	Placed pipet in the urine tube.
		●	Allowed specimen to sit for 1 minute.
		▷	Is able to state the purpose of allowing the specimen to sit.
		●	Properly focused the specimen under low power.
		●	Examined the sediment under low power to scan for the presence of casts.
		●	Properly focused the specimen under high power.
		●	Examined the urine sediment with the high-power objective.
		●	Identified the specific type of cast.
		●	Examined the sediment for the presence of smaller structures (red blood cells, white blood cells, and epithelial cells, bacteria, or crystals).
		●	Examined 10 to 15 high-power fields.
		●	Calculated an average of the high-power fields.
		★	The calculation was performed without a mathematical error.
		●	Turned off the light source.
		●	Removed the slide from the stage.
		●	Disposed of the slide and pipet in a biohazard waste container.
		●	Capped the urine specimen and disposed of it in a biohazard waste container.
		●	Removed gloves and washed hands.
		★	Completed the procedure within 15 minutes.
CHART			
Date			

Evaluation of Student Performance

EVALUATION CRITERIA		
Symbol	**Category**	**Point Value**
★	Critical Step	16 points
●	Essential Step	6 points
▷	Theory Question	2 points

Score calculation: 100 points
− _____ points missed
_____ Score

Satisfactory score: 85 or above

COMMENTS

AAMA/CAAHEP Competency Achieved:
☐ Perform urinalysis.

Notes

Evaluation of Competency

PROCEDURE 16-7: PERFORMING A RAPID URINE CULTURE TEST

Name _____ Date _____

Evaluated By _____ Score_____

Performance Objective

Outcome: Perform a rapid urine culture test.

Conditions: Given the following: disposable gloves, rapid urine culture kit, clean-catch midstream urine specimen, incubator, biohazard waste container.

Standards: Time: 5 minutes

Accuracy: Satisfactory score on the Performance Evaluation Checklist.

Performance Evaluation Checklist

Trial 1	Trial 2	Point Value	Performance Standards
			Preparing the Specimen
		●	Washed hands.
		●	Assembled equipment.
		●	Checked the expiration date on the rapid culture test.
		●	Labeled the vial with the patient's name and date and time of inoculation.
		●	Applied gloves.
		●	Removed the slide from the vial.
		●	Did not touch the culture media.
		●	Completely immersed the slide in urine specimen.
		●	Allowed excess urine to drain from the slide.
		●	Immediately replaced the slide in the vial.
		●	Screwed the cap on loosely.
		●	Placed the vial upright in an incubator.
		▷	Is able to state why the slide should not remain in the incubator for more than 24 hours.

Trial 1	Trial 2	Point Value	Performance Standards
			Reading Test Results
		●	Applied gloves.
		●	Removed the vial from the incubator.
		●	Removed the slide from the vial.
		●	Compared the slide with the reference chart.
		●	Read and interpreted the results.
		★	The results were identical to the evaluator's results.
		●	Charted the results correctly.
		★	Completed the procedure within 5 minutes.

CHART	
Date	

Evaluation of Student Performance

EVALUATION CRITERIA			COMMENTS
Symbol	Category	Point Value	
★	Critical Step	16 points	
●	Essential Step	6 points	
▷	Theory Question	2 points	

Score calculation: 100 points

−＿＿＿＿ points missed

＿＿＿＿ Score

Satisfactory score: 85 or above

AAMA/CAAHEP Competency Achieved:

☐ Perform microbiology testing.

Evaluation of Competency

PROCEDURE 16-8: PERFORMING A URINE PREGNANCY TEST

Name _____   Date _____

Evaluated By _____   Score_____

Performance Objective

Outcome:	Perform a urine pregnancy test.
Conditions:	Given the following: disposable gloves, urine pregnancy testing kit, first-voided morning urine specimen, biohazard waste container.
Standards:	Time: 5 minutes
	Accuracy: Satisfactory score on the Performance Evaluation Checklist.

Performance Evaluation Checklist

Trial 1	Trial 2	Point Value	Performance Standards
			Preparing the Specimen
		●	Washed hands.
		●	Assembled equipment.
		●	Checked the expiration date on the pregnancy test.
		▷	Is able to state why the expiration date should be checked.
		●	Applied gloves.
		●	Removed the test cassette from its pouch.
		●	Placed the test cassette on a clean, dry, level surface.
		●	Added 3 drops of urine to the well on the test cassette.
		●	Disposed of the pipet in a biohazard waste container.
		●	Waited 3 minutes and read the results.
		●	Interpreted the test results.
		★	The results were identical to the evaluator's results.
		▷	Is able to state the appearance of a positive and a negative test result.
		▷	Is able to state what should be done if no result occurred.
		●	Disposed of the test cassette in a biohazard waste container.

Trial 1	Trial 2	Point Value	Performance Standards
		●	Removed gloves and washed hands.
		●	Charted the results correctly.
		★	Completed the procedure within 10 minutes.

CHART	
Date	

Evaluation of Student Performance

EVALUATION CRITERIA			COMMENTS
Symbol	Category	Point Value	
★	Critical Step	16 points	
●	Essential Step	6 points	
▷	Theory Question	2 points	
Score calculation: 100 points			
− _____ points missed			
_____ Score			
Satisfactory score: 85 or above			

AAMA/CAAHEP Competencies Achieved:

☐ Use methods of quality control.

☐ Screen and follow-up test results.

Phlebotomy

NAME _____

Key Terminology Assessment:

Directions: Match each medical term with its definition.

_____ 1. antecubital space
_____ 2. anticoagulant
_____ 3. buffy coat
_____ 4. evacuated tube
_____ 5. hematoma
_____ 6. hemoconcentration
_____ 7. hemolysis
_____ 8. osteochondritis
_____ 9. osteomyelitis
_____ 10. phlebotomist
_____ 11. phlebotomy
_____ 12. plasma
_____ 13. serum
_____ 14. venipuncture
_____ 15. venous reflux
_____ 16. venous stasis

A. The liquid part of blood, consisting of a clear yellowish fluid that makes up approximately 55% of the total blood volume.
B. A substance that inhibits blood clotting.
C. A health professional trained in the collection of a blood specimen.
D. The breakdown of blood cells.
E. A closed glass or plastic tube containing a premeasured vacuum.
F. The temporary cessation or slowing of the venous blood flow.
G. A thin, light-colored layer of white blood cells and platelets that lies between a top layer of plasma and a bottom layer of red blood cells when an anticoagulant has been added to a blood specimen.
H. The surface of the arm in front of the elbow.
I. Inflammation of bone and cartilage.
J. An increase in concentration of the nonfilterable blood components.

K. Plasma from which the clotting factor fibrinogen has been removed.
L. Incision of a vein for the removal or withdrawal of blood.
M. Inflammation of the bone due to bacterial infection.
N. A swelling or mass of coagulated blood caused by a break in a blood vessel.
O. Puncturing of a vein.
P. The backflow of blood into the patient's vein.

Self-Evaluation

Directions: Fill in each blank with the correct answer.

1. List the three major areas of blood collection included in phlebotomy.

    _____

    _____

2. What is the purpose of performing a venipuncture?

    _____

    _____

3. List the three methods that can be used to perform a venipuncture.

    _____

    _____

    _____

4. What are the advantages of using the vacuum tube method of venipuncture?

    _____

    _____

5. When would the butterfly and syringe methods of venipuncture be preferred over the vacuum tube method?

    _____

    _____

    _____

6. Explain how to prevent venous reflux.

    _____

    _____

7. What is the purpose of the tourniquet?

_____

_____

8. After locating a suitable vein for venipuncture, what three qualities should be determined with respect to the vein?

_____

_____

9. Why are the antecubital veins preferred for performing a venipuncture?

_____

_____

_____

10. List four techniques that can be used to make veins more prominent.

_____

_____

_____

_____

11. Why should the veins of the hand be used only as a last resort when performing a venipuncture?

_____

_____

_____

12. How is a serum specimen obtained?

_____

_____

13. How is a whole blood specimen obtained?

_____

_____

14. List the three layers into which the blood separates when it is mixed with an anticoagulant.

_____

_____

15. List the layers into which the blood separates when an anticoagulant is not added to it.

_____

_____

16. List four OSHA safety precautions that must be followed when performing a venipuncture and separating serum or plasma from whole blood.

_____

_____

_____

_____

17. What is the range for the gauge and size of the needle used for the vacuum tube method of venipuncture?

_____

_____

18. What is the purpose of the flange on the plastic holder of the vacuum tube system?

_____

_____

19. What type of additive is present in each of the following evacuated tubes?

red_____

lavender _____

gray_____

light blue _____

green_____

20. What color stopper must be used to collect the blood specimen for each of the tests listed below?

complete blood count _____

prothrombin time _____

glucose tolerance test _____

most blood chemistry tests_____

blood gas determinations _____

21. Why is it important to use the correct order of draw when performing a venipuncture?

_____

_____

22. Why is it important to mix a tube containing an anticoagulant immediately after drawing it?

_____

_____

23. What is the range for the gauge and size of needle used for the butterfly method of venipuncture?

_____

_____

24. List four ways to prevent a blood specimen from becoming hemolyzed.

_____

_____

_____

_____

25. List examples of dissolved substances contained in the serum of blood.

_____

_____

_____

26. What is the purpose of performing laboratory tests on serum?

_____

_____

_____

27. List the proper size tube that must be used to obtain the following serum specimens.

2 ml of serum_____

6 ml of serum_____

4 ml of serum_____

28. What is a fibrin clot and why should it be avoided in a serum specimen?

_____

_____

_____

29. How does a serum separator tube function in the collection of a serum specimen?

_____

_____

_____

30. List four types of solutes contained in the plasma.

_____

_____

_____

_____

31. What is the preferred site for a skin puncture for the following individuals?

a. adult _____

b. infant_____

32. List two examples of microcollection devices.

_____

_____

33. Why shouldn't a finger puncture be performed on the index finger?

_____

_____

Critical Thinking Skills

1. Practice palpating the antecubital veins on at least five persons. Use a tourniquet applied to each person's arm and ask the individual to clench his or her fist. Record the individual's name and which vein would be considered the best to use on each person when performing venipuncture.

NAME   **SUITABLE VEIN**

a. _____

b. _____

c. _____

d. _____

e. _____

2. Using the principles outlined in the vacuum tube venipuncture procedure, state what might happen under the following circumstances:

a. An evacuated tube is used that is past its expiration date.

_____

_____

b. The vacuum tube is not labeled.

_____

_____

c. The tourniquet is not applied tightly enough.

_____

_____

d. The tourniquet is left on for more than 1 minute.

_____

_____

e. The area that has just been cleansed with an antiseptic is not allowed to dry before the venipuncture is made.

_____

_____

f. The evacuated tube is inserted past the indentation in the plastic holder before the vein is entered.

_____

_____

g. An angle of less than 15 degrees is used when performing venipuncture.

_____

_____

h. An angle of more than 15 degrees is used when performing venipuncture.

_____

_____

i. The needle is moved after inserting the needle.

_____

_____

j. Venous reflux occurs when using an EDTA evacuated tube.

_____

_____

k. The vacuum tube is not allowed to fill to the exhaustion of the vacuum.

_____

_____

l. The needle is removed from the arm before the tourniquet has been removed.

_____

_____

m. A gauze pad is not placed over the puncture site before removing the needle.

_____

_____

n. The patient bends the arm at the elbow after the needle is removed.

_____

_____

o. The patient lifts a heavy object after the procedure.

_____

_____

3. You are responsible for performing the venipunctures in your medical office. In the space provided, explain what you would do in each of the following situations:
a. The patient asks you if the venipuncture will hurt.

_____

_____

b. Upon palpating the patient's vein, you find that it feels stiff and hard.

_____

_____

c. You have attempted one venipuncture in a patient with small veins using the vacuum tube method of venipuncture; however, the vein collapsed and you were unable to obtain blood.

_____

_____

d. The patient moves during the procedure causing the needle to come out of his arm.

_____

_____

e. You have inserted the needle in the vein, but notice a sudden swelling around the puncture site.

_____

_____

f. You inadvertently puncture the brachial artery after inserting the needle.

_____

_____

g. The patient begins to sweat and tells you that she feels warm and light-headed.

_____

_____

4. Explain why the following guidelines must be observed while separating serum from whole blood.
   a. Label the transfer tube with the word *serum*.

_____

_____

b. Place the tube in an upright position for 30 to 45 minutes.

_____

_____

c. Do not allow the specimen to stand for more than 1 hour before centrifuging it.

_____

_____

d. Make sure the tube is stoppered during centrifugation.

_____

_____

e. Wear personal protective equipment when transferring serum from whole blood.

_____

_____

f. Do not disturb the cell layer while pipetting the serum.

_____

_____

5. The medical assistant is performing a skin puncture on an adult patient in order to obtain a capillary blood specimen for a hemoglobin test. For each of the following situations, write **C** if the technique is correct and **I** if the technique is incorrect. If the technique is correct, explain the rationale for performing it that way; if incorrect, explain what might happen if the technique were performed in the incorrect manner.

_____a. Before making the puncture, the medical assistant asks the patient to rinse his hand in warm water.

_____

_____

_____b. The puncture is made with the patient in a standing position.

_____

_____

_____c. The site is allowed to dry thoroughly after it is cleansed with an antiseptic wipe.

_____

_____

_____d. The specimen is collected from the lateral part of the tip of the ring finger.

_____

_____

_____e. The puncture is made perpendicular to the lines of the fingerprint.

_____

_____

_____f. The depth of the puncture is 4 mm.

_____

_____

_____g. The first drop of blood is wiped away.

_____

_____

_____h. The puncture site is squeezed in order to obtain the blood specimen.

_____

_____

Practice for Competency

VENIPUNCTURE

Assignment

Vacuum Tube Method.
Practice the procedure for collecting a venous blood specimen using the vacuum tube method. Record the procedure in the chart provided.

Butterfly Method.
Practice the procedure for collecting a venous blood specimen using the butterfly method. Record the procedure in the chart provided.

Syringe Method.
Practice the procedure for collecting a venous blood specimen using the syringe method. Record the procedure in the chart provided.

Separating Serum from Whole Blood.
Separate serum from whole blood and record the procedure in the chart provided.

CHART	
Date	

Practice for Competency

SKIN PUNCTURE

Assignment

Disposable Lancet Method.
Obtain a capillary blood specimen using a disposable lancet. In the space provided below, identify five errors in technique that could lead to contamination or that could affect the quality of the blood specimen.

Disposable Semi-Automatic Lancet Method.
Obtain a capillary blood specimen using a disposable semi-automatic lancet device.

Reusable Semi-Automatic Lancet.
Obtain a capillary blood specimen using a reusable semi-automatic lancet.

ERRORS IN TECHNIQUE

Notes

Evaluation of Competency

PROCEDURE 17-1: VENIPUNCTURE USING THE VACUUM TUBE METHOD

Name_____   Date _____

Evaluated By _____   Score _____

Performance Objective

Outcome:	Perform a venipuncture using the vacuum tube method.
Conditions:	Given the following: disposable gloves, tourniquet, antiseptic wipe, double-pointed needle, plastic holder, evacuated tubes, gauze pads, adhesive bandage, and a biohazard sharps container.
Standards:	Time: 10 minutes
	Accuracy: Satisfactory score on the Performance Evaluation Checklist.

Performance Evaluation Checklist

Trial 1	Trial 2	Point Value	Performance Standards
		●	Washed hands.
		●	Greeted and identified the patient.
		●	Introduced yourself.
		●	Asked patient if he/she prepared properly.
		●	Assembled equipment.
		●	Selected the proper evacuated tubes.
		●	Checked the expiration date of the tubes.
		▷	Is able to state the purpose of checking the expiration date.
		●	Labeled the evacuated tubes.
		●	Completed a laboratory request form, if necessary.
		●	Screwed the needle into the plastic holder and tightened securely.
		●	Opened the gauze packet.
		●	Positioned the evacuated tubes in the correct order of draw.
		●	Tapped evacuated tubes with a powdered additive below the stopper.
		▷	Is able to state the purpose for tapping the tube.
		●	Placed the first tube loosely in the plastic holder.
		●	Placed remaining supplies within comfortable reach of the nondominant hand.

Trial 1	Trial 2	Point Value	Performance Standards
		●	Explained the procedure to the patient and reassured patient.
		●	Performed a preliminary assessment of both arms.
		●	Correctly applied the tourniquet.
		▷	Is able to state the purpose of the tourniquet.
		●	Asked patient to clench fist.
		●	Assessed the veins of both arms.
		●	Determined the best vein to use.
		●	Did not leave the tourniquet on for more than 1 minute.
		▷	Is able to state why the tourniquet should not be left on for more than 1 minute.
		●	Positioned the patient's arm correctly.
		●	Thoroughly palpated the selected vein.
		●	Cleansed area and allowed puncture site to dry.
		▷	Is able to state why the site should be allowed to dry.
		●	Did not touch the site after cleansing.
		●	Applied gloves.
		●	Removed cap from the needle.
		●	Properly held the venipuncture set-up (bevel up) with the dominant hand.
		●	Positioned the tube with the label facing downward.
		●	Grasped the patient's arm and anchored the vein correctly.
		●	Positioned the venipuncture set-up at a 15-degree angle to the arm, with needle pointing in the same direction as the vein to be entered.
		●	Told the patient that a small stick will be felt.
		●	With one continuous motion, entered the skin and then the vein.
		●	The vein was entered approximately $\frac{1}{4}$ inch below the place where the vein is to be entered.
		●	Firmly grasped the plastic holder.
		●	Pushed the tube forward slowly to the end of the holder using the flange.
		●	Did not move the needle once the venipuncture was made.
		●	Allowed evacuated tube to fill to the exhaustion of the vacuum.
		●	Removed the tube from the plastic holder using the flange.
		●	Immediately and gently inverted tube 8 to 10 times if it contains an additive.
		●	Inserted the next tube into the holder using the flange.
		●	Continued until the last tube was filled.

Trial 1	Trial 2	Point Value	Performance Standards
		●	Removed the last tube from the holder.
		▷	Is able to state why the last tube should be removed.
		★	Removed tourniquet at the proper time and asked patient to unclench fist.
		●	Placed gauze pad over puncture site and withdrew the needle slowly and at the same angle as that for penetration.
		●	Applied pressure with gauze after removing needle.
		●	Instructed the patient to apply pressure with the gauze pad for 1 to 2 minutes.
		●	Properly disposed of the venipuncture needle in a biohazard sharps container.
		●	Stayed with patient until bleeding stopped.
		●	Applied adhesive bandage if needed.
		●	Removed gloves and washed hands.
		●	Charted the procedure correctly.
		●	Tested, transferred, or stored the blood specimen according to medical office policy.
		★	Completed the procedure within 10 minutes.

CHART	
Date	

Evaluation of Student Performance

EVALUATION CRITERIA			COMMENTS
Symbol	Category	Point Value	
★	Critical Step	16 points	
●	Essential Step	6 points	
▷	Theory Question	2 points	
Score calculation: 100 points			
−_____ points missed			
_____ Score			
Satisfactory score: 85 or above			

AAMA/CAAHEP Competency Achieved:

☐ Perform venipuncture.

Evaluation of Competency

PROCEDURE 17-2: VENIPUNCTURE USING THE BUTTERFLY METHOD

Name_____ Date _____

Evaluated By _____ Score _____

Performance Objective

Outcome: Perform a venipuncture using the butterfly method.

Conditions: Given the following: disposable gloves, tourniquet, antiseptic wipe, winged-infusion set, plastic holder, evacuated tubes, gauze pads, adhesive bandage, and a biohazard sharps container.

Standards: Time: 10 minutes

Accuracy: Satisfactory score on the Performance Evaluation Checklist.

Performance Evaluation Checklist

Trial 1	Trial 2	Point Value	Performance Standards
		●	Washed hands.
		●	Greeted and identified the patient.
		●	Introduced yourself.
		●	Asked the patient if he/she prepared properly.
		▷	Is able to state why it is important for the patient to prepare properly.
		●	Assembled equipment.
		●	Selected the proper evacuated tubes.
		●	Checked the expiration date on the tubes.
		●	Labeled the evacuated tubes.
		●	Completed a laboratory request form, if necessary.
		●	Removed the winged infusion set from its package.
		●	Extended the tubing.
		▷	Is able to state why the tubing should be extended.
		●	Screwed the plastic holder onto the Luer adapter and tightened securely.
		●	Opened the gauze packet.
		●	Positioned the evacuated tubes in the correct order of draw.
		●	Tapped the evacuated tubes with a powdered additive below the stopper.

Trial 1	Trial 2	Point Value	Performance Standards
		●	Placed the first tube loosely in the plastic holder with label facing downward.
		▷	Is able to state why the label should be facing downward.
		●	Placed remaining supplies within comfortable reach.
		●	Explained procedure and reassured patient.
		●	Performed a preliminary assessment of both arms.
		●	Correctly applied the tourniquet and asked patient to clench fist.
		●	Assessed the veins of both arms.
		●	Determined the best vein to use.
		●	Did not leave the tourniquet on for more than 1 minute.
		●	Positioned the patient's arm correctly.
		●	Thoroughly palpated the selected vein.
		▷	Is able to state the purpose of palpating the vein.
		●	Cleansed area and allowed puncture site to dry.
		●	Did not touch the site after cleansing.
		●	Applied gloves.
		●	Grasped the winged infusion set correctly.
		●	Removed the protective shield.
		●	Positioned the needle with the bevel up.
		▷	Is able to state why the bevel should be up.
		●	Grasped patient's arm and anchored the vein correctly.
		●	Positioned the needle at a 15-degree angle to arm, with needle pointing in the same direction as the vein to be entered.
		●	Told the patient that a small stick will be felt.
		●	With one continuous motion, entered the skin and then the vein.
		▷	Is able to state why a continuous motion should be used.
		●	Decreased the angle of the needle to 5 degrees.
		●	The vein was entered approximately $\frac{1}{4}$ inch below the place where the vein is to be entered.
		●	Seated the needle.
		▷	Is able to state the purpose of seating the needle.
		●	Rested the needle flat against the skin.
		★	Kept the tube and holder in a downward position.
		●	Firmly grasped the holder and slowly pushed the tube forward to the end of the plastic holder using the flange.
		●	Did not move the needle once the puncture was made.

Trial 1	Trial 2	Point Value	Performance Standards
		●	Allowed evacuated tube to fill to the exhaustion of the vacuum.
		▷	Is able to state why the tube should be filled to the exhaustion of the vacuum.
		●	Removed the tube from the holder using the flange.
		●	Immediately and gently inverted evacuated tube 8 to 10 times if it contains an additive.
		▷	Is able to state why a tube with an additive must be inverted immediately.
		●	Inserted the next tube in the holder using the flange.
		●	Continued until the last tube was filled.
		★	Removed the tourniquet and asked the patient to unclench fist.
		▷	Is able to state why the tourniquet must be removed before the needle.
		●	Removed the last tube from the holder.
		●	Placed gauze pad over puncture site and withdrew the needle slowly and at the same angle as that for penetration.
		●	Applied pressure with gauze pad after removing needle.
		●	Instructed the patient to apply pressure with the gauze pad for 1 to 2 minutes.
		●	Properly disposed of needle and tubing in a biohazard sharps container.
		●	Stayed with patient until bleeding stopped.
		●	Applied adhesive bandage if needed.
		●	Removed gloves and washed hands.
		●	Charted the procedure correctly.
		●	Tested, transferred, or stored the blood specimen according to medical office policy.
		★	Completed the procedure within 10 minutes.

CHART

Date	

Evaluation of Student Performance

EVALUATION CRITERIA			COMMENTS
Symbol	Category	Point Value	
★	Critical Step	16 points	
●	Essential Step	6 points	
▷	Theory Question	2 points	

Score calculation: 100 points

− _____ points missed

_____ Score

Satisfactory score: 85 or above

AAMA/CAAHEP Competency Achieved:
☐ Perform venipuncture.

Evaluation of Competency

PROCEDURE 17-3: VENIPUNCTURE USING THE SYRINGE METHOD

Name _____ Date _____

Evaluated By _____ Score _____

Performance Objective

Outcome: Perform a venipuncture using the syringe method.

Conditions: Given the following: disposable gloves, tourniquet, antiseptic wipe, syringe and needle, sterile gauze pads, glass vacuum tube and label, test tube rack, adhesive bandage, and a biohazard sharps container.

Standards: Time: 10 minutes

Accuracy: Satisfactory score on the Performance Evaluation Checklist.

Performance Evaluation Checklist

Trial 1	Trial 2	Point Value	Performance Standards
		●	Washed hands.
		●	Greeted and identified the patient.
		●	Introduced yourself.
		●	Asked the patient if he/she prepared properly.
		●	Assembled equipment.
		●	Selected proper evacuated tubes.
		●	Checked the expiration date on the tubes.
		●	Labeled the evacuated tubes.
		●	Completed a laboratory request form, if necessary.
		●	Prepared the needle and syringe.
		●	Broke the seal on the syringe.
		●	Checked to make sure the tube is screwed tightly into the syringe.
		●	Placed evacuated tubes in a test tube rack in the correct order to be filled.
		●	Tapped evacuated tubes with a powdered additive below the stopper.
		●	Explained procedure and reassured patient.
		●	Correctly applied the tourniquet and asked patient to clench fist.
		●	Assessed the veins of both arms.
		●	Determined the best vein to use.

Trial 1	Trial 2	Point Value	Performance Standards
		●	Did not leave the tourniquet on for more than 1 minute.
		●	Positioned the patient's arm correctly.
		●	Thoroughly palpated the selected vein.
		●	Cleansed area and allowed puncture site to dry.
		●	Applied gloves.
		●	Removed cap from the needle.
		●	Properly held the syringe (bevel up).
		●	Grasped the patient's arm and anchored the vein correctly.
		●	Positioned the needle at a 15-degree angle to patient's arm, with the needle pointing in the same direction as the vein to be entered.
		▷	Is able to state what would happen if an angle of less than 15 degrees or more than 15 degrees were used.
		●	Told the patient that a small stick will be felt.
		●	With one continuous motion, entered the skin and then the vein.
		●	The vein was entered approximately $\frac{1}{4}$ inch below the place where the vein is to be entered.
		●	Did not move the needle once the venipuncture was made.
		●	Removed the desired amount of blood by slowly pulling back the plunger.
		▷	Is able to state why the blood should be withdrawn slowly.
		★	Removed the tourniquet and asked patient to unclench fist.
		▷	Is able to state why the tourniquet should be removed before the needle.
		●	Placed gauze pad over puncture site and withdrew the needle slowly and at the same angle as that for penetration.
		●	Applied pressure with gauze pad after removing needle.
		●	Instructed the patient to apply pressure with the gauze pad for 1 to 2 minutes.
		▷	Is able to state the reason for applying pressure.
		●	Transferred the blood to the evacuated tube as soon as possible.
		▷	Is able to state why the blood should be transferred as soon as possible.
		●	Inserted needle through center of rubber stopper.
		●	Did not apply pressure to the plunger of the syringe.
		●	Did not hold the tube in the hand when transferring blood.
		▷	Is able to state why the tube should not be held in the hand.

Trial 1	Trial 2	Point Value	Performance Standards
		●	Immediately and gently inverted the collection tube 8 to 10 times if it contains an additive.
		▷	Is able to state why the blood should be handled carefully and gently.
		●	Properly disposed of the needle and syringe in a biohazard sharps container.
		●	Stayed with patient until the bleeding stopped.
		●	Applied adhesive bandage if needed.
		●	Removed gloves and washed hands.
		●	Charted the procedure correctly.
		●	Tested, transferred, or stored the blood specimen according to medical office policy.
		★	Completed the procedure within 10 minutes.

CHART	
Date	

Evaluation of Student Performance

EVALUATION CRITERIA			COMMENTS
Symbol	**Category**	**Point Value**	
★	Critical Step	16 points	
●	Essential Step	6 points	
▷	Theory Question	2 points	

Score calculation: 100 points

− _____ points missed

_____ Score

Satisfactory score: 85 or above

AAMA/CAAHEP Competency Achieved:

☐ Perform venipuncture.

Evaluation of Competency

PROCEDURE 17-4: SEPARATING SERUM FROM WHOLE BLOOD

Name_____   Date _____

Evaluated By _____   Score _____

Performance Objective

Outcome:	Separate serum from whole blood.
Conditions:	Given the following: red-stoppered vacuum tube venipuncture set-up, test tube rack, disposable pipet, transfer tube, disposable gloves, face shield or mask and an eye protection device, centrifuge and a biohazard sharps container.
Standards:	Time: 20 minutes
	Accuracy: Satisfactory score on the Performance Evaluation Checklist.

Performance Evaluation Checklist

Trial 1	Trial 2	Point Value	Performance Standards
		●	Collected the blood specimen using venipuncture.
		▷	Is able to explain why a red-stoppered tube should be used.
		●	Placed specimen tube in an upright position for 30 to 45 minutes at room temperature, keeping stopper on specimen tube.
		▷	Is able to state why specimen tube must be placed in an upright position.
		●	Placed specimen tube in the centrifuge, with stopper end up.
		▷	Is able to state why the stopper must remain on specimen tube.
		●	Balanced the specimen with the same type and weight of tube.
		▷	Is able to state the purpose for balancing the centrifuge.
		●	Centrifuged the specimen for 10 to 15 minutes.
		▷	Is able to state the purpose of centrifuging.
		●	Put on a face shield or a mask and an eye-protection device and applied gloves.
		▷	Is able to state the purpose of wearing personal protective equipment.
		●	Removed specimen tube from centrifuge without disturbing the contents.
		▷	Is able to state what must be done if the contents of the tube are disturbed.

Trial 1	Trial 2	Point Value	Performance Standards
		●	Carefully removed the stopper from the tube.
		●	Squeezed bulb of the pipet and placed tip of the pipet against the side of specimen tube approximately $\frac{1}{4}$ inch above the cell layer.
		▷	Is able to state why the bulb should be squeezed before inserting pipet into serum.
		●	Released bulb to suction serum into the pipet.
		●	Transferred serum to transfer tube.
		●	Did not disturb the cell layer.
		●	Continued pipetting until as much serum as possible was removed.
		●	Capped specimen tube tightly and held it up to the light to examine it for hemolysis.
		▷	Is able to explain what should be done if hemolysis is present in the specimen.
		●	Made sure that the proper amount of serum was obtained.
		●	Properly disposed of equipment.
		●	Removed gloves and washed hands.
		●	Tested, transferred, or stored the specimen according to medical office policy.
		★	Completed the procedure within 20 minutes.

Evaluation of Student Performance

EVALUATION CRITERIA			COMMENTS
Symbol	Category	Point Value	
★	Critical Step	16 points	
●	Essential Step	6 points	
▷	Theory Question	2 points	

Score calculation: 100 points

−_____ points missed

_____ Score

Satisfactory score: 85 or above

AAMA/CAAHEP Competency Achieved:
☐ Perform venipuncture.

Evaluation of Competency

PROCEDURE 17-5: SKIN PUNCTURE USING A DISPOSABLE LANCET

Name_____   Date _____

Evaluated By _____   Score _____

Performance Objective

Outcome:	Obtain a capillary blood specimen.
Conditions:	Given the following: disposable gloves, antiseptic wipe, disposable lancet, gauze pads, and a biohazard sharps container.
Standards:	Time: 5 minutes
	Accuracy: Satisfactory score on the Performance Evaluation Checklist.

Performance Evaluation Checklist

Trial 1	Trial 2	Point Value	*Performance Standards*
		●	Washed hands.
		●	Greeted and identified the patient.
		●	Introduced yourself.
		●	Asked patient if he/she prepared properly.
		●	Assembled equipment.
		●	Opened sterile gauze packet.
		●	Explained the procedure to the patient and reassured patient.
		●	Seated patient in chair.
		●	Extended the palmar surface of patient's hand facing up.
		●	Selected a puncture site.
		●	Warmed site if needed.
		●	Cleansed puncture site and allowed it to dry.
		●	Did not touch the site after cleansing.
		●	Applied gloves.
		●	Removed cover from end of lancet without contaminating its tip.
		●	Firmly grasped patient's finger and made puncture with sterile lancet.
		●	Disposed of lancet in biohazard sharps container.
		●	Waited a few seconds to allow blood flow to begin.

Trial 1	Trial 2	Point Value	Performance Standards
		●	Wiped away the first drop of blood with a gauze pad.
		▷	Is able to state why the first drop of blood is wiped away.
		●	Allowed a large well-rounded second drop of blood to form.
		●	Did not squeeze finger to obtain blood.
		▷	Is able to state why finger should not be squeezed.
		●	Collected the blood specimen in the appropriate microcollection device.
		●	Instructed patient to hold a gauze pad over puncture site with pressure.
		●	Remained with patient until bleeding stopped.
		●	Applied an adhesive bandage if needed.
		●	Tested the blood specimen as required by the test being performed.
		●	Removed gloves.
		●	Washed hands.
		★	Completed the procedure within 5 minutes.

Evaluation of Student Performance

EVALUATION CRITERIA			COMMENTS
Symbol	**Category**	**Point Value**	
★	Critical Step	16 points	
●	Essential Step	6 points	
▷	Theory Question	2 points	
Score calculation: 100 points			
− _____ points missed			
_____ Score			
Satisfactory score: 85 or above			

AAMA/CAAHEP Competency Achieved:
☐ Perform capillary puncture.

Evaluation of Competency

PROCEDURE 17-6: SKIN PUNCTURE USING A DISPOSABLE SEMI-AUTOMATIC LANCET

Name_____ Date_____

Evaluated By_____ Score _____

Performance Objective

Outcome: Obtain a capillary blood specimen.

Conditions: Given the following: disposable gloves, antiseptic wipe, microtainer lancet, gauze pads, and a biohazard sharps container.

Standards: Time: 5 minutes

Accuracy: Satisfactory score on the Performance Evaluation Checklist.

Performance Evaluation Checklist

Trial 1	Trial 2	Point Value	Performance Standards
		●	Washed hands.
		●	Greeted and identified the patient.
		●	Introduced yourself.
		●	Asked patient if he/she prepared properly.
		●	Assembled equipment.
		●	Opened sterile gauze packet.
		●	Explained the procedure to the patient and reassured patient.
		●	Seated patient in chair.
		●	Extended the palmar surface of patient's hand facing up.
		●	Selected a puncture site.
		●	Warmed site if needed.
		●	Cleansed puncture site and allowed it to dry.
		●	Did not touch the site after cleansing.
		●	Removed semi-automatic lancet from its plastic packet.
		●	Applied gloves.
		●	Firmly grasped patient's finger.
		●	Placed plastic holder on patient's finger with moderate pressure.
		●	Depressed the plunger and immediately released the plunger.

Trial 1	Trial 2	Point Value	Performance Standards
		●	Disposed of lancet in a biohazard waste container.
		●	Waited a few seconds to allow blood flow to begin.
		●	Wiped away the first drop of blood with a gauze pad.
		●	Allowed a large well-rounded second drop of blood to form.
		●	Did not squeeze finger the obtain blood.
		●	Collected the blood specimen in the appropriate microcollection device.
		●	Instructed patient to hold a gauze pad over puncture site with pressure.
		●	Remained with patient until bleeding stopped.
		●	Applied an adhesive bandage if needed.
		●	Tested the blood specimen as required by the test being performed.
		●	Removed gloves.
		●	Washed hands.
		★	Completed the procedure within 5 minutes.

Evaluation of Student Performance

EVALUATION CRITERIA			COMMENTS
Symbol	Category	Point Value	
★	Critical Step	16 points	
●	Essential Step	6 points	
▷	Theory Question	2 points	

Score calculation: 100 points

− _____ points missed

_____ Score

Satisfactory score: 85 or above

AAMA/CAAHEP Competency Achieved:
☐ Perform capillary puncture.

Evaluation of Competency

PROCEDURE 17-7: SKIN PUNCTURE USING A REUSABLE SEMI-AUTOMATIC LANCET

Name _____ Date _____

Evaluated By _____ Score _____

Performance Objective

Outcome: Perform a venipuncture using the syringe method.

Conditions: Given the following: disposable gloves, antiseptic wipe, Autolet II lancet device, disposable platform, sterile lancet, gauze pads, and a biohazard sharps container.

Standards: Time: 10 minutes

Accuracy: Satisfactory score on the Performance Evaluation Checklist.

Performance Evaluation Checklist

Trial 1	Trial 2	Point Value	Performance Standards
		●	Washed hands.
		●	Greeted and identified the patient.
		●	Introduced yourself.
		●	Asked patient if he/she prepared properly.
		●	Assembled equipment.
		●	Pulled arm of Autolet back until it clicked into place.
		●	Inserted appropriate platform into Autolet.
		▷	Is able to state when to use the standard platform and when to use the super-puncture platform.
		●	Inserted lancet into lancet socket.
		●	Opened the sterile gauze packet.
		●	Explained the procedure to the patient and reassured the patient.
		●	Seated patient in chair.
		●	Extended palmar surface of patient's hand facing up.
		●	Selected a puncture site.
		●	Warmed site if needed.
		▷	Is able to explain how patient's finger can be warmed.
		●	Cleansed puncture site and allowed it to dry.

Trial 1	Trial 2	Point Value	Performance Standards
		●	Applied gloves.
		●	Removed plastic cover from the end of lancet.
		●	Firmly grasped patient's finger.
		●	Placed the platform firmly against puncture site.
		●	Pressed the release button.
		●	Disposed of the platform and lancet in a biohazard waste container.
		●	Allowed a large well-rounded second drop of blood to form.
		●	Wiped away the first drop of blood with a gauze pad.
		▷	Is able to state why finger should not be squeezed.
		●	Collected the blood specimen in the appropriate micrcollection device.
		●	Instructed the patient to hold a gauze pad over puncture site with pressure.
		●	Remained with patient until bleeding stopped.
		●	Applied an adhesive bandage if needed.
		●	Tested the blood specimen as required by the test being performed.
		●	Removed gloves.
		●	Washed hands.
		●	Sanitized and sterilized Autolet.
		●	Stored Autolet with the arm in its resting position.
		★	Completed the procedure within 5 minutes.

Evaluation of Student Performance

EVALUATION CRITERIA			COMMENTS
Symbol	Category	Point Value	
★	Critical Step	16 points	
●	Essential Step	6 points	
▷	Theory Question	2 points	

Score calculation: 100   points

−   _____   points missed

_____   Score

Satisfactory score: 85 or above

AAMA/CAAHEP Competency Achieved:
☐ Perform capillary puncture.

Notes

Notes

Hematology

NAME _____

Key Terminology Assessment:

Directions: Match each medical term with its definition.

C 1. ameboid movement
F 2. anemia
J 3. bilirubin
D 4. diapedesis
H 5. hematology
L 6. hemoglobin
B 7. hemolysis
J 8. leukocytosis
A 9. leukopenia
G 10. oxyhemoglobin
K 11. phagocytosis
E 12. polycythemia

A. An abnormal decrease in the number of white blood cells (below 4,500 per cu mm of blood).

B. The breakdown of erythrocytes with the release of hemoglobin into the plasma.

C. Movement used by leukocytes that permits them to propel themselves from the capillaries out into the tissues.

D. The ameboid movement of blood (especially leukocytes) through the wall of a capillary and out into the tissues.

E. A disorder in which there is an increase in the red cell mass.

F. A condition in which there is a decrease in the number of erythrocytes or in the amount of hemoglobin in the blood.

G. Hemoglobin that has combined with oxygen.

H. The study of blood and blood-forming tissues.

J. An abnormal increase in the number of white blood cells (above 11,000 per cu mm of blood).

J. An orange-colored bile pigment produced by the breakdown of heme from the hemoglobin molecule.

K. The engulfing and destruction of foreign particles, such as bacteria, by special cells called phagocytes.

L. The iron-containing pigment of erythrocytes that transports oxygen in the body.

Self-Evaluation

Directions: Fill in each blank with the correct answer.

1. List the tests generally included in a CBC.

   WBC, RBC, Platelet count
   Hemoglobin, Hematocrit, Dif WBC
   Red Blood cell indices

2. What is the function of plasma?

   to transport nutrients to the
   tissues of the body, to nourish +
   sustain them

3. Where are the erythrocytes formed in the adult? _RB cells_

   In the red bone marrow of
   the ribs, sternum, skull + pelvic bo

4. Describe the shape of an erythrocyte and explain how it acquires this shape.

   immature erythrocyte cantains
   nucleus, as developed it loses nucleus
   + the looks like shape of biconcave disc

5. Describe the normal appearance of arterial and venous blood.

   when oxygen combines c hemoglobin,
   a bright red color (arterial) Venous has a
   darker red color

6. What is the average lifespan of a red blood cell.

   120 days

7. What is the function of leukocytes?

   is to defend the body against
   infection

8. Where do leukocytes do their work?

in the tissues, transported to the site of infection by circulatory system

9. What is the function of platelets?

they participate in the blood clotting mechanism

10. What is the normal range for platelets in an adult?

150,000 to 400,000 per cubic millimeter of blood

11. What is the normal hemoglobin range?
    a. Adult female: 12 to 16 g per 100 ml
    b. Adult male: 14 to 18 g per 100 ml

12. List five conditions that cause a decrease in the hemoglobin level.

anemia, hyperthroidism, cirrhosis of the liver, severe hemorrhaging, hemolytic reactions + certain systemic diseases (leukemia)

13. What is the purpose of the hematocrit?

to seperate blood, to measure the % volume of packed red blood cells in whole blood

14. What is the normal hematocrit range?
    a. Adult female: 37 to 47%
    b. Adult male: 40 to 54%

15. What is the normal range for the white blood count for an adult?

4,500 to 11,000 WB cells per cubic millimeter of blood

16. List examples of conditions which may result in leukocytosis.

appendicitis, chickenpox, diphtheria, infectious mononucleosis, meningitis, + rheumatic fever

17. What is the normal range for the red blood count for an adult?
    a. Adult female: 4 + 5.5 million per cubic millimeter
    b. Adult male: 4.5 to 6.2

18. List the five types of white blood cells and the normal adult range for each.

neutrophils 50 to 70%, Eosinophils 1 to 4%, Basophils 0 to 1%, Lymphocytes 20 to 35% monocytes 3 to 8%

19. Why must the white blood cells be stained when performing a differential cell count?

because white Blood cells are clear + colorless they must be stained c̄ a dye

20. The least numerous white blood cell is the _____ ~~Nongranular leukocyt~~ *Basophils*

21. Why are neutrophils also known as "segs"?

purple, multilobed nucleus that may contain from 3 to 5 lobes or segment

22. What is a band?

Immature forms of leukocytes

23. The largest of the white blood cells is the

~~Eosinophils~~ *monocytes.*

24. What is the function of lymphocytes?

Production of antibodies.

25. List the abbreviation for each of the following tests:
    a. hematocrit _____ *Hct.*
    b. hemoglobin _____ *Hgb or Hb*
    c. differential cell count _____ *diff.*
    d. white blood cell count _____ *WBC*
    e. red blood cell count _____ *RBC*

_____ *Know for Test — up to #25*

Critical Thinking Skills

1. The physician tells you to perform a hematocrit on Suzanne Rudy, age 4 years. As you are assembling the sterile lancet and antiseptic wipe for the finger puncture, Suzanne asks you if it is going to hurt. How would you respond?

No, it just feels like a prick, besides

2. How would the hematocrit be affected (increased or decreased) if the results were read at the top of the buffy coat layer?

Polycythemia, —increased.

3. Label the layers of this microhematocrit capillary tube that has been centrifuged. Place an arrow at the point at which you would take the hematocrit reading.

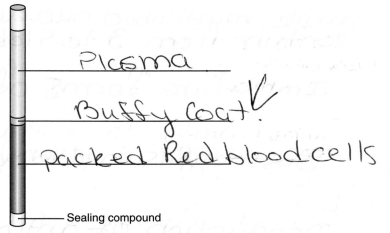

Plcsma

Buffy coat ✓

packed Red blood cells

Sealing compound

4. Observe a well-made blood smear and draw each of the following types of cells in the space provided. Use colored pencils if they are available.

Red Blood Cell:	Platelets:
Neutrophil:	Neutrophilic Band:
Eosinophil:	Basophil:
Lymphocyte:	Monocyte:

5. The following terms may appear on hematology laboratory reports that describe changes in the shape, size, and staining reaction of erythrocytes. Using a reference source, define each in the space provided.

    a. anisocytosis

    Condition in which there is excessive inequality in the size of cells

    b. macrocyte

    Abnormally large erythrocyte exceeding 10 microns in diameter

    c. microcyte

    Small erythrocyte

    d. poikilocyte

    a teardrop or pear-shaped red blood cell, seen in myello-fibrosis + certain anemias

    e. hypochromia

    condition of the blood in which the red blood cells have a reduced hemoglobin content

    f. hyperchromia

    excessive pigmentation or the increased staining capacity of any structure

6. Using a reference source, look up the following pathologic conditions that may affect the blood and give a brief description of each one, including the cause and symptoms associated with it.

    a. iron-deficiency anemia

    resulting from a greater demand on stored iron than can be supplied RBC normal but insufficient hemoglobin

    b. pernicious anemia

    chronic macrocytic anemia, marked by achlorhydria, most often in 40 to 80 yr old northern Europeans of fair skin

c. sickle cell anemia

An inherited disorder transmitted as an autosomal recessive trait that causes an abnormality of the globin genes in hemoglobin.

d. aplastic anemia

Caused by defient red cell production due to bone marrow disorders

e. hemolytic anemia

Anemia as the result of the destruction of Red blood cells by drugs, artificial heart valves, toxins, snake venoms.

f. hemophilia

a group of hereditary bleeding disorders marked by deficiencies of blood-clotting protiens.

g. leukemia

a class of hematological malignancies in which inmortal clones of immature blood cells multiply at the expense of normal blood cells.

Notes

Practice for Competency

HEMATOLOGIC TESTS

Assignment

Hematocrit Determination.
Perform a hematocrit determination in duplicate and record results in the chart provided. Circle any values falling outside of normal range.

Hemoglobin Determination.
Perform a hemoglobin determination using an automated blood analyzer and record results in the chart provided. Circle any values falling outside of normal range.

Blood Smear for a Differential Cell Count.
Prepare a blood smear for a differential white blood cell count.

CHART	
Date	

CHART	
Date	

Evaluation of Competency

HEMOGLOBIN DETERMINATION

Name_____ Date_____

Evaluated By_____ Score _____

Outcome:	Perform a hemoglobin determination.
Conditions:	Using an automated blood analyzer and instruction manual.
	Given the following: personal protective equipment, including disposable gloves, antiseptic wipe, lancet, gauze pads, and a biohazard sharps container.
Standards:	Time: __ minutes (To be provided by the instructor based upon the type of equipment being used.)
	Accuracy: Satisfactory score on the Performance Evaluation Checklist.

Performance Evaluation Checklist

Trial 1	Trial 2	Point Value	Performance Standards
		●	Assembled equipment.
		●	Washed hands.
		●	Greeted and identified patient.
		●	Introduced yourself and explained the procedure.
		●	Put on personal protective equipment, including gloves.
		●	Performed a skin puncture.
		●	Prepared specimen according to manufacturer's instructions.
		●	Inserted specimen into the automated analyzer according to manufacturer's instructions.
		●	Operated the automated analyzer according to manufacturer's instructions.
		●	Read results on the digital display screen.
		●	Properly disposed of used materials.
		●	Removed personal protective equipment, including gloves.
		●	Washed hands.
		●	Charted the test results correctly.

Trial 1	Trial 2	Point Value	Performance Standards
		★	The hemoglobin recording was identical to the reading on the digital display screen.
		★	Completed the procedure within __ minutes.

CHART	
Date	

Evaluation of Student Performance

EVALUATION CRITERIA			COMMENTS
Symbol	Category	Point Value	
★	Critical Step	16 points	
●	Essential Step	6 points	
▷	Theory Question	2 points	
Score calculation: 100 points			
− _____ points missed			
_____ Score			
Satisfactory score: 85 or above			

AAMA/CAAHEP Competency Achieved:
☐ Perform hematology testing.

Evaluation of Competency

PROCEDURE 18-1: HEMATOCRIT DETERMINATION

Name _____ Date _____

Evaluated By _____ Score _____

Outcome: Perform a hematocrit determination.

Conditions: Given the following: personal protective equipment, including disposable gloves, lancet, antiseptic wipe, gauze pads, capillary tubes, sealing compound, microhematocrit centrifuge, and a biohazard sharps container.

Standards: Time: 10 minutes

Accuracy: Satisfactory score on the Performance Evaluation Checklist.

Performance Evaluation Checklist

Trial 1	Trial 2	Point Value	Performance Standards
		●	Assembled equipment.
		●	Washed hands.
		●	Put on personal protective equipment, including gloves.
		●	Greeted and identified the patient.
		●	Introduced yourself and explained the procedure.
		●	Performed a skin puncture and wiped away the first drop of blood.
		●	Properly disposed of the lancet in a biohazard waste container.
		●	Held one end of capillary tube horizontally, but slightly downward next to the free-flowing puncture.
		●	Kept the tip of the pipet in the blood, but did not allow it to press against the skin of the patient's finger.
		●	Filled capillary tube (calibrated tubes filled to the calibration line; un-calibrated tubes filled approximately 3/4 full).
		●	Filled a second capillary tube.
		●	Sealed one end of each capillary tube.
		●	Placed capillary tubes in the microhematocrit centrifuge with the sealed end facing toward the outside.

Trial 1	Trial 2	Point Value	Performance Standards
		▷	Is able to state why the sealed end must face toward the outside.
		●	Balanced one tube with the other tube placed opposite it.
		●	Placed the cover on centrifuge and locked it securely.
		●	Centrifuged blood specimen for 3 to 5 minutes.
		●	Allowed centrifuge to come to a complete stop.
		▷	Is able to state the reason for centrifuging the blood specimen.
		●	Read the results using the appropriate reading device.
		★	The results were within ±1 percent of the evaluator's results.
		●	Averaged the values of the two tubes together to derive the test results.
		★	The calculation was performed without a mathematical error.
		●	Properly disposed of capillary tubes in a biohazard sharps container.
		●	Removed personal protective equipment, including gloves.
		●	Washed hands.
		●	Charted the test results correctly.
		●	Returned equipment.
		★	Completed the procedure within 10 minutes.

CHART	
Date	

Evaluation of Student Performance

EVALUATION CRITERIA			COMMENTS
Symbol	Category	Point Value	
★	Critical Step	16 points	
●	Essential Step	6 points	
▷	Theory Question	2 points	
Score calculation: 100 points			
− _____ points missed			
_____ Score			
Satisfactory score: 85 or above			

AAMA/CAAHEP Competency Achieved:
☐ Perform hematology testing.

Evaluation of Competency

PROCEDURE 18-2: PREPARATION OF A BLOOD SMEAR FOR A DIFFERENTIAL CELL COUNT

Name_____ Date_____

Evaluated By_____ Score_____

Outcome:	Prepare a blood smear for a differential white blood cell count.
Conditions:	Given the following: personal protective equipment, including disposable gloves, supplies to perform a finger puncture or venipuncture, slides with a frosted edge, slide container, and a biohazard sharps container.
Standards:	Time: 10 minutes
	Accuracy: Satisfactory score on the Performance Evaluation Checklist.

Performance Evaluation Checklist

Trial 1	Trial 2	Point Value	Performance Standards
		●	Assembled equipment.
		●	Labeled slides.
		●	Washed hands and put on personal protective equipment, including gloves.
		●	Greeted and identified the patient.
		●	Introduced yourself and explained the procedure.
		●	Performed a venipuncture or finger puncture.
		●	Placed a drop of blood in the middle of each slide approximately $\frac{1}{4}$ inch from the frosted edge of the slide.
		●	Held a spreader slide at 30-degree angle to first slide in front of the drop of blood.
		▷	Is able to state what occurs if the angle is more than 30 degrees or less than 30 degrees.
		●	Moved the spreader slide until it touched the drop of blood.
		●	Spread the blood thinly and evenly across slide using the spreader slide.
		●	Prepared the second blood smear.

Trial 1	Trial 2	Point Value	Performance Standards
		●	Disposed of the spreader slide in a biohazard sharps container.
		●	Quickly dried the blood smears by waving them gently back and forth.
		▷	Is able to state why the blood smears should be dried immediately.
		●	The length of the smear was approximately $1\frac{1}{2}$ inches.
		●	The smear was smooth and even with no ridges, holes, lines, streaks, or clumps.
		●	The smear was not too thick or thin.
		●	There was a feathered edge at the thin end of the smear.
		●	There was a margin on all sides of the smear.
		●	Placed the slides in a protective slide container for transport.
		●	Removed gloves and washed hands.
		★	Completed the procedure within 10 minutes.

Evaluation of Student Performance

EVALUATION CRITERIA			COMMENTS
Symbol	Category	Point Value	
★	Critical Step	16 points	
●	Essential Step	6 points	
▷	Theory Question	2 points	
Score calculation: 100 points			
− points missed			
_____ Score			
Satisfactory score: 85 or above			

AAMA/CAAHEP Competency Achieved:
☐ Use methods of quality control.

## CHAPTER 19

Blood Chemistry and Serology

Blood Chemistry

NAME _____

Key Terminology Assessment:

Directions: Match each medical term with its definition.

C 1. glycogen
D 2. HDL cholesterol
A 3. hyperglycemia
E 4. hypoglycemia
F 5. LDL cholesterol
B 6. lipoprotein

A. An abnormal increase in the glucose level in the blood.

B. A complex molecule consisting of protein and a lipid fraction such as cholesterol. These molecules function in transporting lipids in the blood.

C. The form in which carbohydrate is stored in the body.

D. A lipoprotein consisting of protein and cholesterol that removes excess cholesterol from the cells.

E. An abnormally low level of glucose in the blood.

F. A lipoprotein consisting of protein and cholesterol that picks up cholesterol and delivers it to the cells.

Self-Evaluation

Directions: Fill in each blank with the correct answer.

1. What type of specimen is required for most blood chemistry tests?

   Serum specimen for analysis

2. What is the purpose of quality control?

   consists of methods + means to ensure that the test results are reliable + valid

3. What is the purpose of calibrating a blood chemistry analyzer?

   to check the precision of the blood chemistry analyzer.

4. List two reasons why a control may not fall within its normal range.

   Problems or errors exist, either c̄ the analyzer itself or c̄ the technique used to perform (lipid)

5. What is cholesterol?

   is a white, waxy fatlike substance that is essential for normal functioning of the body

6. List the two main sources of cholesterol in the blood.

   HDL + LDL Cholesterol

7. What is atherosclerosis and why is it a health risk?

   ↑ BP Cholesterol may cause fatty deposits or plaque to build up on walls of arteries

8. Why is LDL cholesterol referred to as "bad" cholesterol and HDL referred to as "good" cholesterol?

   LDL picks up cholesterol from ingested fats + from the liver + delivers it to the blood vessels + muscles, where it is depos in the cells. HDL Removes excess ch

9. What does a total cholesterol test measure?

   a combined measurement of the amount of LDL + HDL in the Blood

10. List the ranges for each of the following cholesterol categories:

    a. Desirable cholesterol level: *under 200*

    b. Borderline cholesterol level: *200 - 239*

    c. High cholesterol level: *240 or ↑*

11. At what level is the HDL cholesterol considered a risk factor for coronary heart disease?

level below 35 has been determined

12. What type of patient preparation is required for a triglyceride test?

Fasting

13. What is the primary use of the cholesterol test?

to diagnosis of ↑ Blood Cholesterol

14. What is the purpose of performing a BUN?

Kidney Function, the ability to excrete the urea properly

15. What is the function of glucose in the body?

end product of carbohydrates metabolism - to serve as the cheif source of energy for the body

16. Explain the function of insulin in the body.

hormone secreted by the beta cells of pancreas - enables glucose to enter the body's cells be converted to energy

17. List the abbreviation for each of the following tests:
    a. fasting blood sugar ___FBS___
    b. 2-hour postprandial glucose ___2 hour PPBS___
    c. glucose tolerance test ___GTT___

18. What type of patient preparation is required for a fasting blood sugar?

Should not have anything to eat or drank except water 12 hrs prior

19. What is the normal range for a fasting blood sugar?

70 + 110

20. List two reasons for performing a fasting blood sugar.

on diagnosised diabetics

21. What type of patient preparation is required for a 2-hour postprandial glucose test?

begin fasting at 12 pm pt must consume 100 grm carbohydrate drink

22. Describe the procedure for performing a 2-hour postprandial glucose test.

blood test before drink + 2 hrs later.

23. What is the purpose of the glucose tolerance test?

provides more detailed info - is body can matabolize glucose.

24. What type of patient preparation is required for the glucose tolerance test?

↑ carbohydrate diet for 3 days 150 grams of carbohydrates/day.

25. Describe the procedure for a glucose tolerance test.

Blood + urine test, glucose drink + Blood is taken every 30 60 + 120 min.

26. Define hypoglycemia and list three conditions that may cause it to occur.

Condition in which the glucose in blood is low Hypothyroidism

27. What are the storage requirements for the blood glucose reagent strips?

Sensitive to heat, light + moisture, Stored in cool area

28. List three advantages of home blood sugar monitoring.

decisions can be made regarding insulin + dietary adjustment. to advoid the extremes of hypoglycemia or hypergleemia

Critical Thinking Skills

1. Using a reference source, list 10 foods that are high in cholesterol. Indicate (in milligrams) the amount of cholesterol in each food.

_____
_____
_____
_____

2. Adam Kranach has been placed on a low-cholesterol diet. Assist him in planning meals for 1 day that are low in cholesterol.

    a. Breakfast

    _____
    _____

    b. Lunch

    _____
    _____

    c. Dinner

    _____
    _____

3. Marty Wolf has arrived at your office for a glucose tolerance test. What should you tell her regarding the following? Explain the reason for each answer.

    a. Consumption of food and fluid

_____

_____

    b. Water consumption

_____

_____

    c. Smoking

_____

_____

    d. Leaving the test site

_____

_____

    e. Activity

_____

_____

4. You are instructing Michael Richardson in the procedure for monitoring blood glucose at home using a glucose meter. In the space provided, state the information that should be emphasized regarding each of the following:

    a. Obtaining the capillary blood specimen

_____

_____

    b. Performing the blood glucose test

_____

_____

    c. Recording results

_____

_____

Notes

Serology

NAME _____

Key Terminology Assessment:

Directions: Match each medical term with its definition.

___D___ 1. agglutination
___K___ 2. antibody
___B___ 3. antigen
___H___ 4. antiserum
___A___ 5. blood antibody
___E___ 6. blood antigen
___I___ 7. donor
___G___ 8. gene
___J___ 9. in vitro
___F___ 10. in vivo
___C___ 11. recipient

A. A protein present in the blood that is capable of combining with its corresponding antigen to produce an antigen-antibody reaction.
B. A substance capable of stimulating the formation of antibodies.
C. One who receives something, such as a blood transfusion, from a donor.
D. Clumping of blood cells.
E. A protein present on the surface of red blood cells that determines the blood type of an individual.
F. Occurring in the living body or organism.
G. A unit of heredity.
H. A serum that contains antibodies.
I. One who furnishes something such as blood, tissue, or organs to be used in another person.
J. Occurring in glass. Refers to tests performed under artificial conditions, as in the laboratory.
K. A substance that is capable of combining with an antigen resulting in an antigen-antibody reaction.

Self-Evaluation

Directions: Fill in each blank with the correct answer.

1. What is the definition of serology?

   the scientific study of the serum of the blood.

2. List three examples of antigens.

   bacteria, viruses, allergens Blood atigens

3. What is the purpose of performing each of the following serologic tests?
   a. rheumatoid factor *younger people*

   blood contains a type of antibody called rheumatoid factor (RF)

   b. antistreptolysin test

   detect the presence of ASO antibodies in the serum.

   c. C-reactive protein

   during inflammation + tissue destruction an abnormal protein called C-reactive protein appears in the blood

   d. ABO and Rh blood typing *RH factor*

   to prevent transfusion + transplant reactions, to identify problems

Pg 652

4. How is infectious mononucleosis transmitted?

   through saliva

5. What are the symptoms of infectious mononucleosis? *VSpleen for enlarg*

   fatigue, swollen lymphnodes vomitting, sorethroat.

6. What happens when a blood antigen and antibody combine?

   Agglutination.

7. Where are the A, B, and Rh antigens located?

Surface of Red Blood cells

8. What is the term used to describe "in glass"?

in vitro

9. Why is agglutination of blood in vivo a threat to life?

Red blood cells can't pass through kidney - Kidney failure

10. If a person has Type A blood, what antigen and what antibody will be present?

_A + B_

11. If a person has Type B blood, what antigens and antibodies will be present?

_B A_

12. If a person has Type AB blood, what antigens and antibodies will be present?

AB, or niether

13. If a person has Type O blood, what antigens and antibodies will be present?

No antigens

14. What is the difference between Rh+ and Rh- blood?

RH + / RH Antigen in Red Blood cells RH → No Antigen

15. What term is used to describe the breakdown of blood?

Hemolysis

Critical Thinking Skills

1. Eryhroblastosis fetalis is a blood disorder of the newborn, usually due to incompatibility between the infant's blood and the mother's blood. Using a reference source, answer the following questions regarding this condition in the space provided:

   a. Explain how an Rh incompatibility between the mother and infant can cause this condition to occur.

   Moms Antigens work against the baby

   b. Describe the symptoms associated with erythroblastosis fetalis.

   liver Jaundice, kidney damage.

   c. Explain the treatment used for this condition.

   transfusion in 2nd baby if it makes it.

   d. How can this condition be prevented?

   mother can get different Antigen before birth - RH testing + Rogam

2. List examples of factors that would disqualify an individual from donating blood.

   HIV +, low hemoglobin, Sick, wt (to small), Anemic Any exposures in foregn countries.

Evaluation of Competency

PERFORMING A BLOOD CHEMISTRY TEST

Name_____   Date_____

Evaluated By_____   Score _____

Performance Objective

Outcome:	Perform a blood chemistry test.
Conditions:	Given the following: personal protective equipment, including disposable gloves, an antiseptic wipe, a lancet, gauze pads, and a biohazard sharps container. Using an automated blood chemistry analyzer and instruction manual.
Standards:	Time: __ minutes. (To be designated by the instructor based upon the automated analyzer being utilized.)
	Accuracy: Satisfactory score on the Performance Evaluation Checklist.

Performance Evaluation Checklist

Trial 1	Trial 2	Point Value	Performance Standards
		●	Assembled equipment.
		●	Washed hands.
		●	Greeted and identified the patient.
		●	Introduced yourself and explained the procedure.
		●	Put on personal protective equipment, including gloves.
		●	Performed a skin puncture.
		●	Prepared the specimen according to manufacturer's instructions.
		●	Inserted the specimen into the automated analyzer according to manufacturer's instructions.
		●	Operated the automated analyzer according to manufacturer's instructions.
		●	Read the results on digital display screen.
		●	Properly disposed of used materials.
		●	Removed gloves.
		●	Washed hands.
		●	Charted the test results correctly.
		★	The recording was identical to the reading on the digital display screen.
		★	Completed the procedure within ___ minutes.

CHART	
Date	

Evaluation of Student Performance

EVALUATION CRITERIA			COMMENTS
Symbol	Category	Point Value	
★	Critical Step	16 points	
●	Essential Step	6 points	
▷	Theory Question	2 points	
Score calculation: 100 points			
− _____ points missed			
_____ Score			
Satisfactory score: 85 or above			

AAMA/CAAHEP Competencies Achieved:

☐ Perform chemistry testing.

☐ Use methods of quality control.

Evaluation of Competency

PROCEDURE 19-1: BLOOD GLUCOSE MEASUREMENT

Name_____ Date_____

Evaluated By_____ Score _____

Performance Objective

Outcome: Perform a fasting blood sugar.

Conditions: Given the following: personal protective equipment, including disposable gloves. ACU-Chek Advantage glucose monitor, reagent strips, lancet, antiseptic wipe, gauze pad, and a biohazard sharps container.

Standards: Time: 10 minutes.
Accuracy: Satisfactory score on the Performance Evaluation Checklist.

Performance Evaluation Checklist

Trial 1	Trial 2	Point Value	Performance Standards
		●	Washed hands.
		●	Assembled equipment.
		●	Checked the expiration date on container of reagent strips.
		●	Greeted and identified the patient.
		●	Introduced yourself and explained the procedure.
		●	Asked the patient if he/she prepared properly.
		●	Asked the patient to wash his/her hands in warm water and thoroughly dry them.
		●	Turned on the monitor.
		●	Checked the code number.
		●	Removed a test strip from the container.
		●	Immediately replaced the lid of the container.
		▷	Is able to state why the lid should be replaced immediately.
		●	Gently inserted the test strip in the yellow target area within 30 seconds.
		●	The yellow target area was facing up.
		●	Cleansed the puncture site with an antiseptic wipe and allowed it to dry.
		●	Put on personal protective equipment including gloves.

Trial 1	Trial 2	Point Value	Performance Standards
		●	Performed a finger puncture.
		●	Disposed of the lancet in the biohazard sharps container.
		●	Wiped away the first drop of blood with a gauze pad.
		▷	Is able to state why the first drop of blood should be wiped away.
		●	Placed the patient's hand in a dependent position and gently squeezed finger until a large drop of blood formed.
		●	Touched the drop of blood to the center of the yellow target area.
		●	Did not smear the blood on the target area.
		●	The entire yellow target area was completely covered with blood.
		●	Had the patient apply pressure with a gauze pad.
		●	Observed digital display of the test results.
		●	Removed the test strip from the monitor and discarded in a biohazard waste container.
		●	Removed personal protective equipment, including gloves, and washed hands.
		●	Charted the test results accurately.
		★	The recording was identical to the reading on the digital display screen.
		●	Properly stored the glucose monitor.
		★	Completed the procedure within 10 minutes.

CHART	
Date	

Evaluation of Student Performance

EVALUATION CRITERIA		
Symbol	**Category**	**Point Value**
★	Critical Step	16 points
●	Essential Step	6 points
▷	Theory Question	2 points

Score calculation: 100 points

− _____ points missed

_____ Score

Satisfactory score: 85 or above

AAMA/CAAHEP Competencies Achieved:

☐ Perform chemistry testing.

☐ Use methods of quality control.

☐ Instruct use and care of patient equipment.

Notes

Practice for Competency

SEROLOGIC TESTS

Assignment

Rapid Mononucleosis Test.
Perform a rapid mononucleosis test and record results in the chart provided.

CHART	
Date	

CHART	
Date	

Evaluation of Competency

RAPID MONONUCLEOSIS TESTING

Name_____   Date_____

Evaluated By_____   Score_____

Performance Objective

Outcome: Perform a rapid mononucleosis test.

Conditions: Given the following: personal protective equipment including gloves, the supplies to perform a finger puncture, a mononucleosis testing kit and a biohazard waste container.

Standards: Time: 10 minutes

Accuracy: Satisfactory score on the Performance Evaluation Checklist.

Performance Evaluation Checklist

Trial 1	Trial 2	Point Value	Performance Standards
		●	Washed hands.
		●	Assembled equipment.
		●	Checked expiration date on the testing kit.
		●	Allowed the reagents to come to room temperature.
		●	Greeted and identified the patient.
		●	Introduced yourself and explained the procedure.
		●	Put on personal protective equipment including gloves.
		●	Ran the test according to the manufacturer's instructions.
		●	Read the results.
		●	Removed personal protective equipment including gloves.
		●	Washed hands.
		●	Charted the results correctly.
		★	The results were identical to the evaluator's results.
		★	Completed the procedure within 10 minutes.

Chart	
Date	

Evaluation of Student Performance

EVALUATION CRITERIA			COMMENTS
Symbol	**Category**	**Point Value**	
★	Critical Step	16 points	
●	Essential Step	6 points	
▷	Theory Question	2 points	
Score calculation: 100 points			
− _____ points missed			
_____ Score			
Satisfactory score: 85 or above			

AAMA/CAAHEP Competency Achieved:

☐ Perform immunology testing.

Medical Microbiology

NAME _____

Key Terminology Assessment:

Directions: Match each medical term with its definition.

_____ 1. bacilli
_____ 2. cocci
_____ 3. colony
_____ 4. contagious
_____ 5. culture
_____ 6. culture medium
_____ 7. fastidious
_____ 8. immunization
_____ 9. incubate
_____ 10. incubation period
_____ 11. infectious disease
_____ 12. inoculate
_____ 13. microbiology
_____ 14. mucous membrane
_____ 15. normal flora
_____ 16. prodrome
_____ 17. resistance
_____ 18. sequelae
_____ 19. smear
_____ 20. specimen
_____ 21. spirilla
_____ 22. susceptible

A. A disease caused by a pathogen that produces harmful effects on its host.
B. The natural ability of an organism to remain unaffected by harmful substances in its environment.
C. A membrane lining body passages or cavities that open to the outside.
D. Capable of being transmitted directly or indirectly from one person to another.
E. The process of becoming protected from a disease through vaccination.
F. The introduction of microorganisms into a culture medium for means of growth and multiplication.
G. Bacteria that have a round shape.
H. A symptom indicating an approaching disease.
I. The scientific study of microorganisms and their activities.
J. Extremely delicate; difficult to culture, therefore involving specialized growth requirements.
K. Material spread on a slide for microscopic examination.

L. A morbid condition occurring as a result of a less serious primary infection.

M. A mixture of nutrients on which microorganisms are grown in the laboratory.

N. A small sample or part taken from the body to show the nature of the whole.

O. The interval of time between invasion by a pathogenic microorganism and the appearance of the first symptoms of the disease.

P. Bacteria that have a spiral shape.

Q. Harmless, nonpathogenic microorganisms that normally reside in many parts of the body but do not cause disease.

R. A mass of bacteria growing on a solid culture medium, which has arisen from the multiplication of a single bacterium.

S. Easily affected; lacking resistance.

T. Bacteria that have a rod shape.

U. The propagation of a mass of microorganisms in a laboratory culture medium.

V. In microbiology, the act of placing a culture in a chamber that provides optimal growth requirements for the multiplication of the organisms, such as the proper temperature, humidity, and darkness.

Self-Evaluation

Directions: Fill in each blank with the correct answer.

1. Explain what happens when a pathogen invades the body.

   _____

   _____

2. How does droplet infection contribute to the transmission of infectious disease?

   _____

   _____

3. What occurs during the prodromal period of an infectious disease?

   _____

   _____

4. List three infectious diseases caused by Staphylococcus aureus.

   _____

   _____

5. List three infectious diseases caused by different types of streptococci.

   _____

   _____

6. List three infectious diseases caused by different types of bacilli.

_____

_____

7. In what part of the body does Escherichia coli normally reside?

_____

_____

8. List for infectious diseases caused by different types of viruses.

_____

_____

9. Explain the purpose of each of the following parts of a microscope:

Stage

where slide is placed on.

Substage condenser

collects + concentrates the lgt rays + directs them up

Iris diaphragm

used to increase or decrease to amount of light

Coarse adjustment

to obtain an approximate focus quickly

Fine adjustment

precise focusing / sharp, clear image

Ocular lens

_____

10. Describe the function of each of the following objective lenses:

Low-power

magnification of 10x

High-power

high dry objective 40x

Oil-immersion

highest power 100x

11. What is the purpose of using oil with the oil-immersion objective?

the oil provides a path for the light to travel on between the slide + the lens

12. List five guidelines that should be followed for proper care of the microscope.

carried c̄ 2 hands, do not touch lens, when not in use, should be covered, cleaned

13. List five common areas of the body from which a microbiologic specimen may be obtained.

_____

_____

14. List two ways to prevent contaminating a specimen with extraneous microorganisms.

_____

_____

15. List two precautions a medical assistant should take to prevent infecting herself or himself with a microbiologic specimen.

_____

_____

16. Why should a specimen be processed as soon as possible after collecting it?

_____

17. What is the purpose of culturing microorganisms?

_____

_____

18. What is the name given to the type of culture that contains two or more different types of microorganisms?

_____

_____

19. Why is it important to diagnose streptococcal pharyngitis as early as possible?

_____

_____

20. What type of reaction is used to identify streptococcus with the direct antigen rapid streptococcus test?

_____

_____

21. When performing a hemolytic reaction and bacitracin susceptibility test, what is observed on the blood agar medium if a patient has streptococcal pharyngitis?

_____

_____

22. What is the purpose of performing a sensitivity test on a bacterial culture?

_____

23. List two reasons for examining a microorganism in the living state.

_____

_____

24. What is the purpose of staining a smear?

_____

_____

25. What color does gram-positive bacteria exhibit in a gram-stained smear?

_____

_____

Critical Thinking Skills

1. Andrew Tyre, age 7, has just come down with a case of chickenpox and cannot understand why he is not permitted to go to school. Using language and terms a child would understand, explain to Andrew why it is important for him to stay at home until he is well.

_____

_____

2. Mrs. Sims wants to know why she cannot have a prescription for an antibiotic for her cold. Respond to her question.

_____

_____

3. You have just taken a wound specimen for culturing and sensitivity testing that will be sent to a local laboratory. Mr. Kibler, the patient, wants to know why it will take 2 days (48 hours) for your medical office to receive the results from the laboratory. How would you respond?

_____

_____

4. List some poor hygienic practices that could lead to the transfer of infectious diseases in the community. Example: not washing the hands before eating.

_____

_____

_____

_____

5. From the following list, select nine infectious diseases. Using a reference source, indicate in the following chart the incubation period, mode of transmission (if applicable), outstanding symptoms, treatment, and prevention (if applicable) for each.

bacillary dysentery	pneumonia
botulism	poliomyelitis
chickenpox (varicella)	rabies
cholera	rheumatic fever
common cold	rubella
diptheria	rubeola
gonorrhea	Salmonella food poisoning
hepatitis	scarlet fever
herpes simplex	smallpox
herpes zoster	staphylococcal food poisoning
impetigo	streptococcal sore throat
infectious mononucleosis	syphilis
influenza	tetanus
mumps	tuberculosis
pertussis	typhoid fever

Infectious Disease	Incubation Period	Mode of Transmission	Symptoms	Treatment	Prevention

Infectious Disease	Incubation Period	Mode of Transmission	Symptoms	Treatment	Prevention

Infectious Disease	Incubation Period	Mode of Transmission	Symptoms	Treatment	Prevention

Practice for Competency

Assignment

Using a Compound Microscope.
Practice using a compound microscope. In the space provided below, indicate each specimen you observed under the microscope and the microscope objective you used for viewing it.

SPECIMEN VIEWED   **OBJECTIVE USED**

Practice for Competency

THROAT CULTURE

Assignment

Throat Specimen.
Obtain a specimen for a throat culture using a sterile cotton swab and/or a collection and transport system. Record the procedure in the chart provided.
Rapid Strep Testing.
Perform a strep test using a rapid strep testing kit and record results in the chart provided.

CHART	
Date	

Practice for Competency

Assignment

Wet Mount.
Prepare a wet mount preparation.
Hanging Drop.
Prepare a hanging drop preparation.
Microbiologic Smear.
Prepare a microbiologic smear.
Gram-Staining.
Observe a gram-stained smear. In the space provided below, indicate each category of gram-stained bacteria observed under the microscope (e.g., gram-positive staphylococci).

TYPE OF GRAM STAINED BACTERIA OBSERVED

Notes

Evaluation of Competency

PROCEDURE 20-1: USING THE MICROSCOPE

Name_____ Date_____

Evaluated By_____ Score _____

Outcome: Use a microscope.

Conditions: Given a microscope, lens paper, immersion oil, xylene, and a soft cloth.

Standards: Time: 15 minutes

Accuracy: Satisfactory score on the Performance Evaluation Checklist.

Performance Evaluation Checklist

Trial 1	Trial 2	Point Value	*Performance Standards*
		●	Cleaned the ocular and objective lenses with lens paper.
		●	Turned on the light source.
		●	Rotated the nosepiece to the low-power objective.
		●	Used the coarse adjustment to provide sufficient working space for placing the slide on the stage.
		●	Placed the slide on the stage specimen side up and secured it.
		●	Positioned the low-power objective until it almost touched the slide using the coarse adjustment.
		●	Observed this step.
		▷	Is able to state why this step should be observed.
		●	Looked through the ocular.
		●	Brought the specimen into coarse focus using the coarse adjustment knob.
		●	Observed the specimen until it came into coarse focus.
		●	Used the fine adjustment knob to bring the specimen into a sharp clear focus.
		●	Adjusted the light as needed using the iris diaphragm.
		●	Rotated the nosepiece to the high-power objective.
		●	Used the fine adjustment knob to bring the specimen into a precise focus.

Trial 1	Trial 2	Point Value	Performance Standards
		●	Did not use the coarse adjustment to focus the high-power objective.
		▷	Is able to state why the coarse adjustment should not be used for focusing at this point.
		●	Examined the specimen as required by the test or procedure being performed.
		●	Turned off the light after use.
		●	Removed the slide from the stage.
		●	Cleaned the stage with a tissue or gauze.
		●	Properly cared for and stored the microscope.
			Using the oil immersion objective:
		●	Rotated the nosepiece to the oil-immersion objective.
		●	Placed the objective to one side.
		●	Placed a drop of immersion oil on the slide directly over the center opening in the stage.
		●	Moved the oil-immersion objective into place.
		●	Made sure the objective did not touch the stage or slide.
		●	Used the coarse adjustment to position the oil-immersion objective.
		●	Brought the objective down until the lens touched the oil but did not come in contact with the slide.
		●	Looked through the eyepiece.
		●	Focused slowly using the coarse objective until the object was visible.
		●	Used the fine adjustment to bring the object into sharp focus.
		●	Adjusted the light as needed using the iris diaphragm.
		●	Examined the specimen as required by the test or procedure being performed.
		●	Turned off the light after use.
		●	Removed the slide from the stage.
		●	Cleaned the oil-immersion objective with lens paper.
		▷	Is able to state why the lens must be cleaned immediately.
		●	Cleaned the oil from the slide by immersing it in xylene and wiping it with a soft cloth.
		★	Completed the procedure within 15 minutes.

Evaluation of Student Performance

EVALUATION CRITERIA			COMMENTS
Symbol	**Category**	**Point Value**	
★	Critical Step	16 points	
●	Essential Step	6 points	
▷	Theory Question	2 points	
Score calculation: 100 points			
− _____ points missed			
_____ Score			
Satisfactory score: 85 or above			

AAMA/CAAHEP Competency Achieved:

☐ Perform microbiology testing.

Notes

Evaluation of Competency

PROCEDURE 20-2: TAKING A SPECIMEN FOR A THROAT CULTURE

Name_____   Date_____

Evaluated By_____   Score_____

Performance Objective

Outcome:	Obtain a specimen for a throat culture.
Conditions:	Given the following: disposable gloves, tongue depressor, sterile swab, and a biohazard waste container.
Standards:	Time: 5 minutes.
	Accuracy: Satisfactory score on the Performance Evaluation Checklist.

Performance Evaluation Checklist

Trial 1	Trial 2	Point Value	Performance Standards
		●	Washed hands.
		●	Assembled equipment.
		●	Greeted and identified the patient.
		●	Introduced yourself and explained the procedure.
		●	Positioned patient and adjusted light.
		●	Applied gloves.
		●	Removed the sterile swab from its peel-apart package, being careful not to contaminate it.
		●	Depressed patient's tongue with tongue depressor.
		●	Placed swab at the back of patient's throat and firmly rubbed it over lesions or white or inflamed areas of mucous membranes of the tonsillar region.
		▷	Is able to explain why swab should be rubbed over these types of areas.
		●	Constantly rotated swab as the specimen was being obtained.
		▷	Is able to state why a rotating motion should be used.
		●	Did not allow swab to touch any area other than throat.
		▷	Is able to state why swab should not be allowed to touch any areas other than throat.
		●	Kept patient's tongue depressed and withdrew swab and removed tongue depressor.

Trial 1	Trial 2	Point Value	Performance Standards
		●	Properly disposed of the tongue depressor.
		●	Processed the swab according to the directions accompanying the rapid strep test.
		●	Removed gloves and washed hands.
		●	Charted the test results correctly.
		★	Completed the procedure within 5 minutes.
			THROAT SPECIMEN—COLLECTION AND TRANSPORT SYSTEM
		●	Completed laboratory request form.
		●	Washed hands and applied gloves.
		●	Checked expiration date on peel-apart envelope.
		●	Peeled open approximately one third of the length of envelope.
		●	Removed plastic collection tube from envelope and labeled it.
		●	Removed the cap/swab unit from tube.
		●	Collected the specimen using aseptic technique.
		●	Did not allow swab to touch any area other than collection site.
		●	Returned the cap/swab unit to plastic tube.
		●	Completely immersed swab in the transport medium.
		●	Removed gloves and washed hands.
		●	Charted the procedure correctly.
		●	Transported the specimen to the laboratory within 72 hours.
		▷	Is able to state why the specimen must be transported within 72 hours.
		★	Completed the procedure within 5 minutes.

CHART		
Date		

Evaluation of Student Performance

EVALUATION CRITERIA			COMMENTS
Symbol	**Category**	**Point Value**	
★	Critical Step	16 points	
●	Essential Step	6 points	
▷	Theory Question	2 points	
Score calculation: 100 points			
− _____ points missed			
_____ Score			
Satisfactory score: 85 or above			

AAMA/CAAHEP Competency Achieved:

☐ Obtain throat specimen for microbiological testing.

Notes

Evaluation of Competency

RAPID STREP TESTING

Name_____ Date_____

Evaluated By_____ Score _____

Outcome:	Perform a rapid strep test.
Conditions:	Given the following: tongue blade, a rapid strep testing kit, and the manufacturer's instructions.
Standards:	Time: __ minutes. (To be designated by the instructor based upon the type of rapid strep test being used.)
	Accuracy: Satisfactory score on the Performance Evaluation Checklist.

Performance Evaluation Checklist

Trial 1	Trial 2	Point Value	Performance Standards
		●	Washed hands.
		●	Assembled equipment.
		●	Greeted and identified the patient.
		●	Introduced yourself and explained the procedure.
		●	Collected a throat specimen.
		●	Performed the testing procedure according to the manufacturer's instructions.
		●	Interpreted the test results.
		★	The results were identical to the evaluator's results.
		●	Properly disposed of used materials.
		●	Washed hands.
		●	Recorded results in patient's chart.
		★	Completed the procedure within __ minutes.

CHART	
Date	

Evaluation of Student Performance

EVALUATION CRITERIA			COMMENTS
Symbol	**Category**	**Point Value**	
★	Critical Step	16 points	
●	Essential Step	6 points	
▷	Theory Question	2 points	
Score calculation: 100 points			
− _____ points missed			
_____ Score			
Satisfactory score: 85 or above			

AAMA/CAAHEP Competency Achieved:
☐ Perform microbiology testing.

Evaluation of Competency

PROCEDURE 20-3: WET MOUNT AND HANGING DROP PREPARATION METHODS

Name_____ Date_____

Evaluated By_____ Score _____

Outcome: Prepare a wet mount and a hanging drop preparation.

Conditions: 1. WET MOUNT METHOD:
Given the following: disposable gloves, a drop of fluid containing the microbiologic specimen, glass slide, coverslip, petroleum jelly, microscope, and a biohazard container.

2. HANGING DROP PREPARATION:
Given the following: disposable gloves, a drop of fluid containing the microbiologic specimen, a hanging drop slide, coverslip, petroleum jelly, microscope, and a biohazard container.

Standards: Time: 10 minutes.

Accuracy: Satisfactory score on the Performance Evaluation Checklist.

Performance Evaluation Checklist

Trial 1	Trial 2	Point Value	Performance Standards
			WET MOUNT METHOD
		●	Applied gloves and placed a drop of fluid containing the organism on glass slide.
		●	Ringed coverslip with petroleum jelly.
		▷	Is able to state the purpose of ringing coverslip with petroleum jelly.
		●	Placed coverslip over the specimen on glass slide.
		●	Placed slide under the microscope.
		●	Examined the specimen with the high-power objective.
		●	Diminished the intensity of light by partially closing diaphragm.
		●	Properly disposed of slide coverslip.
			HANGING DROP PREPARATION
		●	Spread a small amount of petroleum jelly around the edge of coverslip.
		●	Placed coverslip on a clean, dry surface with the petroleum jelly facing up.

Trial 1	Trial 2	Point Value	Performance Standards
		●	Applied gloves and transferred a drop of the specimen to the center of coverslip.
		●	Placed the hanging drop slide over coverslip so that the center of the depression lay directly over the drop.
		●	Applied slight pressure to slide to ensure good contact.
		●	Inverted slide quickly so that drop to be examined hung from the bottom of coverslip.
		●	Placed slide under the microscope.
		●	Examined the specimen with the high-power objective.
		●	Reduced light by partially closing the diaphragm.
		●	Properly disposed of slide and coverslip.
		★	Completed the procedure within 10 minutes.

CHART	
Date	

Evaluation of Student Performance

EVALUATION CRITERIA			COMMENTS
Symbol	**Category**	**Point Value**	
★	Critical Step	16 points	
●	Essential Step	6 points	
▷	Theory Question	2 points	
Score calculation: 100 points			
− _____ points missed			
_____ Score			
Satisfactory score: 85 or above			

AAMA/CAAHEP Competency Achieved:

☐ Perform microbiology testing.

Evaluation of Competency

PROCEDURE 20-4: PREPARING A SMEAR

Name_____ Date_____

Evaluated By_____ Score _____

Performance Objective

Outcome: Prepare a microbiologic smear.

Conditions: Given the following: disposable gloves, a microbiologic specimen, slide forceps, a Bunsen burner, sterile swab or inoculating needle, clean slide, and a biohazard container.

Standards: Time: 40 minutes

Accuracy: Satisfactory score on the Performance Evaluation Checklist.

Performance Evaluation Checklist

Trial 1	Trial 2	Point Value	Performance Standards
		●	Washed hands.
		●	Assembled equipment.
		●	Labeled slide.
		●	Applied gloves and held the edge of slide between thumb and index finger.
		●	Started at the right side of slide, used a rolling motion, and gently and evenly spread the material from the specimen over slide.
		▷	Is able to state why the material should not be rubbed over slide.
		●	Allowed the smear to air dry.
		●	Is able to state why heat should not be applied at this point.
		●	Held slide with slide forceps and heat-fixed the smear.
		▷	Is able to state purpose of heat-fixing the smear.
		●	Allowed the slide to cool completely.
		●	Examined or stained the smear according to medical office policy.
		★	Completed the procedure within 40 minutes.

Evaluation of Student Performance

EVALUATION CRITERIA			COMMENTS
Symbol	**Category**	**Point Value**	
★	Critical Step	16 points	
●	Essential Step	6 points	
▷	Theory Question	2 points	
Score calculation: 100 points			
− _____ points missed			
_____ Score			
Satisfactory score: 85 or above			

AAMA/CAAHEP Competency Achieved:

☐ Perform microbiology testing.

Emergency Medical Procedures

NAME _____

Key Terminology Assessment:

Directions: Match each medical term with its definition.

_____ 1. burn
_____ 2. cardiac arrest
_____ 3. crash cart
_____ 4. crepitus
_____ 5. dislocation
_____ 6. emergency medical services
_____ 7. first aid
_____ 8. fracture
_____ 9. hypothermia
_____10. poison
_____11. pressure point
_____12. seizure
_____13. shock
_____14. splint
_____15. sprain
_____16. strain
_____17. wound

A. A network of community resources, equipment, and personnel that provides care to victims of injury or sudden illness.
B. Any substance that causes illness, injury, or death if it enters the body.
C. An injury to the tissues caused by exposure to thermal, chemical, electrical, or radioactive agents.
D. Any item that will immobilize a body part.
E. A grating sensation caused by fractured bone fragments rubbing against each other.
F. A sudden episode of involuntary muscular contractions and relaxation, often accompanied by a change in sensation, behavior, and level of consciousness.

G. A situation in which the heart has stopped beating or beats too irregularly to circulate blood effectively through the body.

H. A stretching or tearing of muscles or tendons caused by trauma.

I. The immediate care that is administered to an individual who is injured or suddenly becomes ill before complete medical care can be obtained.

J. A break in the continuity of an external or internal surface caused by physical means.

K. A specially equipped cart for holding and transporting medications, equipment, and supplies needed for performing life-saving procedures in an emergency.

L. Any break in a bone.

M. The failure of the cardiovascular system to deliver enough blood to all the vital organs of the body.

N. An injury in which one end of a bone making up a joint is separated or displaced from its normal position.

O. A life-threatening condition in which the temperature of the entire body falls to a dangerously low level.

P. A site on the body where an artery lies close to the surface of the skin and can be compressed against an underlying bone.

Self-Evaluation

Directions: Fill in each blank with the correct answer.

1. What is the purpose of first aid?

    _____

    _____

    _____

    _____

2. What is the purpose of the office crash cart?

    _____

    _____

    _____

    _____

3. What is the difference between an EMT-Basic and a paramedic?

    _____

    _____

    _____

4. What are the responsibilities of an emergency medical dispatcher?

_____

_____

_____

5. List five OSHA Standards which should be followed when administering first aid.

_____

_____

_____

_____

_____

6. What questions must be answered when performing the primary assessment?

_____

_____

_____

_____

_____

7. According to the American Heart Association, what should be done if the patient is found to be unresponsive?

_____

_____

8. a. What methods can be used to open the airway?

_____

_____

   b. Which of these methods should be used with a patient who has suffered a head, neck, or spinal injury?

_____

_____

9. What is the reason for performing each of the following during an emergency situation?

   a. Remaining calm and speaking in a normal tone of voice.

_____

_____

   b. Making sure it is safe before approaching the patient.

_____

_____

   c. Following the OSHA Standard when providing emergency care.

_____

_____

d. Activating the emergency medical services.

_____

_____

e. Not moving the patient unnecessarily.

_____

_____

f. Checking the patient for a medical alert tag.

_____

_____

10. What are the signs of respiratory arrest?

_____

_____

_____

_____

11. List five conditions which can result in respiratory arrest.

_____

_____

_____

_____

_____

12. What is the purpose of rescue breathing?

_____

_____

_____

13. What factors increase the likelihood of a foreign object becoming lodged in the airway?

_____

_____

14. What is the difference between a complete and a partial airway obstruction?

_____

_____

15. What is the universal distress signal for choking?

_____

_____

16. How does the Heimlich maneuver help relieve an airway obstruction?

_____

_____

17. What are the symptoms of asthma?

_____

_____

18. What is emphysema?

_____

_____

19. What are the symptoms of hyperventilation?

_____

_____

20. What conditions may cause cardiac arrest?

_____

_____

21. What is the purpose of CPR?

_____

_____

22. What is the purpose of defibrillation?

_____

_____

23. What are the symptoms of a heart attack?

_____

_____

24. What are the symptoms of a stroke?

_____

_____

25. What is the cause of the following types of shock?
    a. hypovolemic

_____

_____

    b. cardiogenic

_____

_____

    c. neurogenic

_____

_____

    d. anaphylactic

_____

_____

e. psychogenic

_____

_____

26. What are the characteristics of each of the following types of external bleeding?
    a. capillary

_____

_____

    b. venous

_____

_____

    c. arterial

_____

_____

27. What is the difference between an open wound and a closed wound?

_____

_____

28. What are the signs and symptoms of a fracture?

_____

_____

29. What are the characteristics of each of the following types of fractures?
    a. impacted

_____

_____

    b. greenstick

_____

_____

    c. transverse

_____

_____

    d. oblique

_____

_____

    e. comminuted

_____

_____

    f. spiral

_____

_____

30. What are the characteristics of each of the following types of burns?

a. superficial

_____

_____

b. partial thickness

_____

_____

c. full thickness

_____

_____

31. What is the difference between a partial seizure and a generalized seizure?

_____

_____

32. List two examples of each of the following types of poisoning:

a. ingested

_____

_____

b. inhaled

_____

_____

c. absorbed

_____

_____

d. injected

_____

_____

33. What spiders (found in the United States) have bites that can result in serious or life-threatening reactions?

_____

_____

34. What species of snakes (found in the United States) are poisonous?

_____

_____

35. What animals tend to have a high incidence of rabies?

_____

_____

36. What factors place an individual at higher risk for developing heat- and cold-related

injuries?

_____

_____

37. What areas of the body are most susceptible to frostbite?

_____

_____

38. What is the difference between Type I diabetes and Type II diabetes?

_____

_____

39. What is insulin shock and what causes it to occur?

_____

_____

40. What is diabetic coma and what causes it to occur?

_____

_____

Critical Thinking Skills

1. You are assembling a first aid kit. What supplies should be included in your kit? Identify one use for each of the supplies you list.

_____

_____

_____

_____

_____

_____

_____

_____

_____

_____

_____

2. Jeff Stickler suddenly develops weakness of his left arm and leg, has difficulty in speaking, a severe headache and dizziness. You immediately call the EMS. What information should you be prepared to relay to the emergency medical dispatcher?

_____

_____

3. In which of the following emergency situations would you be legally permitted to administer first aid? Explain your answers.

    a. A patient is unconscious and bleeding profusely.

_____

_____

    b. You identify yourself and state your level of training and what you plan to do. You ask the patient if it is alright to administer emergency care. The patient responds by saying, "Yes, please help me."

_____

_____

    c. You ask the patient if you can administer emergency care but the patient refuses your help.

_____

_____

4. Holly Murphy falls while roller skating. She comes down hard on her left arm which begins to swell and discolor. Holly guards her arm and complains of intense pain. What would you do in this situation?

_____

_____

_____

_____

5. John Phillips is mowing the grass and mows over a yellow jacket nest. He is stung twice and soon afterwards, starts complaining of intense itching and exhibits erythema and hives on his arms, torso, and face. What would you do in this situation?

_____

_____

_____

_____

6. Steve Williams complains of severe indigestion and squeezing pain in the chest. He is short of breath and perspiring profusely. What would you do in this situation?

_____

_____

_____

_____

7. Clara Miller is playing basketball and is accidentally hit in the face with the ball. Her nose begins bleeding profusely. What would you do in this situation?

_____

_____

_____

_____

8. Debbie Carter, age 4, finds some children's chewable vitamins that have been left open on a table. She chews up about ten of them. What would you do in this situation?

_____

_____

_____

_____

9. Rita Preston accidentally cuts her finger with a knife while preparing dinner. Her finger begins bleeding profusely. What would you do in this situation?

_____

_____

_____

_____

10. Brad Graves is eating lunch and suddenly starts choking on a piece of meat. He grabs his throat and is unable to speak or breathe. What would you do in this situation?

_____

_____

_____

_____

11. Jose Perez is jogging on a cinder track. He falls and scrapes his left knee on the cinders. What would you do in this situation?

_____

_____

_____

_____

12. Charlotte Lambert is getting ready to perform a piano recital for her entire church congregation. Suddenly she starts breathing very rapidly and deeply and complains that she feels light-headed and dizzy. What would you do in this situation?

_____

_____

_____

_____

13. Bruce Jones is a diabetic. He is in a hurry and forgets to eat breakfast. He begins exhibiting behavior similar to that of someone who is intoxicated. What would you do in this situation?

_____

_____

_____

_____

_____

_____

14. Debra Murray is delivering newspapers and is bitten by a strange dog. The bite causes several puncture marks and slight bleeding. What would you do in this situation?

_____

_____

_____

_____

15. Tanya Howe is playing tennis on a hot and humid day and begins to feel weak and nauseous. Her skin feels cold and clammy and she is sweating profusely and complains of dizziness. What would you do in this situation?

_____

_____

_____

_____

Notes

Appendix A

Virtual Medical Office Challenge CD-ROM

Virtual Medical Office Challenge CD-ROM is designed to be used in conjunction with the 5th Edition of the W.B. Saunders textbook *Clinical Procedures for Medical Assistants*, by Kathy Bonewit-West. Through the use of case studies, the program allows students to practice the application of information provided in the textbook, and to use problem-solving, decision-making, and critical thinking skills. In addition, for specific clinical competencies, the learner's ability to use critical thinking and priority-setting skills during a clinical procedure can be challenged. This Appendix contains information on how to install and use the program. It also contains materials and forms used throughout the program, should students wish to refer to printed documents or complete any forms manually.

Minimum System Requirements		
PC and PC-Compatible:	Computer:	80486/66, or Pentium CPU
	System:	Windows 95 or 98/Windows NT
	Memory:	24 MB RAM
	Other:	4x CD-ROM Drive
		256-color mode
		Sound card/speakers
		Mouse
		SVGA, or higher graphics
		640 x 480 screen resolution
Macintosh:	Computer:	Power PC Processor
	System:	7.6x, or higher
	Memory:	24 MB RAM
	Other:	4x CD-ROM Drive
		256-color mode
		Mouse
		640 x 480 screen resolution

LOGGING ON TO THE VIRTUAL MEDICAL OFFICE CHALLENGE

Logging on for the first time

To record the challenges that they complete, students will enter their first initial and last name as a single word (e.g., tsmith). See Figure 1. Students will then click **ENTER**. If students do not wish to record their progress, they will simply click **BYPASS LOGIN** and advance to the **MAIN MENU**.

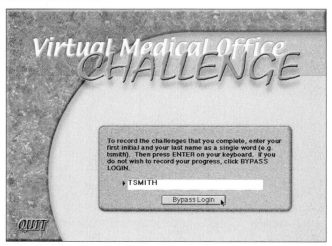

Figure 1

Logging on after the first time

If students have entered their names during the first log-on, the program will keep track of the challenges they have attempted, and those they have completed. If students enter their names the same way every time, the program will recognize them and give them the option to review the status of those challenges they have completed, or attempted, to date. Students can either review this status information or go straight to the **MAIN MENU**.

- **Storing bookmarking to the hard disk.** If the installation is configured to store students' bookmarking on the hard drive, then the students will not need to insert a floppy into the diskette drive and can simply proceed to the **MAIN MENU** after selecting the hard drive option and logging on.

- **Storing bookmarking to a floppy disk.** If the installation is configured to store student bookmarking on data diskettes, the data diskette must be inserted into the diskette drive before logging on. If no diskette is detected, the program will prompt for it. *Note:* The program will accept blank, formatted data diskettes as student data diskettes. After inserting the data diskette into the floppy drive, students can then proceed to the **MAIN MENU** after selecting the A:\drive option and logging on.

USING THE MAIN MENU

The **MAIN MENU** is the navigational front door to the *Virtual Medical Office Challenge.* Through it, students can select to explore any one of four patient case scenarios, or go directly to the Clinical Skills Building section (see Figure 2). Students also have an option to check Challenge Status, which is a log of what interactions they have either completed or partially explored.

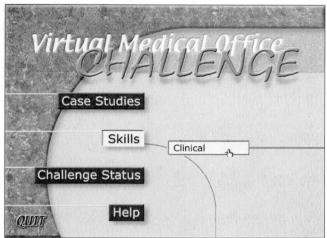

Figure 2

Selecting CASE STUDIES. By selecting **CASE STUDIES** on the **MAIN MENU,** students will be directed to the Patient Cases screen, which allows them to select a particular case by patient name (see Figure 3). When the cursor rolls over the patient's name, a description of that case, and the clinical competencies that are challenged within that case, appears in the dialog box below. Students can then select a case by clicking on a patient case file folder, which will automatically advance them to the beginning of that case. A new case can be accessed at any time from anywhere in the program by first selecting **MAIN MENU,** then selecting **CASE STUDIES,** and a new case folder from the Patient Cases screen.

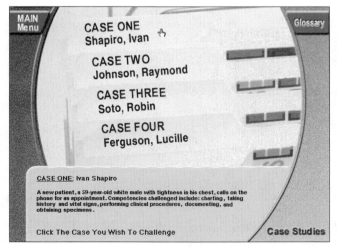

Figure 3

- **Selecting SKILLS.** Selecting **SKILLS** on the **MAIN MENU** will take students through all the skills, or they can select an individual skill to explore. Skills can be selected from anywhere in the program by first selecting **MAIN MENU**, then selecting **SKILLS**.

- **Selecting CHALLENGE STATUS.** *The Virtual Medical Office Challenge* will keep track of where students have been in the program, and what areas are still left to be challenged. Selecting **Challenge Status** on the **MAIN MENU** will bring up a list of what sections of the program have been partially completed and which have been fully completed. Separate screens will then show students what portions of the four patient cases have been completed, or partially completed (see Figure 4), and what portions of the **Clinical Skills** have been fully, or partially, challenged (see Figure 5). Partially completed sections are marked with a circle that is filled in with color. Fully completed sections are filled in with the same color and marked with an X within the circle. The **CHALLENGE STATUS** can be accessed at any point in the program by first selecting **MAIN MENU**, then selecting **CHALLENGE STATUS.**

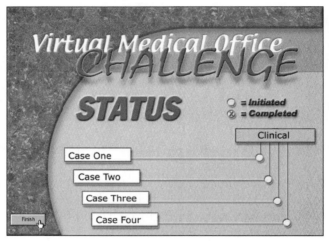

Figure 4

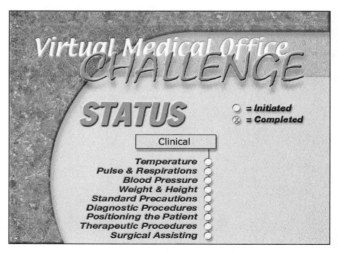

Figure 5

PATIENT CASE SCENARIOS

Four patient case scenarios are presented in the *Virtual Medical Office Challenge* (see Table 1). Combined with the **CLINICAL SKILLS** section, they represent most of the key clinical competencies students will need to master, as identified by the American Association of Medical Assistants (AAMA) in their entry-level Medical Assisting Curriculum. In each of the cases, students will play the role of a certified medical assistant working in the clinical area of a busy general practice medical office. The practice, which is called Blackburn Primary Care Associates, has three doctors and a broad mixture of patients with varying situations and needs. Students will be asked to respond to simulated, realistic medical office situations. Students will receive feedback based on the choices they make, and can explore that feedback further to understand the rationale behind their correct or incorrect responses.

When you enter a patient case for the first time, you will start at the beginning of that case. If at any time during that case you wish to return to the main menu, click **MAIN** when you see the icon in the top left corner of the screen. This icon will appear each time you begin a new challenge throughout the case. If you have worked through part of the case previously, the program will bookmark which portions, or portion, you have completed. When you return to that case, it will ask you whether you would like to start at the **BEGINNING**, or your **PREVIOUS LOCATION**, which is the last challenge location you completed the last time you worked in that case.

To make the program as realistic as possible, all the patient situations have been selected from the files of practicing physicians. For confidentiality, all names, dates, places, and any other identifiable characteristics of physicians and patients have been carefully deleted, or changed. All forms are replicas of forms in current use. The four patient cases are described in Table 1.

Table 1: Patient Case Studies

CASE ONE: Ivan Shapiro

A new patient, a 57-year-old white male with tightness in his chest, calls on the phone for an appointment. Competencies challenged include: prioritizing information, taking history and vital signs, performing clinical procedures, documenting, obtaining specimens.

CASE TWO: Raymond Johnson

An established 32-year-old white male patient has an exacerbation of his asthma and calls on the phone for an appointment. Competencies challenged include: responding to emergencies, taking history and vital signs, preparing and giving medications, performing procedures, documenting.

CASE THREE: Robin Soto

A 4 1/2-month-old Hispanic child is brought in for her immunizations after a missed appointment. Also she has not been given her vitamins for a week. Competencies challenged include: taking history and vital signs, performing developmental assessment, giving immunizations and patient instruction.

CASE FOUR: Lucille Ferguson

A 75-year-old black widow seeks her first appointment in the medical office. Due to her age and state of health, she is having difficulty functioning independently. Competencies challenged include: taking history and vital signs, positioning, examination procedures, performing diagnostic tests, patient instruction.

CLINICAL SKILLS

In addition to the four patient cases, students can select to work on individual clinical skills. These can be accessed through the **MAIN MENU** by selecting **SKILLS**, then selecting which skill they wish to explore.

- CLINICAL SKILLS. Individual clinical skills presented in this part of the program include:

  Temperature

  Pulse and Respirations

  Blood Pressure

  Weight and Height

  Diagnostic Procedures

  Standard Precautions

  Positioning the Patient

  Therapeutic Procedures

  Surgical Assisting

USING THE GLOSSARY

The **Glossary** can be accessed from all screens in the software once students have selected an activity from the **MAIN MENU.** It can be accessed in one of two ways, either by clicking on any word in red type that appears within a dialog box, or by clicking on the **Glossary** icon button. A word can be selected within the **Glossary** from the alphabetical list provided by scrolling to search for a word. The definition appears in the Definition Box, and students can hear the word pronounced by selecting the **Pronunciation** button (see Figure 6). Clicking on the **RETURN** button on the **Glossary** screen returns students to their previous location.

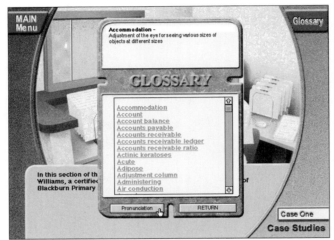

Figure 6

PATIENT FORMS AND REFERENCE MATERIALS

The following forms are available to students who prefer to reference information or complete any forms manually. These forms and reference materials are exact duplicates of the forms and reference materials used throughout the *Virtual Medical Office Challenge* program.

FORMS:

Form 1: Health History Questionnaire for Ivan Shapiro

Form 2: Progress Note Form for documenting Ivan Shapiro's visit

Form 3: Progress Note Form for documenting Raymond Johnson's visit

Form 4: Infant Growth and Development Chart for documenting
          Robin Soto's visit

Form 5: Progress Note Form for documenting Robin Soto's height and weight

Form 6: Health History Questionnaire for Lucille Ferguson

Form 7: Progress Note Form for documenting Lucille Ferguson's visit

Form 8: Blank Progress Note Form for practice

Form 1

ANDRUS/CLINI-REC® HEALTH HISTORY QUESTIONNAIRE

Chart No. _____

Today's Date _____

Identification Information

Name __Shapiro, Ivan__ Date of Birth __3/6/45__

Occupation __Carpenter__ Marital Status __Married__

PART A – PRESENT HEALTH HISTORY

I. CURRENT MEDICAL PROBLEMS

Please list the medical problems for which you came to see the doctor. About when did they begin?

Problems / Date Began

Chest pain when exercising

What concerns you most about these problems?

If you are being treated for any other illness or medical problems by another physician, please describe the problems and write the name of the physician or medical facility treating you.

Illness or Medical Problem / Physician or Medical Facility / City

II. MEDICATIONS

Please list all medications you are now taking, including those you buy without a doctor's prescription (such as aspirin, cold tablets or vitamin supplements).

III. ALLERGIES AND SENSITIVITIES

List anything that you are allergic to such as certain foods, medications, dust, chemicals or soaps, household items, pollens, bee stings, etc., and indicate how each affects you.

Allergic To: __Penicillin__ Effect: __Hives__ Allergic To: _____ Effect: _____

IV. GENERAL HEALTH, ATTITUDE AND HABITS

How is your overall health now?................... Health now: Poor ___ Fair ___ Good __X__ Excellent ___
How has it been most of your life?............... Health has been: Poor ___ Fair ___ Good __X__ Excellent ___

In the past year:
Has your appetite changed?.................. Appetite: Decreased ___ Increased ___ Stayed same __X__
Has your weight changed?.................... Weight: Lost ___ lbs. Gained __10__ lbs. No change ___
Are you thirsty much of the time?............. Thirsty: No __X__ Yes ___
Has your overall pep changed?............... Pep: Decreased ___ Increased ___ Stayed same __X__
Do you usually have trouble sleeping?............ Trouble sleeping: No ___ Yes __X__
How much do you exercise?.................... Exercise: Little or none ___ Less than I need ___ All I need __X__
Do you smoke?................................ Smokes: No __X__ Yes ___ If yes, how many years? ___
How many each day?.......................... ___ Cigarettes ___ Cigars ___ Pipesfull
Have you ever smoked?....................... Smoked: No ___ Yes __X__ If yes, how many years? __15__
How many each day?.......................... __20__ Cigarettes ___ Cigars ___ Pipesfull
Do you drink alcoholic beverages?............ Alcohol: No ___ Yes __X__ I drink ___ Beers ___ Glasses of wine ___ Drinks of hard liquor - per day __Socially__
Have you ever had a problem with alcohol?......... Prior problem: No __X__ Yes ___
How much coffee or tea do you usually drink?....... Coffee/Tea: __2__ cups of coffee or tea a day
Do you regularly wear seatbelts?.................. Seatbelts: No ___ Yes __X__

DO YOU:	Rarely/Never	Occasionally	Frequently	DO YOU:	Rarely/Never	Occasionally	Frequently
Feel nervous?	X			Ever feel like committing suicide?	X		
Feel depressed?	X						
Find it hard to make decisions?	X			Feel bored with your life?	X		
Lose your temper?		X		Use marijuana?	X		
Worry a lot?	X			Use hard drugs?	X		
Tire easily?		X		Do you want to talk to the doctor about a personal matter? No __X__ Yes ___			
Have trouble relaxing?		X					
Have any sexual problems?	X						

CONFIDENTIAL

rm 1

PART A – PRESENT HEALTH HISTORY (continued)

IV. GENERAL HEALTH, ATTITUDE AND HABITS (continued)

Have you recently had any changes in your:

If yes, please explain:

Marital status?	No __X__ Yes_____	
Job or work?	No_____ Yes _X_	Self employed
Residence?	No_____ Yes _X_	Moved from LA CA
Financial status?	No _X_ Yes_____	
Are you having any legal problems or trouble with the law?	No _X_ Yes_____	

PART B – PAST HISTORY

I. FAMILY HEALTH

Please give the following information about your immediate family:

Relationship	Age, if Living	Age At Death	State of Health Or Cause of Death
Father	_____	78	Lung cancer
Mother	_____	45	Heart disease
Brothers and Sisters	38	_____	good
	_____	_____	_____
	_____	_____	_____
Spouse	51	_____	good
Children	22	_____	good
	25	_____	good
	_____	_____	_____
	_____	_____	_____

Have any **blood relatives** had any of the following illnesses? If so, indicate relationship (mother, brother, etc.)

Illness	Family Members
Asthma	_____
Diabetes	_____
Cancer	Father
Blood Disease	_____
Glaucoma	_____
Epilepsy	_____
Rheumatoid Arthritis	Aunt
Tuberculosis	_____
Gout	_____
High Blood Pressure	Mother
Heart Disease	Mother
Mental Problems	_____
Suicide	_____
Stroke	Grandmother
Alcoholism	_____
Rheumatic Fever	_____

II. HOSPITALIZATIONS, SURGERIES, INJURIES

Please list all times you have been hospitalized, operated on, or seriously injured.

Year	Operation, Illness, Injury	Hospital and City
1990	Appendix removed	LA CA
_____	_____	_____
_____	_____	_____

III. ILLNESS AND MEDICAL PROBLEMS

Please mark with an (X) any of the following illnesses and medical problems you have or have had and indicate the year when each started. If you are not certain when an illness started, write down an approximate year.

Illness	(x)	(Year)	Illness	(x)	(Year)
Eye or eye lid infection	____	_____	Hernia	____	_____
Glaucoma	____	_____	Hemorrhoids	____	_____
Other eye problems	____	_____	Kidney or bladder disease	____	_____
Ear trouble	____	_____	Prostate problem (male only)	____	_____
Deafness or decreased hearing	____	_____	Mental problems	____	_____
Thyroid trouble	____	_____	Headaches	____	_____
Strep throat	____	_____	Head injury	____	_____
Bronchitis	____	_____	Stroke	____	_____
Emphysema	____	_____	Convulsions, seizures	____	_____
Pneumonia	____	_____	Arthritis	____	_____
Allergies, asthma or hay fever	____	_____	Gout	____	_____
Tuberculosis	____	_____	Cancer or tumor	____	_____
Other lung problems	____	_____	Bleeding tendency	____	_____
High blood pressure	____	_____	Diabetes	____	_____
Heart attack	____	_____	Measles/Rubeola	____	_____
High cholesterol	____	_____	German measles/Rubella	____	_____
Arteriosclerosis	____	_____	Polio	____	_____
(Hardening of arteries)	____	_____	Mumps	____	_____
Heart murmur	____	_____	Scarlet fever	____	_____
Other heart condition	____	_____	Chicken pox	____	_____
Stomach/duodenal ulcer	____	_____	Mononucleosis	____	_____
Diverticulosis	____	_____	Eczema	____	_____
Colitis	____	_____	Psoriasis	____	_____
Other bowel problems	____	_____	Venereal disease	____	_____
Hepatitis	____	_____	Genital herpes	____	_____
Liver trouble	____	_____	HIV test	____	_____
Gallbladder trouble	____	_____	AIDS	____	_____

' 1979, 1983 Bibbero Systems International, Inc.   To Order Call:800-BIBBERO (800 242-2376)
(REV. 8/95)   Or Fax: (800 242-9330)   STOCK NO. 19-742-4   8/95

e 2

Form 1

PART C – BODY SYSTEMS REVIEW

Please answer all of the following questions.

Circle any questions you find difficult to answer.

<u>MEN:</u>	Please answer questions 1 through 12, then skip to question 18.
<u>WOMEN:</u>	Please start on question 6.

<u>MEN ONLY</u>

1. Have you had or do you have prostate trouble? .... No **X** ____ Yes ____
2. Do you have any sexual problems or a problem with impotency? .... No **X** ____ Yes ____
3. Have you ever had sores or lesions on your penis? .... No **X** ____ Yes ____
4. Have you ever had any discharge from your penis? .... No **X** ____ Yes ____
5. Do you ever have pain, lumps or swelling in your testicles? .... No **X** ____ Yes ____

Check here if you wish to discuss any special problems with the doctor .... [ ]

<u>MEN & WOMEN</u>

		Rarely/Never	Occasionally	Frequently
6.	Is it sometimes hard to start your urine flow?	**X**		
7.	Is urination ever painful?	**X**		
8.	Do you have to urinate more than 5 times a day?	**X**		
9.	Do you get up at night to urinate?	**X**		
10.	Has your urine ever been bloody or dark colored?	**X**		
11.	Do you ever lose urine when you strain, laugh, cough or sneeze?	**X**		
12.	Do you ever lose urine during sleep?	**X**		

<u>WOMEN ONLY</u>
Do you:

			Rarely/Never	Occasionally	Frequently
13.	a.	Have any menstrual problems?			
	b.	Feel rather tense just before your period?			
	c.	Have heavy menstrual bleeding?			
	d.	Have painful menstrual periods?			
	e.	Have any bleeding between periods?			
	f.	Have any unusual vaginal discharge or itching?			
	g.	Ever have tender breasts?			
	h.	Have any discharge from your nipples?			
	i.	Have any hot flashes?			

14.	How many times, if any, have you been pregnant?	_____
15.	How many children born alive?	_____
16.	Are you taking birth control pills?	No____ Yes____
17.	Do you examine your breasts monthly for lumps?	No____ Yes____
17a.	What was the date of your last menstrual period?	Date____

Check here if you wish to discuss any special problem with the doctor .... [ ]

<u>MEN & WOMEN</u>

		Rarely/Never	Occasionally	Frequently
18.	In the past year have you had any:			
	a. Severe shoulder pain?	**X**		
	b. Severe back pain?	**X**		
	c. Muscle or joint stiffness or pain due to sports, exercise or injury?		**X**	
	d. Pain or swelling in any joints not due to sports, exercise or injury?	**X**		

19.	Do you have dry skin or brittle fingernails?	No **X** Yes____
20.	Do you bruise easily?	No **X** Yes____
21.	Do you have any moles that have changed in color or in size?	No **X** Yes____
22.	Do you have any other skin problems?	No **X** Yes____
23.	In the last 3 months have you had:	
	a. A fever that lasted more than one day?	No **X** Yes____
	b. Sores or cuts that were hard to heal?	No **X** Yes____
	c. Any cold sores (fever blisters)?	No **X** Yes____
	d. Any lumps in your neck, armpits or groin?	No **X** Yes____
	e. Do you ever have chills or sweat at night?	No **X** Yes____
24.	Have you traveled out of the country in the last 2 years?	No **X** Yes, Traveled in:____

25. Write in the dates for the shots you have had: ....
{ Measles ____   Smallpox ____
  Mumps ____   Tetanus ____
  Polio ____   Typhoid ____ }

26.	Have you had a tuberculin (TB) skin test?	No____ Yes **X** Date _2003_
	If so, was it negative or positive?	Neg **X** Pos____
27.	Have you had an HIV test for AIDS?	No **X** Yes____ Date____
	If so, was it negative or positive?	Neg____ Pos____

' 1979, 1983 Bibbero Systems International, Inc.   **PLEASE TURN THIS PAGE**   STOCK NO. 19-742-4   8/95   **Page 3**

CONFIDENTIAL

Form 1

BODY SYSTEMS REVIEW

VISION / HEARING

#	Question	No	Yes		Label
28.	Do you wear eyeglasses?	X			Wears eyeglasses
29.	Do you wear contact lenses?	X			Wears contacts
30.	Has your vision changed in the last year?	X			Vision changes in last year

#	Question	Rarely/Never	Occasionally	Frequently	Label
31.	How often do you have:				
a.	Double vision?	X			Double vision
b.	Blurry vision?	X			Blurred vision
c.	Watery or itchy eyes?	X			Watery/itchy eyes
32.	Do you ever see colored rings around lights?	X			Sees halos
33.	Do others tell you you have a hearing problem?	X			Hearing problem
34.	Do you have trouble keeping your balance?	X			Loses balance
35.	Do you have any discharge from your ears?	X			Discharge from ears
36.	Do you ever feel dizzy or have motion sickness?	X			Dizzy / motion sickness

#	Question	No	Yes		Label
37.	Do you have any problems with your hearing?	X			Hearing Problems
38.	Do you ever have ringing in your ears?	X			Ringing in ears

NOSE / THROAT / RESPIRATORY

#	Question	Rarely/Never	Occasionally	Frequently	Label
39.	How often do you have:				
a.	Head colds?		X		Head colds
b.	Chest colds?		X		Chest colds
c.	Runny nose?		X		Runny nose
d.	Stuffed up nose?		X		Head congestion
e.	Sore/hoarse throat?	X			Sore / hoarse throat
f.	Bad coughing spells?	X			Coughing spells
g.	Sneezing spells?	X			Sneezing spells
h.	Trouble breathing?	X			Trouble breathing
i.	Nose bleeds?	X			Nose bleeds
j.	Cough blood?	X			Cough blood

#	Question	No	Yes	Label
40.	Have you ever worked or spent time:			
a.	On a farm?		X	Worked on a farm
b.	In a mine?	X		Worked in a mine
c.	In a laundry or mill?	X		Worked in a laundry/mill
d.	In very dusty places?	X		Worked in high dust concentrations
e.	With or near toxic chemicals?	X		Exposed to toxic chemicals
f.	With or near radioactive materials?	X		Exposed to radioactive materials
g.	With or near asbestos?	X		Exposed to asbestos

CARDIOVASCULAR

#	Question	Rarely/Never	Occasionally	Frequently	Label
41.	Do you get out of breath easily when you are active (like climbing stairs)?	X			Out of breath quickly when exercising
42.	Do you ever feel light-headed or dizzy?		X		Dizziness
43.	Have you ever fainted or passed out?	X			Fainted
44.	Do you sometimes feel your heart is racing or beating too fast?		X		Rapid heartbeat
45.	When you exercise do you ever get pains in your chest or shoulders?			X	Chest/shoulder pains in exercise
46.	Do you have any leg cramps or pain in your thighs or legs when walking?	X			Pain in thighs or legs when walking
47.	Do you ever have to sit up at night to breathe easier?	X			Sits up at night to breathe easier
48.	Do you use two pillows at night to help you breathe easier?	X			Breathing problems during sleep
49.	Would you say you are a restless sleeper?		X		Restless sleeper
50.	Are you bothered by leg cramps at night?	X			Leg cramps at night
51.	Do you sometimes have swollen ankles or feet?	X			Swollen ankles/feet

DIGESTIVE

#	Question	Rarely/Never	Occasionally	Frequently	Label
52.	How often, if ever:				
a.	Are you nauseated (sick to your stomach)?	X			Nauseated
b.	Do you have stomach pains?	X			Stomach pains
c.	Do you burp a lot after eating?	X			Burps after eating
d.	Do you have heartburn?		X		Heartburn
e.	Do you have trouble swallowing your food?	X			Trouble swallowing food
f.	Have you vomited blood?	X			Vomited blood
g.	Are you constipated?	X			Constipated
h.	Do you have diarrhea (watery stools)?	X			Diarrhea
i.	Are your bowel movements painful?	X			Painful bowel movements
j.	Are your bowel movements bloody?	X			Bloody bowel movements
k.	Are your bowel movements dark or black?	X			Dark bowel movements

#	Question	No	Yes	Date	Label
53.	Have you ever had a sigmoidoscopy?	X			Date of last sigmoidoscopy?

PLEASE TURN TO BACK PAGE AND COMPLETE QUESTIONS ON NUTRITION.

' 1979, 1983 Bibbero Systems International, Inc.

Form 1

Andrus/Clini-Rec®
BIBBero **SYSTEMS, INC.**

COMPREHENSIVE
PHYSICAL EXAMINATION
MALE OR FEMALE
NEW OR ESTABLISHED PATIENT
CPT # 99201 - 99215

(For Office Use Only)

NAME Shapiro, Ivan AGE 59 YRS. OLD	TODAY'S DATE 1/5/05
	DATE OF BIRTH 3/6/45

Key: [O] Neg. Findings [+] Positive Findings [X] Omitted [✔] See Notes/CIRCLE WORDS OF IMPORTANCE & EXPLA

1	GEN. APPEARANCE	[ ]	Apparent Age/Nutrition/Development/Mental & Emotional Status/Gait/Posture/Distress/Speech
2	HEAD / SCALP	[ ]	Size/Shape/Tender over Sinuses/Hair/Alopecia/Eruption/Masses/Bruit –
3	EYES	[ ]	Conjunct/Sclerae/Cornea/Pupils/EOM'S/Arcus/Ptosis/Fundi/Tension/Eyelids/Pallor/Light/Bruit –
4	EARS	[ ]	Ext. Canal/TM's/Perforation/Discharge/Tophi/Hearing Problem/Weber/Rinne –
5	NOSE / SINUSES	[ ]	Septum/Obstruction/Turbinates/Discharge –
6	MOUTH / THROAT	[ ]	Odor/Lips/Tongue/Tonsils/Teeth/Dentures/Gums/Pharynx –
7	NECK	[ ]	Adenopathy/Thyroid/Carotids/Trachea/Veins/Masses/Spine/Motion/Bruit –
8	BACK	[ ]	Kyphosis/Scoliosis/Lordosis/Mobility/CVA/Bone/Tenderness –
9	THORAX	[ ]	Symmetry/Movement/Contour/Tender –
10	BREASTS	[ ]	Size/Size-Consistency/Nipples/Areolar/Palpable Mass/Discharge/Tenderness/Nodes/Scars –
11	HEART	[ ]	Rate/Rhythm/Apical Impulse/Thrills/Quality of Sound/Intensity/Splitting/Extra Sounds/ Murmurs –
12	CHEST / LUNGS	[ ]	Excursion/Dullness or Hyperresonance to Percussion/Quality of Breath Sounds/Rales/Wheez Rhonchi/Diaphragm/Rubs/Bruit –
13	ABDOMEN	[ ]	Bowel Sounds/Appearance/Liver/Spleen/Masses/Hernias/Murmurs/Contour/Tenderness/Bruit/ ING Nodes –
14	GROIN	[ ]	Hernia/Inguinal Nodes/Femoral Pulses –
15	MALE GENITALIA	[ ]	Penis/Testes/Scrotum Epididymis/Varicocele/Scars/Discharge –
16	FEMALE GENITALIA	[ ]	Vuvla/Vagina/Cervix/Uterus/Adnexae/Rectocele/Cystocele/Bartholin Gland/Urethra/ Discharge – Pap Smear (if done ✔) ☐
17	EXTREMITIES	[ ]	Deformity/Clubbing/Cyanosis/Edema/Nails/Peripheral Pulses/Calf Tenderness/Joints for Swel ROM –
18	SKIN	[ ]	Color/Birthmarks/Scars/Texture/Rash/Eczema/Ulcers –
19	NEUROLOGICAL	[ ]	DTR's/Babinski/Cranial Nerves/Motor Abnormalities/Tremor/Paralysis/Sensory Exam – (touch, pin prick, vibration)/Coordination/Romberg –
20	MUSCULAR SYSTEM	[ ]	Strength/Wasting/Development –
21	RECTAL EXAM	[ ]	Sphincter Tone/Hemorrhoids/Fissures/Masses/Prostate/Stool Guaiac (if done ✔) ☐ Pos ☐ N

Impression: ☐ Check If Normal Physical Examination
Summary: _____

_____
Signature _____   Date _____

Page 4   ' 1979, 1983 Bibbero Systems International, Inc.

n 1

COMPREHENSIVE
PHYSICAL EXAMINATION
(continued)

(For Office Use Only)

PHYSICIAN'S NOTES:

dy Area
umber   REMARKS:

R   L   L   R

R   L

VISION

GHT_____

GHT_____

_D _____

SE _____

P. _____

P. _____

Without Glasses

Far	R	20/	L	20/
Near	R	20/	L	20/

With Glasses

R	20/	L	20/
R	20/	L	20/

Tonometry R_____ L_____

Colorvision_____

Peripheral Fields R_____ L_____

AUDIOMETRIC TESTING

	250	500	1000
R	_____	_____	_____
L	_____	_____	_____

	2000	4000	8000
R	_____	_____	_____
L	_____	_____	_____

Gross Hearing _____

BLOOD PRESSURE

Sitting

R   /   L   /

Standing

R   /   L   /

Lying

R   /   L   /

gnostic Test: Results:

pace below is provided for additional information when these data are being forwarded to a hospital, insurance company, a referral physician, etc.

nificant Comments / Recommendations:

Physician's Name _____

Address _____

Telephone (area code) _____

3 Bibbero Systems International, Inc.

Page 5

Form 1

NUTRITION AND DIET

1. How many meals do you eat each day? .... __3__ Meals each day
2. Do you usually eat breakfast? .... ☐ No ☒ Yes Breakfast
3. Do you diet frequently and/or are you now dieting? .... ☒ No ☐ Yes Diets
4. Do you consider yourself .... ☐ Underweight ☐ Overweight ☒ Just right? Weight
5. Do you snack? .... ☐ More than once a day ☒ Usually daily ☐ Rarely? Snacks
6. Do you add salt to your food at the table? ..... ☐ Almost always ☐ Sometimes ☒ Rarely Salts food
7. Check the frequency you eat the following types of foods:

	More than once daily	Daily	3 times weekly	Once weekly	Twice monthly	Le or n
a. Whole grain or enriched bread or cereal	X					
b. Milk, cheese, or other dairy products		X				
c. Eggs				X		
d. Meat, Poultry, Fish			X			
e. Beans, Peas, or other legumes		X				
f. Citrus	X					
g. Dark green or deep yellow vegetables		X				

List any food supplements or vitamins you take regularly: *One a day vitamins*

Additional Patient Comments:

Thanks for completing this questionnaire. Please review for skipped questions, sign your name on the space to the right and return it to the physician or assistant. If you wish to add any information, please write it in the spaces provided above.

Patient s Signature _____

Physician s Notes: _____

CONFIDENTIAL

To order, call or write:
Bibbero Systems, Inc.
1300 N. McDowell Blvd., Petaluma, CA 94
Toll Free: 800-BIBBERO (800 242-2376)
Or Fax: 800-242-9330
STOCK NO. 19-742-4   8/95

Page 6
' 1979, 1983 Bibbero Systems International, Inc.

Form 2

OUTLINE FORMAT PROGRESS NOTES

Patient Name ___Shapiro, Ivan___

Prob. No. or Letter	DATE	S Subjective	O Objective	A Assess	P Plans	Page 3

Start each Progress Note (Subjective, Objective, through the intervening columns to the right   Assessment and Plans) at the appropriate margin of the page.   shaded column to create an outline form. Write

ANDRUS/CLINI-REC PRIMARY CARE CHARTING SYSTEM FORM NO. 26-7115, '1976 BIBBERO SYSTEMS, INC., PETALUMA, CA.

Courtesy of Bibbero Systems, Inc., Petaluma, California.

Form 3

OUTLINE FORMAT PROGRESS NOTES

Patient Name ___Johnson, Raymond___

Prob. No. or Letter	DATE	S Subjective	O Objective	A Assess	P Plans	Page___3

Start each Progress Note (Subjective, Objective, through the intervening columns to the right

Assessment and Plans) at the appropriate margin of the page.

shaded column to create an outline form

ANDRUS/CLINI-REC□ PRIMARY CARE CHARTING SYSTEM FORM NO. 26-7115, '1976 BIBBERO SYSTEMS, INC., PETALUMA, CA.

Courtesy of Bibbero Systems, Inc., Petaluma, California.

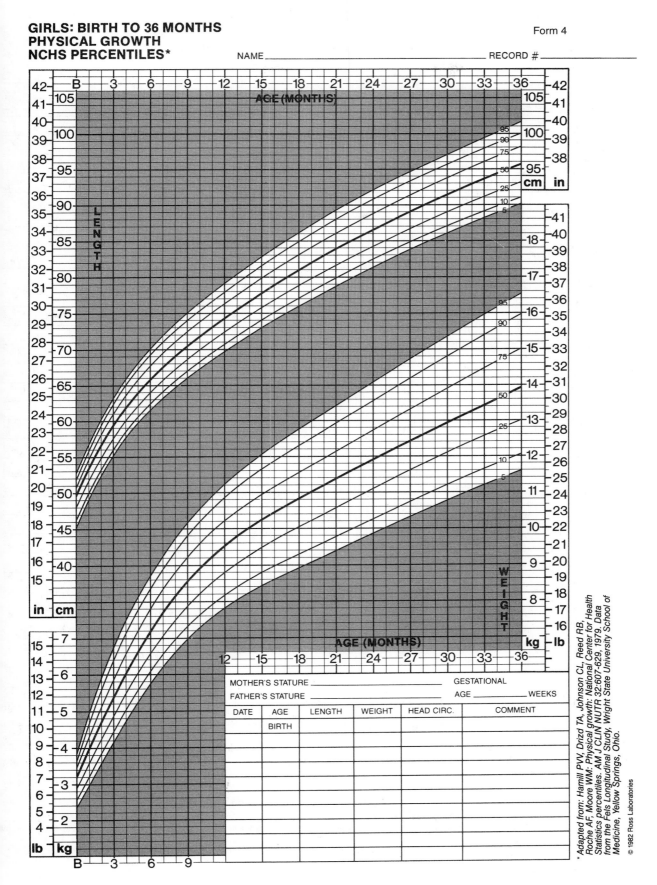

GIRLS: BIRTH TO 36 MONTHS
PHYSICAL GROWTH
NCHS PERCENTILES*

Form 4

NAME_____ RECORD #_____

MOTHER'S STATURE _____ GESTATIONAL
FATHER'S STATURE _____ AGE _____ WEEKS

DATE	AGE	LENGTH	WEIGHT	HEAD CIRC.	COMMENT
	BIRTH				

* Adapted from: Hamill PVV, Drizd TA, Johnson CL, Reed RB, Roche AF, Moore WM: Physical growth: National Center for Health Statistics percentiles. AM J CLIN NUTR 32:607-629, 1979. Data from the Fels Longitudinal Study, Wright State University School of Medicine, Yellow Springs, Ohio.
© 1982 Ross Laboratories

Form 5

OUTLINE FORMAT PROGRESS NOTES

Patient Name _Soto, Robin_

Page___2___

Prob. No. or Letter	DATE	**S** Subjective	**O** Objective	**A** Assess	**P** Plans	

Start each Progress Note (Subjective, Objective, through the intervening columns to the right   Assessment and Plans) at the appropriate margin of the page.   shaded column to create an outline form.

ANDRUS/CLINI-REC□ PRIMARY CARE CHARTING SYSTEM FORM NO. 26-7115, '1976 BIBBERO SYSTEMS, INC., PETALUMA, CA.

Courtesy of Bibbero Systems, Inc., Petaluma, California.

rm 6

ANDRUS/CLINI-REC® HEALTH HISTORY QUESTIONNAIRE

Chart No. _____

entification Information

Today s Date __1/15/05__

ame __Lucille Ferguson__　　　　Date of Birth __6/21/30__

ccupation _____　　　　Marital Status __Widowed__

PART A – PRESENT HEALTH HISTORY

I. CURRENT MEDICAL PROBLEMS

Please list the medical problems for which you came to see the doctor. About when did they begin?

Problems	Date Began
Pain when urinating	1 wk ago
Fever	Yesterday

What concerns you most about these problems?

If you are being treated for any other illness or medical problems by another physician, please describe the problems and write the name of the physician or medical facility treating you.

Illness or Medical Problem	Physician or Medical Facility	City
Osteoarthritis		

II. MEDICATIONS

Please list all medications you are now taking, including those you buy without a doctor s prescription (such as aspirin, cold tablets or vitamin supplements).

III. ALLERGIES AND SENSITIVITIES

List anything that you are allergic to such as certain foods, medications, dust, chemicals or soaps, household items, pollens, bee stings, etc., and indicate how each affects you.

Allergic To:	Effect	Allergic To:	Effect
None			

IV. GENERAL HEALTH, ATTITUDE AND HABITS

How is your overall health now?. . . . . Health now: Poor _____ Fair _____ Good _✓_ Excellent _____

How has it been most of your life?. . . . . Health has been: Poor _____ Fair _____ Good _✓_ Excellent _____

In the past year:

Has your appetite changed?. . . . . Appetite: Decreased _✓_ Increased _____ Stayed same _____

Has your weight changed?. . . . . Weight: Lost _____lbs. Gained _____lbs. No change _✓_

Are you thirsty much of the time?. . . . . Thirsty: No _✓_ Yes _____

Has your overall pep changed?. . . . . Pep: Decreased _____ Increased _____ Stayed same _✓_

Do you usually have trouble sleeping?. . . . . Trouble sleeping: No _____ Yes _✓_

How much do you exercise?. Exercise: Little or none _____ Less than I need _✓_ All I need _____

Do you smoke?. . . . . Smokes: No _✓_ Yes _____ If yes, how many years? _____

How many each day?. . . . . _____ Cigarettes _____ Cigars _____ Pipesfull

Have you ever smoked?. . . . . Smoked: No _____ Yes _✓_ If yes, how many years? _15_

How many each day?. . . . . _30_ Cigarettes _____ Cigars _____ Pipesfull

Do you drink alcoholic beverages?. . . . . Alcohol: No _____ Yes _✓_ I drink _____ Beers _✓_ Glasses of wine _2_ Drinks of hard liquor - per day

Have you ever had a problem with alcohol?. . . . . Prior problem: No _✓_ Yes _____

How much coffee or tea do you usually drink?. . . . . . . Coffee/Tea: _1_ cups of coffee or tea a day

Do you regularly wear seatbelts?. . . . . Seatbelts: No _____ Yes _✓_

DO YOU:	Rarely/Never	Occasionally	Frequently	DO YOU:	Rarely/Never	Occasionally	Frequently
Feel nervous?	X			Ever feel like committing suicide?	X		
Feel depressed?	X						
Find it hard to make decisions?	X			Feel bored with your life?	X		
Lose your temper?	X			Use marijuana?	X		
Worry a lot?	X			Use hard drugs ?	X		
Tire easily?		X		Do you want to talk to the doctor about a personal matter? No X Yes _____			
Have trouble relaxing?	X						
Have any sexual problems?	X						

ted and Developed by Medical Economics Professional Systems

yright ' 1979, 1983 Bibbero Systems International, Inc.

STOCK NO. 19-742-4   8/95   **P**age 1

tesy of Bibbero Systems, Inc., Petaluma, California.

Form 6

PART A – PRESENT HEALTH HISTORY (continued)

IV. GENERAL HEALTH, ATTITUDE AND HABITS (continued)

Have you recently had any changes in your: If yes, please explain:

Marital status?   No __X__ Yes _____

Job or work?   No __X__ Yes _____

Residence?   No __X__ Yes _____

Financial status?   No __X__ Yes _____

Are you having any legal problems
or trouble with the law? No __X__ Yes _____

PART B – PAST HISTORY

C O N F I D E N T I A L

I. FAMILY HEALTH

Please give the following information about your immediate family:

Relationship	Age, if Living	Age At Death	State of Health Or Cause of Death
Father		95	excellent
Mother		unknown	cancer
Brothers and Sisters	68		multiple sclerosis
Spouse			
Children			

Have any **blood relatives** had any of the following illnesses? If so, indicate relationship (mother, brother, etc.)

Illness	Family Members
Asthma	Brother
Diabetes	
Cancer	Breast cancer-Mom
Blood Disease	
Glaucoma	
Epilepsy	
Rheumatoid Arthritis	
Tuberculosis	
Gout	
High Blood Pressure	
Heart Disease	
Mental Problems	
Suicide	
Stroke	
Alcoholism	Uncle
Rheumatic Fever	

II. HOSPITALIZATIONS, SURGERIES, INJURIES

Please list all times you have been hospitalized, operated on, or seriously injured.

Year	Operation, Illness, Injury	Hospital and City
1976	Appendix taken out	Mercy Hospital

III. ILLNESS AND MEDICAL PROBLEMS

Please mark with an (X) any of the following illnesses and medical problems you have or have had and indicate the year when each started. If you are not certain when an illness started, write down an approximate year.

Illness	(x)	(Year)	Illness	(x)	(Year)
Eye or eye lid infection			Hernia		
Glaucoma			Hemorrhoids	X	1955
Other eye problems			Kidney or bladder disease		
Ear trouble			Prostate problem (male only)		
Deafness or decreased hearing			Mental problems		
Thyroid trouble			Headaches		
Strep throat	X	as child	Head injury		
Bronchitis	X	several	Stroke		
Emphysema			Convulsions, seizures		
Pneumonia			Arthritis	X	now
Allergies, asthma or hay fever			Gout		
Tuberculosis			Cancer or tumor		
Other lung problems			Bleeding tendency		
High blood pressure			Diabetes		
Heart attack			Measles/Rubeola	X	child
High cholesterol	X	1991	German measles/Rubella		
Arteriosclerosis			Polio	X	child
(Hardening of arteries)			Mumps	X	child
Heart murmur			Scarlet fever		
Other heart condition			Chicken pox	X	child
Stomach/duodenal ulcer			Mononucleosis		
Diverticulosis			Eczema		
Colitis			Psoriasis		
Other bowel problems			Venereal disease		
Hepatitis			Genital herpes		
Liver trouble			HIV test		
Gallbladder trouble			AIDS		

' 1979, 1983 Bibbero Systems International, Inc.   To Order Call:800-BIBBERO (800 242-2376)
(REV. 8/95)   Or Fax: (800 242-9330)

Page 2   STOCK NO. 19-742-4   8/95

rm 6

PART A – PRESENT HEALTH HISTORY (continued)

IV. GENERAL HEALTH, ATTITUDE AND HABITS (continued)

Have you recently had any changes in your:　　　　　If yes, please explain:

	No	Yes
Marital status?	X	
Job or work?	X	
Residence?	X	
Financial status?	X	
Are you having any legal problems or trouble with the law?	X	

PART B – PAST HISTORY

I. FAMILY HEALTH

Please give the following information about your immediate family:

Relationship	Age, if Living	Age At Death	State of Health Or Cause of Death
Father		95	excellent
Mother		unknown	cancer
Brothers and Sisters	68		multiple sclerosis
Spouse			
Children			

Have any **blood relatives** had any of the following illnesses? If so, indicate relationship (mother, brother, etc.)

Illness	Family Members
Asthma	Brother
Diabetes	
Cancer	Breast cancer-Mom
Blood Disease	
Glaucoma	
Epilepsy	
Rheumatoid Arthritis	
Tuberculosis	
Gout	
High Blood Pressure	
Heart Disease	
Mental Problems	
Suicide	
Stroke	
Alcoholism	Uncle
Rheumatic Fever	

II. HOSPITALIZATIONS, SURGERIES, INJURIES

Please list all times you have been hospitalized, operated on, or seriously injured.

Year	Operation, Illness, Injury	Hospital and City
1976	Appendix taken out	Mercy Hospital

III. ILLNESS AND MEDICAL PROBLEMS

Please mark with an (X) any of the following illnesses and medical problems you have or have had and indicate the year when each started. If you are not certain when an illness started, write down an approximate year.

Illness	(x)	(Year)	Illness	(x)	(Year)
Eye or eye lid infection			Hernia		
Glaucoma			Hemorrhoids	X	1955
Other eye problems			Kidney or bladder disease		
Ear trouble			Prostate problem (male only)		
Deafness or decreased hearing			Mental problems		
Thyroid trouble			Headaches		
Strep throat	X	as child	Head injury		
Bronchitis	X	several	Stroke		
Emphysema			Convulsions, seizures		
Pneumonia			Arthritis	X	now
Allergies, asthma or hay fever			Gout		
Tuberculosis			Cancer or tumor		
Other lung problems			Bleeding tendency		
High blood pressure			Diabetes		
Heart attack			Measles/Rubeola	X	child
High cholesterol	X	1991	German measles/Rubella		
Arteriosclerosis			Polio	X	child
(Hardening of arteries)			Mumps	X	child
Heart murmur			Scarlet fever		
Other heart condition			Chicken pox	X	child
Stomach/duodenal ulcer			Mononucleosis		
Diverticulosis			Eczema		
Colitis			Psoriasis		
Other bowel problems			Venereal disease		
Hepatitis			Genital herpes		
Liver trouble			HIV test		
Gallbladder trouble			AIDS		

' 1979, 1983 Bibbero Systems International, Inc.　To Order Call:800-BIBBERO (800 242-2376)
(REV. 8/95)　　　　Or Fax: (800 242-9330)　　　　STOCK NO. 19-742-4　　8/95

e 2

Form 6

PART C – BODY SYSTEMS REVIEW

Please answer all of the following questions.

Circle any questions you find difficult to answer.

MEN: Please answer questions 1 through 12, then skip to question 18.

WOMEN: Please start on question 6.

MEN ONLY

1. Have you had or do you have prostate trouble? . . . . No _____ Yes _____
2. Do you have any sexual problems or a problem with impotency? . . . . No _____ Yes _____
3. Have you ever had sores or lesions on your penis? . . . . No _____ Yes _____
4. Have you ever had any discharge from your penis? . . . . No _____ Yes _____
5. Do you ever have pain, lumps or swelling in your testicles? . . . . No _____ Yes _____

Check here if you wish to discuss any special problems with the doctor . . . . [ ]

MEN & WOMEN	Rarely/ Never	Occasionally	Frequently
6. Is it sometimes hard to start your urine flow?	X		
7. Is urination ever painful?			X
8. Do you have to urinate more than 5 times a day?	X		
9. Do you get up at night to urinate?	X		
10. Has your urine ever been bloody or dark colored?	X		
11. Do you ever lose urine when you strain, laugh, cough or sneeze?	X		
12. Do you ever lose urine during sleep?	X		

WOMEN ONLY
Do you:

		Rarely/ Never	Occasionally	Frequently
13.	a. Have any menstrual problems?	X		
	b. Feel rather tense just before your period?	X		
	c. Have heavy menstrual bleeding?	X		
	d. Have painful menstrual periods?	X		
	e. Have any bleeding between periods?	X		
	f. Have any unusual vaginal discharge or itching?	X		
	g. Ever have tender breasts?	X		
	h. Have any discharge from your nipples?	X		
	i. Have any hot flashes?	X		

14. How many times, if any, have you been pregnant? 3
15. How many children born alive? 3
16. Are you taking birth control pills? . . . . No X Yes _____
17. Do you examine your breasts monthly for lumps? . . . . No _____ Yes _Sometimes_
17a. What was the date of your last menstrual period? . . . . Date ____1980____

Check here if you wish to discuss any special problem with the doctor . . . . [ ]

MEN & WOMEN	Rarely/ Never	Occasionally	Frequently
18. In the past year have you had any:			
a. Severe shoulder pain?	X		
b. Severe back pain?	X		
c. Muscle or joint stiffness or pain due to sports, exercise or injury?	X		
d. Pain or swelling in any joints not due to sports, exercise or injury?	X		

19. Do you have dry skin or brittle fingernails? . . . . No X Yes _____
20. Do you bruise easily? . . . . No X Yes _____
21. Do you have any moles that have changed in color or in size? . . . . No X Yes _____
22. Do you have any other skin problems? . . . . No X Yes _____

23. In the last 3 months have you had:
    a. A fever that lasted more than one day? . . . . No _____ Yes X
    b. Sores or cuts that were hard to heal? . . . . No X Yes _____
    c. Any cold sores (fever blisters)? . . . . No X Yes _____
    d. Any lumps in your neck, armpits or groin? . . . . No X Yes _____
    e. Do you ever have chills or sweat at night? . . . . No X Yes _____

24. Have you traveled out of the country in the last 2 years? . . . . No X Yes, Traveled in: _____

25. Write in the dates for the shots you have had: . . . .

Measles _____		Smallpox _____
Mumps _____		Tetanus _____
Polio _____		Typhoid _____

26. Have you had a tuberculin (TB) skin test? . . . . No X Yes _____ Date _____
    If so, was it negative or positive? . . . . Neg _____ Pos _____
27. Have you had an HIV test for AIDS? . . . . No X Yes _____ Date _____
    If so, was it negative or positive? . . . . Neg _____ Pos _____

' 1979, 1983 Bibbero Systems International, Inc.   **PLEASE TURN THIS PAGE**   STOCK NO. 19-742-4   8/95   **Page 3**

Form 6

BODY SYSTEMS REVIEW

VISION / HEARING

#	Question	No	Yes	Description
28.	Do you wear eyeglasses?	No___	Yes _X_	Wears eyeglasses
29.	Do you wear contact lenses?	No_X_	Yes___	Wears contacts
30.	Has your vision changed in the last year?	No___	Yes_X_	Vision changes in last year

#	Question	Rarely/Never	Occasionally	Frequently	Description
31.	How often do you have:				
a.	Double vision?	___	X	___	Double vision
b.	Blurry vision?	___	X	___	Blurred vision
c.	Watery or itchy eyes?	___	___	X	Watery/itchy eyes
32.	Do you ever see colored rings around lights?	X	___	___	Sees halos
33.	Do others tell you you have a hearing problem?	___	X	___	Hearing problem
34.	Do you have trouble keeping your balance?	X	___	___	Loses balance
35.	Do you have any discharge from your ears?	X	___	___	Discharge from ears
36.	Do you ever feel dizzy or have motion sickness?	X	___	___	Dizzy / motion sickness

#	Question	No	Yes	Description
37.	Do you have any problems with your hearing?	No_X_	Yes___	Hearing Problems
38.	Do you ever have ringing in your ears?	No_X_	Yes___	Ringing in ears

NOSE / THROAT / RESPIRATORY

#	Question	Rarely/Never	Occasionally	Frequently	Description
39.	How often do you have:				
a.	Head colds?	___	X	___	Head colds
b.	Chest colds?	___	X	___	Chest colds
c.	Runny nose?	___	X	___	Runny nose
d.	Stuffed up nose?	___	X	___	Head congestion
e.	Sore/hoarse throat?	___	X	___	Sore / hoarse throat
f.	Bad coughing spells?	X	___	___	Coughing spells
g.	Sneezing spells?	X	___	___	Sneezing spells
h.	Trouble breathing?	X	___	___	Trouble breathing
i.	Nose bleeds?	X	___	___	Nose bleeds
j.	Cough blood?	X	___	___	Cough blood

#	Question	No	Yes	Description
40.	Have you ever worked or spent time:			
a.	On a farm?	No___	Yes _X_	Worked on a farm
b.	In a mine?	No_X_	Yes___	Worked in a mine
c.	In a laundry or mill?	No_X_	Yes___	Worked in a laundry/mill
d.	In very dusty places?	No_X_	Yes___	Worked in high dust concentrations
e.	With or near toxic chemicals?	No_X_	Yes___	Exposed to toxic chemicals
f.	With or near radioactive materials?	No_X_	Yes___	Exposed to radioactive materials
g.	With or near asbestos?	No_X_	Yes___	Exposed to asbestos

CARDIOVASCULAR

#	Question	Rarely/Never	Occasionally	Frequently	Description
41.	Do you get out of breath easily when you are active (like climbing stairs)?	X	___	___	Out of breath quickly when exercising
42.	Do you ever feel light-headed or dizzy?	X	___	___	Dizziness
43.	Have you ever fainted or passed out?	X	___	___	Fainted
44.	Do you sometimes feel your heart is racing or beating too fast?	X	___	___	Rapid heartbeat
45.	When you exercise do you ever get pains in your chest or shoulders?	X	___	___	Chest/shoulder pains in exercise
46.	Do you have any leg cramps or pain in your thighs or legs when walking?	X	___	___	Pain in thighs or legs when walking
47.	Do you ever have to sit up at night to breathe easier?	X	___	___	Sits up at night to breathe easier
48.	Do you use two pillows at night to help you breathe easier?	X	___	___	Breathing problems during sleep
49.	Would you say you are a restless sleeper?	X	___	___	Restless sleeper
50.	Are you bothered by leg cramps at night?	X	___	___	Leg cramps at night
51.	Do you sometimes have swollen ankles or feet?	X	___	___	Swollen ankles/feet

DIGESTIVE

#	Question	Rarely/Never	Occasionally	Frequently	Description
52.	How often, if ever:				
a.	Are you nauseated (sick to your stomach)?	X	___	___	Nauseated
b.	Do you have stomach pains?	X	___	___	Stomach pains
c.	Do you burp a lot after eating?	X	___	___	Burps after eating
d.	Do you have heartburn?	X	___	___	Heartburn
e.	Do you have trouble swallowing your food?	X	___	___	Trouble swallowing food
f.	Have you vomited blood?	X	___	___	Vomited blood
g.	Are you constipated?	X	___	___	Constipated
h.	Do you have diarrhea (watery stools)?	X	___	___	Diarrhea
i.	Are your bowel movements painful?	X	___	___	Painful bowel movements
j.	Are your bowel movements bloody?	X	___	___	Bloody bowel movements
k.	Are your bowel movements dark or black?	X	___	___	Dark bowel movements

#	Question	No	Yes	Description
53.	Have you ever had a sigmoidoscopy?	No_X_	Yes___ Date_____	Date of last sigmoidoscopy?

PLEASE TURN TO BACK PAGE AND COMPLETE QUESTIONS ON NUTRITION.

' 1979, 1983 Bibbero Systems International, Inc.

Form 6

Andrus/Clini-Rec®

BIBBERO **SYSTEMS, INC.**

COMPREHENSIVE
PHYSICAL EXAMINATION
MALE OR FEMALE
NEW OR ESTABLISHED PATIENT
CPT # 99201 - 99215

(For Office Use Only)

TODAY'S DATE _____	
NAME _____ AGE _____ YRS. OLD	DATE OF BIRTH _____

Key: [O] Neg. Findings [+] Positive Findings [X] Omitted [✔] See Notes/CIRCLE WORDS OF IMPORTANCE & EXPLAIN

C O N F I D E N T I A L

1	GEN. APPEARANCE	[ ]	Apparent Age/Nutrition/Development/Mental & Emotional Status/Gait/Posture/Distress/Speech –
2	HEAD / SCALP	[ ]	Size/Shape/Tender over Sinuses/Hair/Alopecia/Eruption/Masses/Bruit –
3	EYES	[ ]	Conjunct/Sclerae/Cornea/Pupils/EOM'S/Arcus/Ptosis/Fundi/Tension/Eyelids/Pallor/Light/Bruit –
4	EARS	[ ]	Ext. Canal/TM's/Perforation/Discharge/Tophi/Hearing Problem/Weber/Rinne –
5	NOSE / SINUSES	[ ]	Septum/Obstruction/Turbinates/Discharge –
6	MOUTH / THROAT	[ ]	Odor/Lips/Tongue/Tonsils/Teeth/Dentures/Gums/Pharynx –
7	NECK	[ ]	Adenopathy/Thyroid/Carotids/Trachea/Veins/Masses/Spine/Motion/Bruit –
8	BACK	[ ]	Kyphosis/Scoliosis/Lordosis/Mobility/CVA/Bone/Tenderness –
9	THORAX	[ ]	Symmetry/Movement/Contour/Tender –
10	BREASTS	[ ]	Size/Size-Consistency/Nipples/Areolar/Palpable Mass/Discharge/Tenderness/Nodes/Scars –
11	HEART	[ ]	Rate/Rhythm/Apical Impulse/Thrills/Quality of Sound/Intensity/Splitting/Extra Sounds/ Murmurs –
12	CHEST / LUNGS	[ ]	Excursion/Dullness or Hyperresonance to Percussion/Quality of Breath Sounds/Rales/Wheezing/ Rhonchi/Diaphragm/Rubs/Bruit –
13	ABDOMEN	[ ]	Bowel Sounds/Appearance/Liver/Spleen/Masses/Hernias/Murmurs/Contour/Tenderness/Bruit/ ING Nodes –
14	GROIN	[ ]	Hernia/Inguinal Nodes/Femoral Pulses –
15	MALE GENITALIA	[ ]	Penis/Testes/Scrotum Epididymis/Varicocele/Scars/Discharge –
16	FEMALE GENITALIA	[ ]	Vuvla/Vagina/Cervix/Uterus/Adnexae/Rectocele/Cystocele/Bartholin Gland/Urethra/ Discharge – Pap Smear (if done ✔) ☐
17	EXTREMITIES	[ ]	Deformity/Clubbing/Cyanosis/Edema/Nails/Peripheral Pulses/Calf Tenderness/Joints for Swelling/ ROM –
18	SKIN	[ ]	Color/Birthmarks/Scars/Texture/Rash/Eczema/Ulcers –
19	NEUROLOGICAL	[ ]	DTR's/Babinski/Cranial Nerves/Motor Abnormalities/Tremor/Paralysis/Sensory Exam – (touch, pin prick, vibration)/Coordination/Romberg –
20	MUSCULAR SYSTEM	[ ]	Strength/Wasting/Development –
21	RECTAL EXAM	[ ]	Sphincter Tone/Hemorrhoids/Fissures/Masses/Prostate/Stool Guaiac (if done ✔) ☐ Pos ☐ Neg –

Impression: ☐ Check If Normal Physical Examination
Summary: _____
_____

Signature _____ Date _____

Form 6

COMPREHENSIVE
PHYSICAL EXAMINATION
(continued)

(For Office Use Only)

Body Area Number	REMARKS:	**PHYSICIAN'S NOTES:**

C O N F I D E N T I A L

HEIGHT_____

WEIGHT_____

BUILD _____

PULSE _____

RESP. _____

TEMP. _____

VISION

Without Glasses
Far   R ^{20}/   L ^{20}/
Near   R ^{20}/   L ^{20}/

With Glasses
       R ^{20}/   L ^{20}/
       R ^{20}/   L ^{20}/

Tonometry R_____ L_____

Colorvision_____

Peripheral Fields R_____ L_____

AUDIOMETRIC TESTING

	250	500	1000
R	____	____	____
L	____	____	____
	2000	4000	8000
R	____	____	____
L	____	____	____

Gross Hearing _____

BLOOD PRESSURE

Sitting
R   /   L   /

Standing
R   /   L   /

Lying
R   /   L   /

Diagnostic Test:	Results:

The space below is provided for additional information when these data are being forwarded to a hospital, insurance company, a referral physician, etc.

Significant Comments / Recommendations:
_____
_____
_____
_____

Physician's Name _____

Address _____
_____

Telephone (area code) _____

, 1983 Bibbero Systems International, Inc.

Page 5

Form 6

C O N F I D E N T I A L

NUTRITION AND DIET

1. How many meals do you eat each day? . . . . _____ Meals each day

2. Do you usually eat breakfast? . . . . □ No □ Yes Breakfast

3. Do you diet frequently and/or are you now dieting? . . . . □ No □ Yes Diets

4. Do you consider yourself . . . . □ Underweight □ Overweight □ Just right? Weight

5. Do you snack? . . . . □ More than once a day □ Usually daily □ Rarely? Snacks

6. Do you add salt to your food at the table? . . . . . □ Almost always □ Sometimes □ Rarely Salts food

7. Check the frequency you eat the following types of foods:

	More than once daily	Daily	3 times weekly	Once weekly	Twice monthly	Less or never
a. Whole grain or enriched bread or cereal						
b. Milk, cheese, or other dairy products						
c. Eggs						
d. Meat, Poultry, Fish						
e. Beans, Peas, or other legumes						
f. Citrus						
g. Dark green or deep yellow vegetables						

List any food supplements or vitamins you take regularly: _____

Additional Patient Comments: _____

_____

_____

_____

_____

_____

_____

_____

Thanks for completing this questionnaire. Please review for skipped questions, sign your name on the space to the right and return it to the physician or assistant. If you wish to add any information, please write it in the spaces provided above.

Patient's Signature _____

Physician's Notes: _____

_____

_____

_____

_____

_____

To order, call or write:
Bibbero Systems, Inc.
1300 N. McDowell Blvd., Petaluma, CA 94954-1180
Toll Free: 800-BIBBERO (800 242-2376)
Or Fax: 800-242-9330
STOCK NO. 19-742-4   8/95

© 1979, 1983 Bibbero Systems International, Inc.

m 7

OUTLINE FORMAT PROGRESS NOTES

Patient Name ___Ferguson, Lucille___

b. or ter	DATE	**S** Subjective	**O** Objective	**A** Assess	**P** Plans	

Page___3___

t each Progress Note (Subjective, Objective,   Assessment and Plans) at the appropriate   shaded column to create an outline form. Write
ugh the intervening columns to the right   margin of the page.

ANDRUS/CLINI-REC◻ PRIMARY CARE CHARTING SYSTEM FORM NO. 26-7115, '1976 BIBBERO SYSTEMS, INC., PETALUMA, CA.

esy of Bibbero Systems, Inc., Petaluma, California.

Form 8

OUTLINE FORMAT PROGRESS NOTES

Patient Name _____

Prob. No. or Letter	DATE	S Subjective	O Objective	A Assess	P Plans	Page_____

Start each Progress Note (Subjective, Objective, Assessment and Plans) at the appropriate shaded column to create an outline form. through the intervening columns to the right margin of the page.

ANDRUS/CLINI-REC® PRIMARY CARE CHARTING SYSTEM FORM NO. 26-7115, '1976 BIBBERO SYSTEMS, INC., PETALUMA, CA.

Courtesy of Bibbero Systems, Inc., Petaluma, California.